Subscriptions:

CNS & Neurological Disorders - Drug Targets ISSN: 1871-5273; eISSN: 1996-3181

Vol. 16, 10 issues, 2017

Corporate subscription, print or online: $ 4,140.00
Academic subscription, print or online: $ 2,280.00
Personal subscription, print only: $ 540.00

Subscription orders are paid in US dollar currency and include airmail postage. The corporate rate applies for all corporations and the academic rate applies for academic and government institutions. For corporate clients who want to order a combined print and online subscription, there is an additional 20% surcharge to the stated print or online subscription rate and a 10% surcharge for academic clients. The personal subscription rate, which includes both print and online subscriptions, applies only when the subscription is strictly for personal use, and the subscriber is not allowed to distribute the journals for use within a corporation or academic institution.

Subscription orders and single issue orders and enquiries should be sent to either address: Bentham Science Publishers, Executive Suite Y-2, P.O. Box 7917, Saif Zone, Sharjah, U.A.E., Tel: (+971) 65571132, Fax: (+971) 65571134, E-mail: subscriptions@benthamscience.org Bentham Science Publishers, P.O. Box 446, Oak Park, IL 60301, USA, Fax: 312 996-7107, E-mail: subscriptions@benthamscience.org

Visit the journal's homepage at: **http://benthamscience.com/journals/cnsnddt**

Aims and Scope

CNS & Neurological Disorders - Drug Targets aims to cover all the latest and outstanding developments on the medicinal chemistry, pharmacology, molecular biology, genomics and biochemistry of contemporary molecular targets involved in neurological and central nervous system (CNS) disorders e.g. disease specific proteins, receptors, enzymes, genes.

CNS & Neurological Disorders - Drug Targets publishes guest edited thematic issues written by leaders in the field covering a range of current topics of CNS & neurological drug targets. The journal also accepts for publication original research articles, letters, reviews and drug clinical trial studies.

As the discovery, identification, characterization and validation of novel human drug targets for neurological and CNS drug discovery continues to grow; this journal is essential reading for all pharmaceutical scientists involved in drug discovery and development.

Editorial Policies

The editorial policies of Bentham Science Publishers on publication ethics, peer-review, plagiarism, copyrights/ licenses, errata/ corrections, and article retraction/ withdrawal can be viewed at http://www.benthamscience.com/editorial-policies-main.php

Journal Instructions for Authors

For the journal Instructions for Authors please refer either to the first published issue of each year or the journal's website at www.benthamscience.com

Multiple Journal Subscriptions & Global Online Licenses

For multiple journal subscriptions, possible discounts and global online licenses please contact our special sales department at E-mail: subscriptions@benthamscience.org

Advertising

To place an advertisement in this journal please contact the advertising department at E-mail: ads@benthamscience.org

Journal Sample Copies

A free online sample issue can be viewed at the journal's internet homepage. Alternatively a free print sample issue may be requested, please send your request to E-mail: sample.copy@benthamscience.org

CNS & Neurological Disorders - Drug Targets

Volume 16, Number 8, 2017

Contents

Thematic Issues
Unmet Needs in Modern Psychiatry
Guest Editors: Maurizio Pompili and Andrea Fiorillo

Review Articles

Research Article

Contd....

General Articles

Review Articles

Conference Report

The cover illustration shows scheme showing key assumptions and rationale underlying cognitive remediation in schizophrenia. Source: Wykes T, Reeder C (eds) (2005). Cognitive remediation therapy for schizophrenia. Theory and Practice. Routledge, London.

*Editor's Choice

Graphical Abstracts

CNS & Neurological Disorders - Drug Targets, **2017**, *Vol. 16, No. 8*   **858**

Potential Novel Treatments for Bipolar Depression: Ketamine, Fatty Acids, Anti-inflammatory Agents, and Probiotics

Gustavo H. Vázquez, Sebastián Camino, Leonardo Tondo and Ross J. Baldessarini[*]

[*]*International Consortium for Bipolar & Psychotic Disorder Research, Mailman Research Center, McLean Hospital, Belmont, Massachusetts 02478, USA*

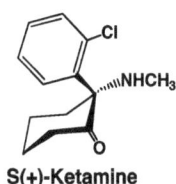

S(+)-Ketamine

Ketamine represents an innovative, rapidly acting, experimental treatment for bipolar depression with practical limitations. Unsaturated fatty acids and anti-inflammatory agents have inconsistent support; probiotic treatments lack evidence. These innovative approaches require much more clinical investigation.

CNS & Neurological Disorders - Drug Targets, **2017**, *Vol. 16, No. 8*   **870**

Unmet Needs in Schizophrenia

Maurizio Pompili[*], Gloria Giordano, Mario Luciano, Dorian A. Lamis, Valeria Del Vecchio, Gianluca Serafini, Gaia Sampogna, Denise Erbuto, Peter Falkai and Andrea Fiorillo

[*]*Department of Neurosciences, Mental Health and Sensory Organs, Suicide Prevention Center, Sant'Andrea Hospital, Sapienza University of Rome, Italy*

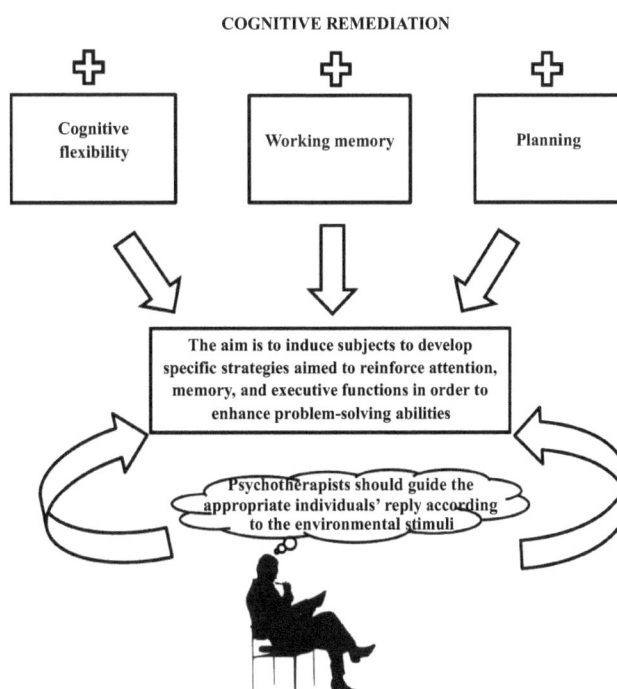

CNS & Neurological Disorders - Drug Targets, **2017**, *Vol. 16, No. 8*   **885**

Older and Newer Strategies for the Pharmacological Management of Agitation in Patients with Bipolar Disorder or Schizophrenia

Giovanni Amodeo*, Andrea Fagiolini, Gabriele Sachs and Andreas Erfurth

Department of Molecular Medicine, University of Siena School of Medicine, Viale Bracci 1, Siena 53100, Italy

Pharmacologic treatment of agitation should be based on an assessment of the most likely cause of the agitation. The use for treatment of acute agitation in patients with schizophrenia and bipolar disease of a variety of first-generation antipsychotic drugs, second-generation antipsychotic drugs, benzodiazepines and the newer inhaled antipsychotic loxapine, is reviewed and commented.

CNS & Neurological Disorders - Drug Targets, **2017**, *Vol. 16, No. 8*   **891**

Pharmacological Treatment of Cognitive Symptoms in Major Depressive Disorder

Zihang Pan, Radu C. Grovu, Danielle S. Cha, Nicole E. Carmona, Mehala Subramaniapillai, Margarita Shekotikhina, Carola Rong, Yena Lee and Roger S. McIntyre*

Mood Disorders Psychopharmacology Unit, University Health Network, Toronto, ON, Canada

Cognitive dysfunction in MDD is a principal determinant of patient-reported outcomes (*e.g.*, psychosocial function). Healthcare providers are encouraged to screen for cognitive dysfunction in MDD and familiarize themselves with the efficacy profiles of antidepressants on disparate cognitive domains.

CNS & Neurological Disorders - Drug Targets, **2017**, *Vol. 16, No. 8*   **900**

New Trends in the Treatment of Schizophrenia

Herbert Y. Meltzer*

Department of Psychiatry and Behavioral Sciences, Northwestern Feinberg School of Medicine, 303 East Chicago Ave, Ward Building 7-101, Chicago, Il 60611, USA

The heterogeneity of the pathophysiology of the various domains of schizophrenia require a diversity of treatments that are best met by the expert use of AAPDs at the current time. Pharmacogenetic efforts are consistent with new evidence that multiple genes are involved in the risk for schizophrenia and the effectiveness of AAPDs.

Graphical Abstracts

CNS & Neurological Disorders - Drug Targets, **2017**, *Vol. 16, No. 8* **858**

Potential Novel Treatments for Bipolar Depression: Ketamine, Fatty Acids, Anti-inflammatory Agents, and Probiotics

Gustavo H. Vázquez, Sebastián Camino, Leonardo Tondo and Ross J. Baldessarini[*]

[*]*International Consortium for Bipolar & Psychotic Disorder Research, Mailman Research Center, McLean Hospital, Belmont, Massachusetts 02478, USA*

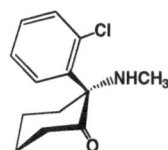

S(+)-Ketamine

Ketamine represents an innovative, rapidly acting, experimental treatment for bipolar depression with practical limitations. Unsaturated fatty acids and anti-inflammatory agents have inconsistent support; probiotic treatments lack evidence. These innovative approaches require much more clinical investigation.

CNS & Neurological Disorders - Drug Targets, **2017**, *Vol. 16, No. 8* **870**

Unmet Needs in Schizophrenia

Maurizio Pompili[*], Gloria Giordano, Mario Luciano, Dorian A. Lamis, Valeria Del Vecchio, Gianluca Serafini, Gaia Sampogna, Denise Erbuto, Peter Falkai and Andrea Fiorillo

[*]*Department of Neurosciences, Mental Health and Sensory Organs, Suicide Prevention Center, Sant'Andrea Hospital, Sapienza University of Rome, Italy*

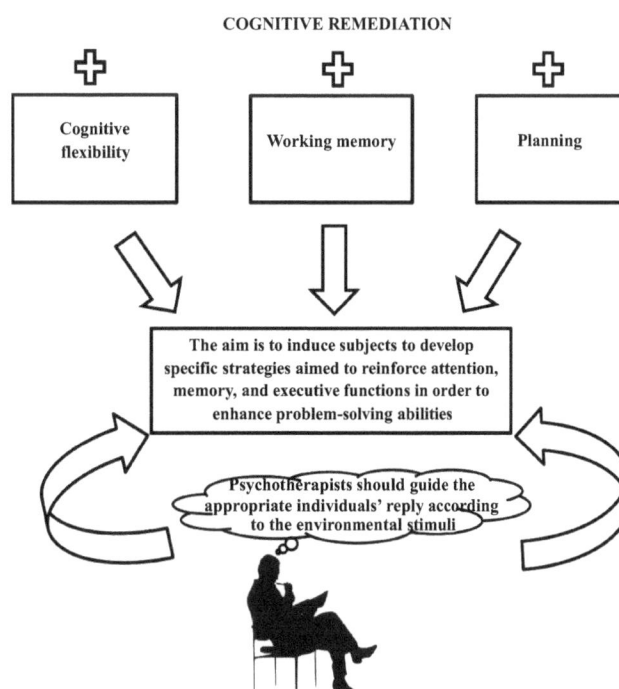

CNS & Neurological Disorders - Drug Targets, **2017**, *Vol. 16, No. 8*   **885**

Older and Newer Strategies for the Pharmacological Management of Agitation in Patients with Bipolar Disorder or Schizophrenia

Giovanni Amodeo[*], Andrea Fagiolini, Gabriele Sachs and Andreas Erfurth

[*]*Department of Molecular Medicine, University of Siena School of Medicine, Viale Bracci 1, Siena 53100, Italy*

Pharmacologic treatment of agitation should be based on an assessment of the most likely cause of the agitation. The use for treatment of acute agitation in patients with schizophrenia and bipolar disease of a variety of first-generation antipsychotic drugs, second-generation antipsychotic drugs, benzodiazepines and the newer inhaled antipsychotic loxapine, is reviewed and commented.

CNS & Neurological Disorders - Drug Targets, **2017**, *Vol. 16, No. 8*   **891**

Pharmacological Treatment of Cognitive Symptoms in Major Depressive Disorder

Zihang Pan, Radu C. Grovu, Danielle S. Cha, Nicole E. Carmona, Mehala Subramaniapillai, Margarita Shekotikhina, Carola Rong, Yena Lee and Roger S. McIntyre[*]

[*]*Mood Disorders Psychopharmacology Unit, University Health Network, Toronto, ON, Canada*

Cognitive dysfunction in MDD is a principal determinant of patient-reported outcomes (*e.g.*, psychosocial function). Healthcare providers are encouraged to screen for cognitive dysfunction in MDD and familiarize themselves with the efficacy profiles of antidepressants on disparate cognitive domains.

CNS & Neurological Disorders - Drug Targets, **2017**, *Vol. 16, No. 8*   **900**

New Trends in the Treatment of Schizophrenia

Herbert Y. Meltzer[*]

[*]*Department of Psychiatry and Behavioral Sciences, Northwestern Feinberg School of Medicine, 303 East Chicago Ave, Ward Building 7-101, Chicago, Il 60611, USA*

The heterogeneity of the pathophysiology of the various domains of schizophrenia require a diversity of treatments that are best met by the expert use of AAPDs at the current time. Pharmacogenetic efforts are consistent with new evidence that multiple genes are involved in the risk for schizophrenia and the effectiveness of AAPDs.

CNS & Neurological Disorders - Drug Targets, **2017**, *Vol. 16, No. 8* **907**

Neural Correlates in Patients with Major Affective Disorders: An fMRI Study

Gianluca Serafini, Maurizio Pompili[*], Andrea Romano, Denise Erbuto, Dorian A. Lamis, Marta Moraschi, Maria Camilla Rossi Espagnet, Mario Amore, Paolo Girardi and Alessandro Bozzao

[*]*Department of Neurosciences, Suicide Prevention Center, Sant'Andrea Hospital, University of Rome, Rome, Italy*

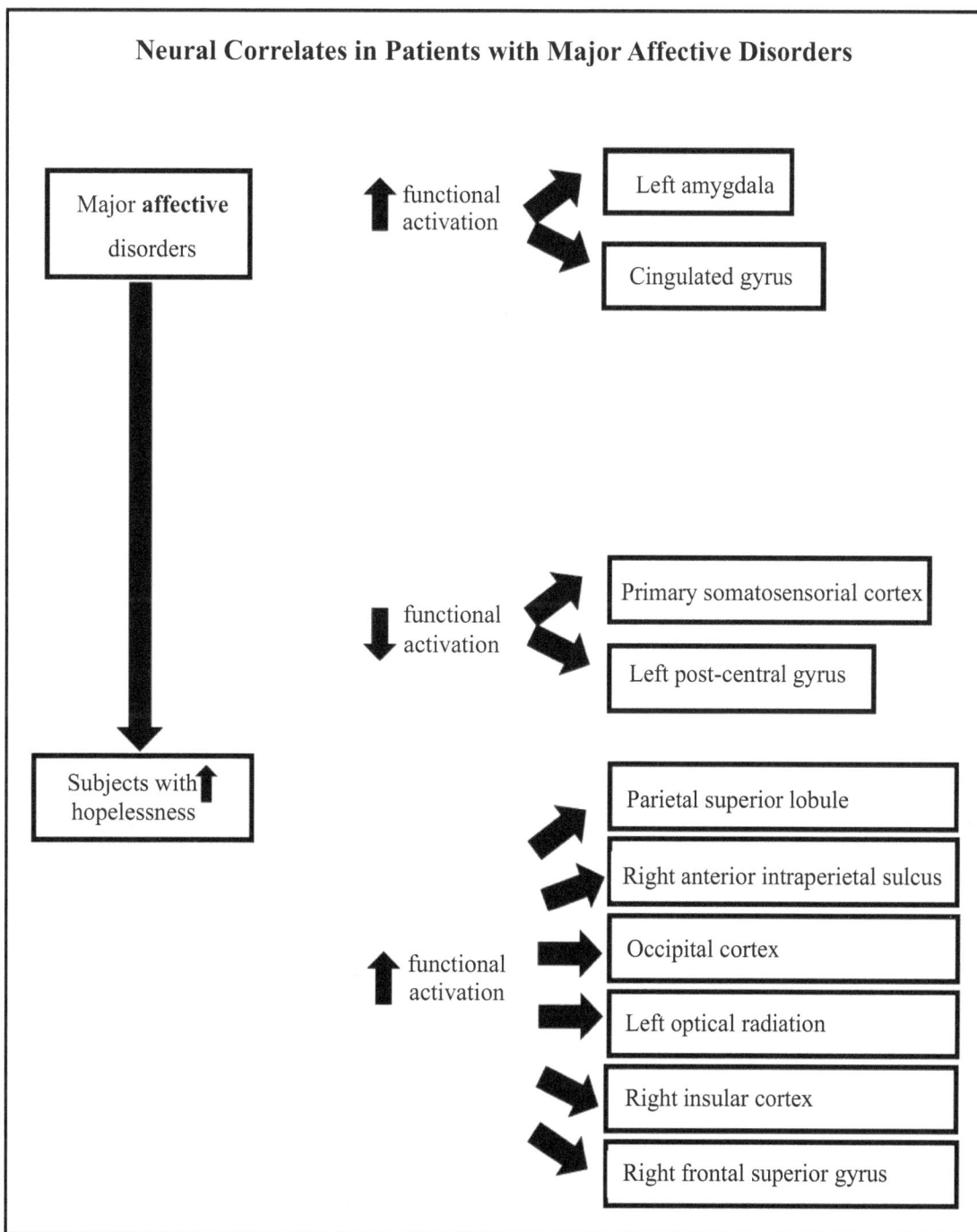

Neural Correlates in Patients with Major Affective Disorders

CNS & Neurological Disorders - Drug Targets, **2017**, *Vol. 16, No. 8*   **915**

Neural Stem Cells and Human Induced Pluripotent Stem Cells to Model Rare CNS Diseases

Lidia De Filippis[*], Cristina Zalfa and Daniela Ferrari

[*]*Casa Sollievo della Sofferenza, San Giovanni Rotondo (FG), Italy*

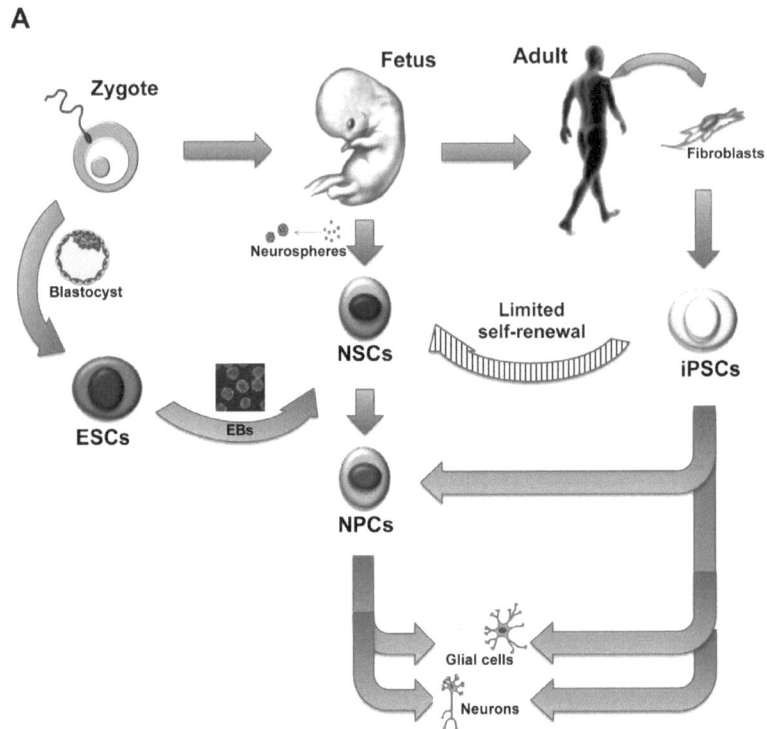

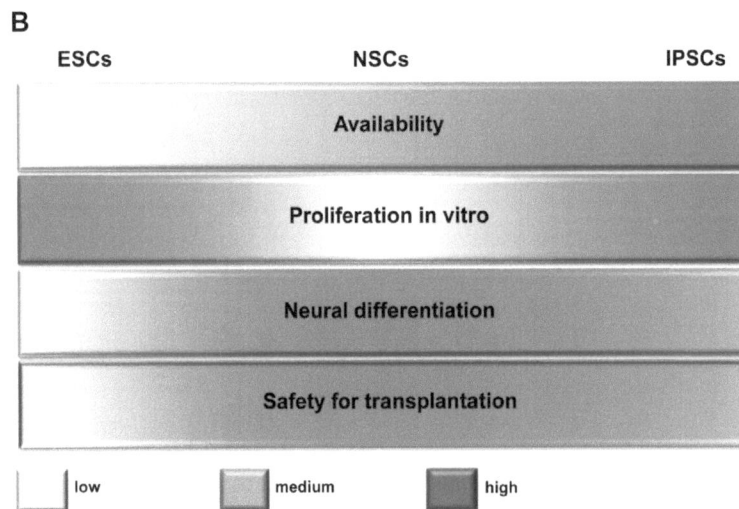

Cell modeling of rare CNS diseases. **A)** Diagram showing developmental evolution from pluripotent stem cells (ESC from the blastocyst or iPS from adult somatic cells) to fetal neural stem cells to neural progenitors (NPC) to neural phenotypes. **B)** Diagram showing colorimetric index of different stem cell properties required to define a reliable cell modeling system in ESC, NSC and iPSC.

CNS & Neurological Disorders - Drug Targets, **2017**, *Vol. 16, No. 8*   **927**

Leber's Hereditary Optic Neuropathy: Novel Views and Persisting Challenges

Jasna Jančić, Janko Samardžić[*], Stevan Stojanović, Amalija Stojanović, Ana Marija Milanović, Blažo Nikolić, Nikola Ivančević and Vladimir Kostić

[*]*Institute of Pharmacology, Clinical Pharmacology and Toxicology, Medical Faculty, University of Belgrade, Belgrade, Serbia*

The aim of this review is to provide an overview of literature regarding the epidemiology, etiology, pathogenesis, clinical features, diagnostics and possible treatment options and drug targets, as well as presenting challenges related to the disease and proposing a diagnostic algorithm based on current clinical experience.

CNS & Neurological Disorders - Drug Targets, **2017**, *Vol. 16, No. 8*   **936**

Immunomodulatory Strategies for Huntington's Disease Treatment

Gabriela D. Colpo[*], Natalia P. Rocha, Erin Fur Stimming and Antonio L. Teixeira

[*]*Neuropsychiatry Program, Department of Psychiatry and Behavioral Sciences, McGovern Medical School, The University of Texas Health Science Center at Houston, Houston, TX, USA*

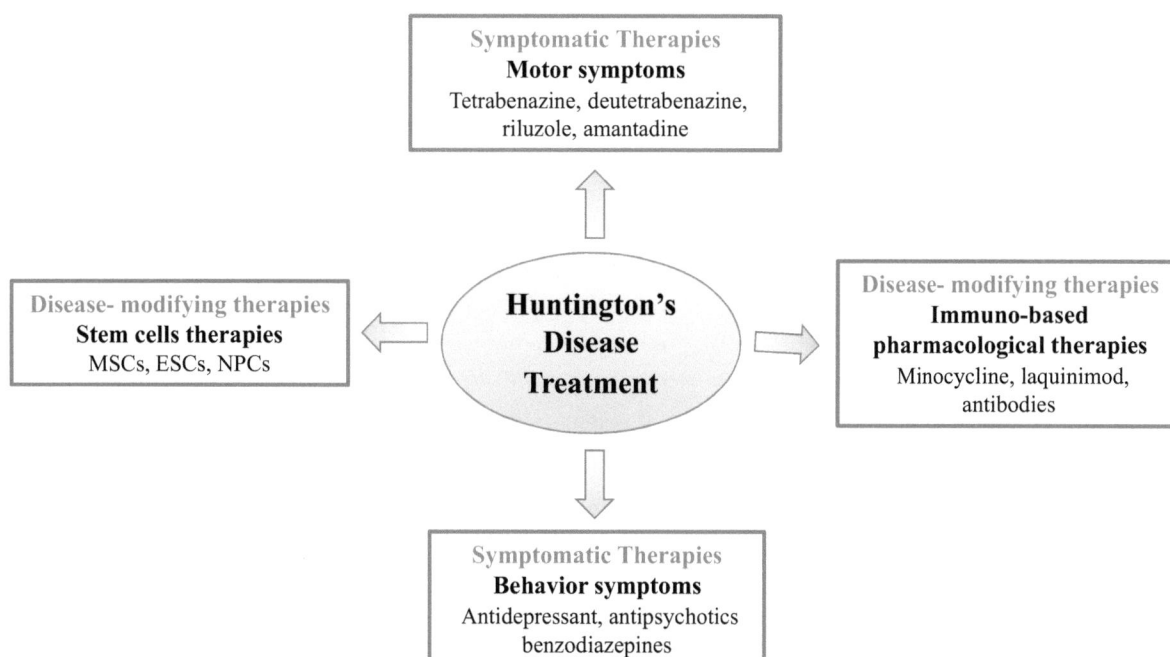

CNS & Neurological Disorders - Drug Targets, **2017**, *Vol. 16, No. 8*   **945**

Interrelationships Among Gut Microbiota and Host: Paradigms, Role in Neurodegenerative Diseases and Future Prospects

Javier Caballero-Villarraso, Alberto Galván, Begoña María Escribano and Isaac Túnez[*]

[*]*Departmento de Bioquimica y Biologia Molecular, Facultad de Medicina y Enfermeria, Universdiad de Cordoba, Spain*

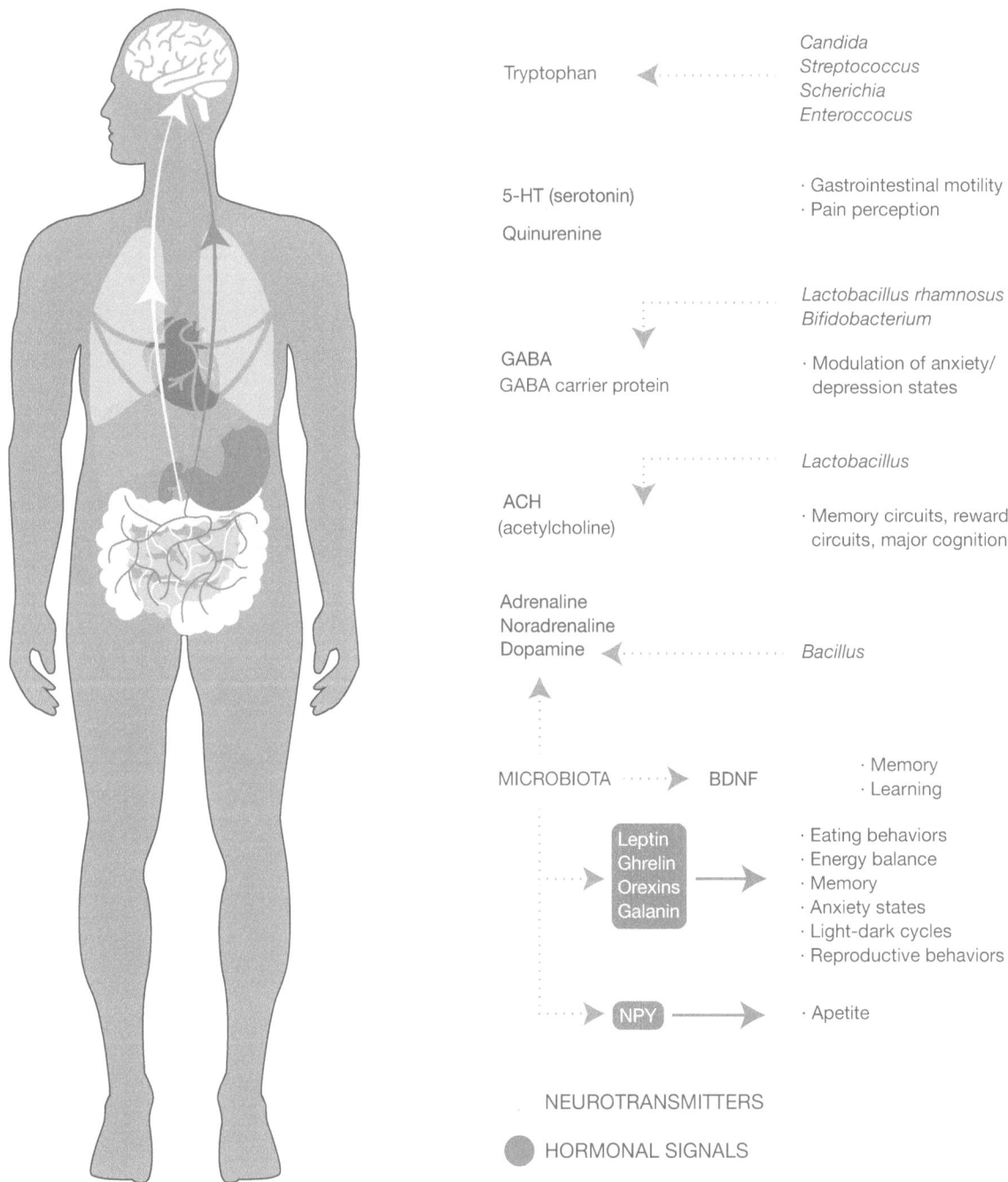

Meet Our Editorial Board Member

Dr. Beth Levant
University of Kansas Medical Center,
Kansas City, USA

Dr. Beth Levant, Ph.D., M.P.A. is a Professor with Tenure in the Department of Pharmacology, Toxicology and Therapeutics at the University of Kansas Medical Center. She is also a Scientist in the Kansas Intellectual and Developmental Disabilities Research Center.

Dr. Levant's research focuses on the role of polyunsaturated fatty acids in neuronal functional and neuropsychiatric disorders, and drugs and diseases affecting the CNS dopamine systems. Major research interests are the role of brain polyunsaturated fatty acid composition in postpartum depression and the role of developmental docosahexaenoic acid deficiency in attention deficit-hyperactivity disorder, Parkinson's disease, and traumatic brain injury. Her key research accomplishments in this area include demonstration that adult rats can experience a loss of DHA from brain phospholipids

Beth Levant

under certain nutritional and/or physiological circumstances, notably pregnancy and lactation. This loss of DHA from the adult brain results in neurochemical, physiological, and behavioral effects that suggest a contributory role for decreased brain DHA levels in the etiology of depression. Moreover, in female rats, this effect interacts with reproductive status such that a greater number of neurochemical alterations are present in postpartum dams when compared to virgin females with decreased brain DHA. This observation, combined with the vulnerability of the maternal brain to experience a loss of DHA, suggests a particular role for decreased brain DHA in postpartum depression. With respect to the role of DHA in neurodevelopment, Dr. Levant has shown that n-3 fatty acid deficiency during pre- and postnatal life results in altered numbers of dopamine neurons and behaviors relevant to activity and attention, supporting a contributory role for low dietary n-3 fatty acids in the etiology of ADHD and Parkinson's disease. She has also shown that higher tissue DHA levels, or the acute administration of n-3 fatty acids, produce beneficial effects on traumatic brain injury-induced sensorimotor deficits in a rat model of juvenile brain injury.

Additional interests include the D_3 dopamine receptor as a therapeutic target for schizophrenia, drug addiction, and Parkinson's disease. Dr. Levant's notable findings include the identification of a discrete population of D_3 receptors in cerebellum, determination of the pharmacological profile of the D_3 receptor, and demonstration of function and regulation of the D_3 receptor in native brain tissue. She also contributed to a drug discovery program that resulted in the design, synthesis, and demonstration of *in vivo* activity of D_3 agonists, partial agonists, and antagonists, some with greater than 1,000-fold selectivity. Recent studies have characterized dopaminergic cell numbers and morphology in the 6-hydroxydopamine model of Parkinson's disease.

Dr. Levant has published 75 peer-reviewed research reports and 31 reviews and book chapters on these topics.

In addition to her research, Dr. Levant teaches extensively in medical and graduate pharmacology courses, has held a variety of leadership roles in faculty governance, and is active in research on medical education practices.

Dr. Levant has received research support from the National Institutes of Health and a variety of private foundations. Her work has been recognized by a number of awards including a Kansas IDeA Research Excellence Faculty Scholar Award and the American College of Neuropsychopharmacology/Mead Johnson Travel Award. She has served as a chartered member on the National Institutes of Health Developmental Brain Disorders study section, as President of the local chapter of Sigma Xi, and as Treasurer of the Society for Neuroscience Kansas City Chapter.

Dr. Levant earned a B.S. in Zoology from the University of California, Davis and a Ph.D in Pharmacology from Duke University. She then undertook postdoctoral training in neuropharmacology at the DuPont Merck Pharmaceutical Co. She also holds a M.P.A. with emphases in health services administration and higher education from the University of Missouri-Kansas City.

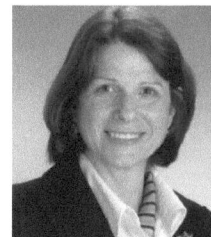

SELECTED PUBLICATIONS

[1]   Bancroft GN, Morgan KA, Flietstra RJ, Levant B. Binding of [^{3}H]PD 128907, a putatively selective ligand for the D_3 dopamine receptor, in rat brain: a receptor binding and quantitative autoradiographic study. Neuropsycho-pharmacology 1998; 18: 305-16.
[2]   Levant B, Radel JD, Carlson SE. Decreased brain docosahexaenoic acid during development alters dopamine-related behaviors in adult rats that are differentially affected by dietary remediation. Behav Brain Res 2004; 152: 49-57.
[3]   Levant B, Radel JD, Carlson SE. Reduced brain DHA content after a single reproductive cycle in female rats fed a diet deficient in n-3 polyunsaturated fatty acids. Biol Psychiatry 2006; 60: 987-90.

1871-5273/17 $58.00+.00   © 2017 Bentham Science Publishers

[4] Levant B, Ozias MK, Davis PF, Winter M, Russell KL, Carlson SE, Reed GA, McCarson KE. Decreased brain docosahexaenoic acid content produces neurobiological effects associated with depression: interactions with reproductive status in female rats. Psychoneuroendocrinology 2008; 33: 1279-92.

[5] Levant B, Zarcone TJ, Fowler SC. Developmental effects of dietary n-3 fatty acid content on activity and response to spatial novelty. Physiol Behav 2010; 101: 176-83.

[6] Russell KL, Berman NEJ, Levant B. Low brain DHA content worsens sensorimotor outcomes after TBI and decreases TBI-induced Timp-1 expression in juvenile rats. Prostaglandins Leukot Essent Fatty Acids 2013; 89: 97-105.

[7] Russell KL, Berman NEB, Gregg PRA, Levant B. Fish oil improves motor function, limits blood-brain barrier disruption, and reduces MMP9 gene expression in a rat model of juvenile traumatic brain injury. Prostaglandins Leukot Essent Fatty Acids 2014; 90: 5-11.

[8] Healy-Stoffel M, Ahmad SO, Stanford JA, Levant B. Differential effects of intrastriatal 6-hydroxydopamine on cell number and morphology in midbrain dopaminergic subregions of the rat. Brain Res 2014; 1574: 113-9.

[9] Pes R, Godar SC, Fox, AT, *et al.* Pramipexole enhances disadvantageous decision-making: lack of relation to changes in phasic dopamine release. Neuropharmacology 2017; 114: 77-87.

Editorial

Unmet Needs in Modern Psychiatry

According to the World Health Organization (2016), mental disorders dramatically contribute to the social and financial burden across countries. Specifically, they negatively impact the quality of life among those affected and their families as well are a source of economic consequences around the world.

Despite efforts spent for caring for psychiatric patients and treating mental disorders, there are still many unmet needs in several domains of mood disorders, schizophrenia, and suicide risk. For example, treatment resistance, nonadherence, and adverse effects are some of the more essential unmet needs.

It has been repeatedly shown that the needs of patients, relatives, the community at large and those of the governmental bodies only partially overlap. For instance, patients and their families are more concerned about quality of life, treatment, autonomy, independent living and so on; governmental stakeholders are typically more concerned about relapse prevention and reduction of hospitalizations.

A decisive step in the management of patients suffering from psychiatric illness is nowadays arising, leading to identify the most common needs of those affected, describe the type of aid, and determine the associated variables to unmet needs. Recent research has underlined a number of unmet needs in patients suffering from schizophrenia with the urgent call to action to deliver new therapeutic options to target both symptoms and side effects reduction.

Although patient management, in every branch of medicine, encounters the problem of non-adherence to treatment, its impact in the psychiatric context assumes significant proportions, especially considering the burden that mental illness - especially major depressive disorder, and bipolar disorder.

The impact of non-adherence to treatment is a significant phenomenon, especially in MDD, whose management continues to be a challenge for psychiatrists. In fact, there is not a general consensus as to the most effective treatment for this pathology and, in many cases, more than one approach is necessary to achieve clinical remission. At the functional level, there is now evidence that disability persists also when patients are symptom-free; recent studies have pointed out the need for patients to achieve a full functional recovery, that is the complete return to a satisfactory life and the achievement of a good daily functioning. As part of MDD, another clinical challenge is relapse, which is due to the lack of medication adherence. Moreover, delays and/or interference in the treatment also contribute to decreased adherence and poor prognosis, especially in MDD.

In addition to the need for timely treatment and long-term oriented depressive symptoms, a future challenge, which involves both patient and doctors, appears to be the recognition and management of cognitive impairment (CI) in MDD and other mood disorders. Among mood disorders, there are several available treatments to address CI and reduce the burden of this condition. However, these are symptoms that have partial benefit from available treatments and recurrence may ensue when stabilization is achieved. New treatment options are therefore needed and one of the papers included in this issue will focus on this topic. Furthermore, suicide is a major public health issue with more 800,000 people dying annually. Pharmacological treatment for reducing suicide risk is still limited to a few medications that have shown promising results; clinicians are looking for new perspectives for preventing suicide.

Treatment of agitation still represents a major clinical challenge especially because initial verbal methods often fail to calm the patient and medications become necessary. Acute agitation is common and may occur across a range of somatic, psychiatric, and substance abuse disorders, and a diagnosis is often still unclear when rapid intervention is necessary.

We are pleased to have collected papers for the present issue of CNS & Neurological Disorders-Drug Targets written by opinion leaders in the treatment of psychiatric disorders. We are particularly thankful to the authors of this Special Issue, who are all leaders in their field and have contributed their work relevant to the important topic of "unmet needs in modern psychiatry". We are also grateful to the Editor, who invited us to focus on neglected areas of psychiatric practice. We hope that the readers of CNS & Neurological Disorders-Drug Targets will find these papers as interesting as we did.

Guest Editors
Maurizio Pompili, M.D., Ph.D.
Department of Neurosciences,
Mental Health and Sensory Organs,
Suicide Prevention Center
Sant'Andrea Hospital, Sapienza University of Rome, Rome, Italy
E-mail: maurizio.pompili@uniroma1.it

Andrea Fiorillo, MD, PhD
Department of Psychiatry
University of Campania "Luigi Vanvitelli"
Naples, Italy
E-mail: andrea.fiorillo@unicampania.it

1871-5273/17 $58.00+.00   © 2017 Bentham Science Publishers

CNS & Neurological Disorders - Drug Targets, 2017, *16*, 858-869

REVIEW ARTICLE

Potential Novel Treatments for Bipolar Depression: Ketamine, Fatty Acids, Anti-inflammatory Agents, and Probiotics

Gustavo H. Vázquez[1,2], Sebastián Camino[3], Leonardo Tondo[1,4,5] and Ross J. Baldessarini[1,4,*]

[1]*International Consortium for Bipolar & Psychotic Disorder Research, Mailman Research Center, McLean Hospital, Belmont, Massachusetts 02478, USA;* [2]*Department of Psychiatry, Queens University School of Medicine, Kingston, Ontario, K7L-2V7, Canada;* [3]*"Dr. Braulio A. Moyano" Neuropsychiatric Hospital, Ciudad de Buenos Aires, Argentina;* [4]*Department of Psychiatry, Harvard Medical School, Boston, Massachusetts 02115, USA;* [5]*Lucio Bini Mood Disorder Centers, Cagliari and Rome, Italy*

Abstract: *Background*: Treatments for depression in bipolar disorder (BD) are far less well developed than for unipolar major depressive disorder. Several innovative and experimental approaches have been emerging recently, including use of the dissociative anesthetic ketamine and other antagonists of central NMDA glutamate receptors, as well as unsaturated fatty acids, anti-inflammatory agents, and possibly probiotic methods.

Method: We reviewed relevant reports from the past decade.

Findings: Ketamine, a phencyclidine-like NMDA-glutamate receptor antagonist, has emerged as a highly innovative, experimental treatment for treatment-resistant unipolar major depression, possibly in bipolar depression, and with brief antisuicidal effects. Its limitations include poor bioavailability, rapid but short-lived effects, and little information about long-term benefits and safety of repeated administration. Polyunsaturated fatty acids critical for the structure and functioning of neuronal and other cell membranes have some evidence of benefit as experimental treatments for depression including in BD. There also is evidence of altered expression of peptides associated with inflammation in mood disorder patients, encouraging experimental treatment with anti-inflammatory agents; of these, the COX-II inhibitor celecoxib has shown some evidence of benefit. The concept of altering intestinal flora with probiotic treatments to treat mood disorders remains speculative.

Conclusion: Ketamine represents an innovative, rapidly acting, experimental treatment for bipolar depression with practical limitations. Unsaturated fatty acids and anti-inflammatory agents have inconsistent support; probiotic treatments lack evidence. These innovative approaches require much more clinical investigation.

ARTICLE HISTORY

Received: January 03, 2017
Revised: July 11, 2017
Accepted: July 11, 2017

DOI:
10.2174/1871527316666170728165648

Keywords: Anti-inflammatory, bipolar disorder, depression, ketamine, inflammation, NMDA receptor, polyunsaturated fatty acids, probiotics.

1. INTRODUCTION

Research aimed at developing effective and safe treatments for depressive episodes of bipolar disorder (BD) remains remarkably less well developed than for unipolar major depressive disorder [1]. In part, this status may reflect an uncritical assumption that treatments proved to be effective and tolerated for unipolar depression would be similarly useful in depressive phases of BD as well. However, standard antidepressants (tricyclics, serotonin- and mixed amine-reuptake inhibitors, and monoamine oxidase inhibitors) have produced inconsistent evidence of efficacy in acute bipolar depression [2-4] and risk induction of mania and affective instability [5]. Alternatives include reliance on mood-stabilizing agents including lithium and certain anticonvulsants, which have limited and inconsistent evidence for efficacy in acute bipolar depression and for its long-term prevention [1, 6]. In addition several atypical or second-generation antipsychotic agents (including lurasidone, olanzapine with fluoxetine, and quetiapine) have emerged as effective treatments for acute bipolar depression, and they extend the range of utility of these nominally antipsychotic or antimanic drugs [5, 7, 8].

It is particularly striking that relatively little research has been reported on the treatment of depression in BD, specifically, in contrast to a massive literature collected since the

*Address correspondence to this author at the Mailman Research Center 306, McLean Hospital, 115 Mill Street, Belmont, MA 02478-9106 USA;
Tel: 1-617-855-3203; Fax: 1-617-855-3479;
E-mail: rbaldessarini@mclean.harvard.edu.

late 1950s pertaining to unipolar major depression [1]. The result is that better treatments for the common, potentially disabling or fatal syndrome bipolar depression remain very much needed [9]. Some progress has been emerging in recent years. The present overview considers a series of innovative treatments that are unusual but show some encouraging findings including from controlled treatment trials. Specifically, we consider treatment of acute bipolar depression with ketamine or other emerging glutamate NMDA receptor antagonists, certain poly-unsaturated fatty acids (PUFAs), anti-inflammatory agents (including aspirin, acetaminophen, COX-II inhibitors, other nonsteroidal agents, N-acetylcysteine, minocycline, and pregnanolone), and comment briefly on proposals that modifying intestinal flora, by administering "probiotic" bacteria including lactobacilli, may be of interest.

2. KETAMINE

2.1. Introduction

Recent studies support the potential of ketamine and emerging new glutamate excitatory receptor antagonist agents to provide effective and rapid benefits for depression, even in BD after failure of standard treatments, and with high risks of suicide [10-16]. Among biological treatments for severe depression, including in BD, ketamine represents a rare and salutary innovation.

2.2. Pharmacology

Ketamine, a chiral arylcyclohexylamine derivative, was first synthesized in 1962 in efforts to develop a safer agent than phencyclidine by chemist Calvin Stevens at Wayne State University in Detroit, Michigan, Phencylidine was used as a dissociative anesthetic-analgesic since 1970, and is listed as a Schedule III substance of abuse (along with androgenic-anabolic steroids) by the US Drug Enforcement Administration (DEA; Fig. 1). It has a complex pharmacology, marked notably by noncompetitive antagonism of N-methyl-D-aspartate (NMDA) glutamate receptors in the central nervous system, targeted at a receptor sub-site favored by phencyclidine, of which ketamine is an analog (Fig. 1). Like phencyclidine, ketamine has hallucinogenic and depersonalizing effects that encourage its abuse for recreational purposes in addition to useful clinical indications as a veterinary and human analgesic and anesthetic, usually as the racemic product, R,S-ketamine (Ketalar® and others, and generic) [17, 18].

In addition to its actions as an NMDA antagonist, ketamine has weak interactions with AMPA glutamate receptors, as well as with mu (μ) and kappa (κ) opioid receptors with little antagonism by naloxone; it can also block voltage-gated Na^+ and L-type Ca^{2+} ion channels, inhibit nitric oxide (NO) synthase, modulate nicotinic acetylcholine (ACh_n) receptors, exert weak agonistic effects on γ-aminobutyric acid type A ($GABA_A$) receptors, as well as showing some inhibitory effect at transporters for norepinephrine (NET), serotonin (SERT), and dopamine (DAT), and weak D_2 dopamine receptor agonism. Ketamine may also have neuroprotective actions. It can slowly modify the morphology of neurons, including increases of neuronal spines, probably mediated by effects on the expression of genes for proteins that stimulate

and modulate neuronal morphology, including brain-derived neurotrophic factor (BDNF) and the phosphatidylinositol 3-kinase mTOR (the protein "mammalian or mechanistic target of rapamycin") [19-22].

How these various pharmacodynamic actions may contribute to the apparent antidepressant effects of ketamine and its metabolic by-products remains uncertain, but NMDA antagonism is unlikely to be the only relevant effect [23, 24]. It is likely that slowly-evolving molecular or neuroanatomical changes contribute to clinical effects that continue for days after clearance of ketamine. Finally, ketamine is highly reinforcing based on self-administration animal models and by producing dependency and withdrawal reactions after repeated use may represent a clinical risk factor [25].

The ketamine molecule occurs as optically active isomers, with 3-4-times higher potency at NMDA receptors of the S(+) than the R(-) enantiomer [17, 18, 22, 23]. The S(+) enantiomer has twice the analgesic-anesthetic potency of racemic, R,S-ketamine, and is more rapidly cleared metabolically, although isomeric differences in antidepressant potency remain untested [22]. Ketamine is poorly bioavailable orally (<20%), somewhat better sublingually or intranasally (25%-50%), well absorbed ($\geq$90%) by intramuscular injection, and best tested for depression by intravenous infusion. It is very rapidly cleared, with a human elimination half-life of 2-3 hours. It undergoes rapid N-dealkylation by hepatic microsomal oxidative enzymes (especially CYP-3A4) to norketamine, a prominent, pharmacologically active by-product with somewhat slower elimination, and plasma concentrations typically thrice those of ketamine itself. Norketamine, in turn, is further oxidized, including to 6-hydroxynorketamine (HNK), the 2-R,6-R isomeric form of which (2R,6R-HNK) may have antidepressant activity, based on behavioral effects in animal models (Fig. 1) [24]. The therapeutic index (LD_{50}/ED_{50}) or margin of safety of ketamine is low ($\leq$2.5, and even lower for the less active R[-] enantiomer) when given at anesthetic doses much higher than those employed to treat depression [17, 18, 22, 23].

Doses of R,S-ketamine used for antidepressant effects typically are 0.10-0.50 mg/kg, infused slowly intravenously (IV) over 40-100 minutes to avoid adverse effects, sometimes repeated daily for several days, or twice or thrice weekly for several weeks. Analgesic effects are achieved at 0.20-0.75 mg/kg, IV, overlapping the range for antidepressant effects, whereas anesthetic doses average 1.0-4.5 mg/kg, IV. Doses for hallucinatory effects or recreational use of ketamine ("Special K") are much higher, typically 60-250 mg by inhalation [18, 22, 26, 27].

2.3. Experimental Alternatives to R,S-ketamine

The short clinical action (typically less than one hour for anesthesia, but mood-elevating effects can last up to one week), poor oral bioavailability, abuse potential, and low margin of safety of racemic ketamine have encouraged efforts to develop more conveniently dosed and safer NMDA glutamate receptor antagonists [14, 16]. Racemic ketamine can be given sublingually, though at somewhat higher doses than are given by intravenous injection [18]. Intravenous S[+]-ketamine (esketamine), in doses as low as 0.2 mg/kg, has antidepressant effects [28], and intranasal S[+]-ketamine

(Ketanest-S®, Janssen) is under investigation as an antidepressant [29], but the R[-] enantiomer has not been studied. Norketamine has antidepressant-like effects in animal models [30]. Interestingly, ketamine has been used as an anesthetic for electroconvulsive treatment (ECT), with inconsistent claims of increased antidepressant effects compared to ECT with short-acting barbiturates or propofol for anesthesia [31-33].

A series of novel compounds are in development which may provide alternatives to ketamine [14, 16, 34]. Most act at the glycine site in the NMDA receptor (unlike ketamine and phencyclidine) or other sites in the receptor complex; some appear to lack hallucinogenic or dissociative effects and should be safer to use clinically. Several such compounds have at least preliminary clinical findings that indicate antidepressant activity. They include 4-chloro-kynurinine (VistaGen Corporation), CERC-301 (Cerecor) for intravenous administration, rapastinel (GLYX-13; Allergan), and apimostinel (NRX-1074; Naurex) which is orally active and quite potent (Fig. **1**). Another NMDA-antagonist with some antidepressant activity and apparently low risk of psychotomimetic effects is lanicemine (AZD-6765; AstraZeneca) [35]. They all require evaluation of efficacy, dosing, and safety in controlled trials for major depression, including in BD. Clinical development of another NMDA-antagonist, traxoprodil (CP-101696; Pfizer) has been discontinued due to toxic effects. In addition, the anti-dementia agent memantine (Eli Lilly) is an NMDA antagonist which may have beneficial effects in BD [36] but does not appear to be effective for treating bipolar depression [13].

2.4. Clinical Evidence of Efficacy of Ketamine for Depression

An early suggestion that ketamine might have antidepressant effects was the anecdotal self-report of a Detroit patient who had taken ketamine as an illicit, unprescribed drug in ca. 1980, as reported by Edward Domino [37]. The first, small but controlled clinical trial of R,S-ketamine as an antidepressant was reported in 2000 [38], based rationally on pharmacological theory and animal modeling [25, 39]. A considerable amount of clinical research has been reported on the use of ketamine for treatment of unipolar major depression, including several dozen case reports, case series, and uncontrolled trials [8, 25, 40, 41]. Additional reports are emerging that include or focus on depressed patients diagnosed with BD [11-13, 15, 42-45]. Most of the findings are encouraging in finding at least short-term benefits of ketamine treatment in bipolar depression, often after failure of other treatments, but usually with gradual loss of benefits over the following 1-2 weeks. Little research has addressed long-term use of ketamine to maintain antidepressant effects in either unipolar or bipolar depression, and such efforts may encounter difficulties in maintaining double-blind conditions, with uncertain risks of abuse of the drug [46].

Two uncontrolled, anecdotal reports include 56 cases of bipolar depression and found strong clinical responses in 51.8% (29/56), usually within the initial hours or first day after IV or sublingual administration of ketamine [47, 48]. However, well-controlled, randomized trials for bipolar depression remain very few. We found only two, short-term, double-blind, cross-over, placebo-controlled trials of ketamine for previously treatment-resistant, bipolar depression [49, 50]. In these trials, among a total of 33 participants at the US National Institute of Mental Health (NIMH), response rate (≥50% improvement of symptom ratings) averaged 60.6% (20/33) at 24 hours, compared to no response during crossover, add-on treatment with placebo [49, 50]. These findings included reductions in suicide items (mainly suicidal ideation) on standard depression rating scales [49, 50]. An additional uncontrolled study from the same investi-

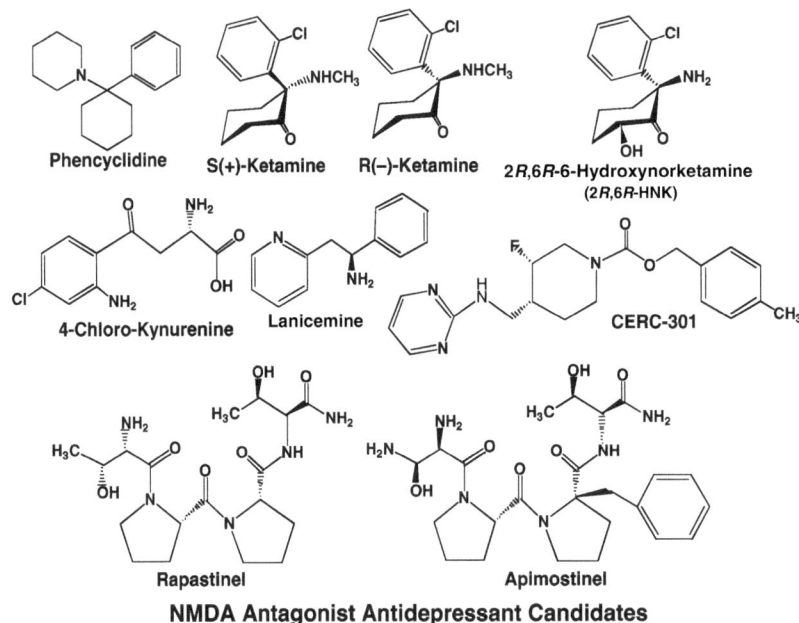

NMDA Antagonist Antidepressant Candidates

Fig. (1). NMDA Antagonist antidepressant candidates.

gators found that ketamine was similarly effective among depressed BD subjects with and without prominent anxiety, with maximum benefits found at seven days after acute, add-on treatment [51]. In a recent review that includes comparisons of unipolar and bipolar depressed trial participants, overall symptomatic improvements (1-7 days, with between-diagnosis matching for outcome measures) averaged 35.6% less among BD subjects [25]. This finding may suggest lesser benefits in bipolar than in unipolar depression, but the selection criteria, outcome measures, and assessment times varied considerably across trials, leaving the question of relative efficacy unresolved. Although the matter has not been adequately evaluated other than in short-term use of ketamine, it has only rarely been associated with switching of mood into hypomania or mania [16, 44, 45]. If true, this is a major benefit for a treatment aimed at bipolar depression.

2.5. Comments about Ketamine

The discovery of rapid mood-elevating effects of low doses of the phencyclidine-like NMDA antagonist ketamine is an historically intriguing development, particularly since there has been very little that is fundamentally new for the biological treatment of severe depression since the development of ECT in the 1930s, monoamine oxidase (MAO) inhibitors in the mid-1950s, monoamine transport-inhibitors since the late 1950s, and recent applications of some second-generation antipsychotic agents to the treatment of unipolar and bipolar depression [1]. Interest in ketamine includes the hope that its pharmacodynamic actions may lead the way to other, novel and rapidly acting antidepressant drugs [21]. Despite growing evidence for at least short-term antidepressant effects of ketamine in bipolar as well as unipolar major depression, including in cases resistant to other treatments, and perhaps including temporary reduction of suicidal thinking, many questions and challenges remain. Ketamine presents an unusual situation in that it has regulatory approval for use as an anesthetic or analgesic, legally allowing its increasing "off-label" use in various clinical settings, even though many aspects of its clinical pharmacology, efficacy, dosing and optimal routes of administration, long-term use, safety and abuse potential in mood-disorder patients remain uncertain [25, 52-56].

Tension between pressure to make early use of a promising treatment for difficult clinical problems and to address the usual requirements for evaluating a new treatment is high. To date, despite many reports and reviews of ketamine for depression, much of the research carried out has involved small and highly selected samples, controls of uncertain validity, varied outcome measures, and short-term evaluations. Such treatment has often appeared to provide beneficial responses with few adverse outcomes or toxic effects. However, the benefits inevitably wear off over times greater than one week, with high rates of relapse, leaving uncertainties about how to maintain or regain benefits in typically enduring or highly recurrent depressive illnesses.

Controlled trials of ketamine for bipolar depression are particularly infrequent, have been carried out by relatively few investigators, and often involve cross-over rather than preferred parallel-group trial designs. Controls typically involve use of IV saline or sometimes a short-acting sedative-anesthetic such as midazolam, but lacking are comparisons of effects of ketamine to euphoriants such as amphetamine or cocaine, or to an opioid [53]. Moreover, most of the reported experience with ketamine for treating depression has occurred in relatively closely controlled academic and research environments with highly selected subjects. It is uncertain how well such circumstances may translate to safe and effective clinical applications of this controlled and potentially toxic substance in more typical settings, although clinical applications have been expanding.

Problems and limitations in the use of ketamine to treat depression include its poor oral bioavailability, short duration of action (perhaps a week, compared to a short elimination half-life of 2-3 hours), lack of data about optimal doses, routes of administration, and timing of initial and subsequent treatments, adverse effects, and potential for abuse and dependency [25, 54, 56]. Adverse effects notably include acutely increased blood pressure and pulse rate, and later risk of cystitis and other adverse urological effects (possibly through local toxic effects on bladder tissue), cognitive impairment, dependency and withdrawal reactions that can include psychosis [18, 56].

Many of the shortcomings of ketamine may be minimized by further development of novel agents that follow the lead of ketamine, which is widely assumed to act primarily as an NMDA glutamate receptor antagonist (Fig. 1). Some such agents currently in development appear to have antidepressant effects, but to lack the dose-dependent psychotomimetic effects of ketamine and perhaps to be better tolerated. Agents that can be administered in a more convenient way than ketamine and can be used repeatedly, safely and effectively are needed. In general, the major significance of ketamine for depression is as a model or lead agent that has opened a new era in developing effective antidepressants with novel actions, following limited success of such efforts over the past half-century [1].

3. FATTY ACIDS

3.1. Introduction and Chemistry of Fatty Acids

Long-chain fatty acids are important constituents of cell membranes, including neuronal membranes in the central nervous system [57, 58] (Fig. 2). Their availability depends on endogenous synthesis from two essential (requiring dietary intake) fatty acid precursors. Linoleic acid, an 18-carbon chain, omega (ω)-6-unsaturated molecule (double-bond at carbons 6 and 7 from the methyl terminus) is required to synthesize arachidonic acid, a 20-carbon chain, ω-6-unsaturated product. The essential fatty acid α-linolenic acid, an 18-carbon chain, ω-3-unsaturated molecule (double-bond at carbons 3 and 4) is the precursor of eicosapentaenoic (EPA; 20-carbon, ω-3 unsaturated) and docosahexaenoic (DHA; 22-carbon, ω-3 unsaturated) acids. Although EPA and DHA can be biosynthesized in the body from α-linolenic acid by elongation and oxidative desaturation, the process is inefficient, so that some dietary supplementation with the polyunsaturated fatty acids (PUFAs) EPA and DHA is needed to maintain physiological concentrations in brain and other tissues. Common dietary sources include oily fish and some oily nuts and seeds (such as linseed or flaxseed).

Omega-3 Fatty Acids   **Omega-6 Fatty Acids**

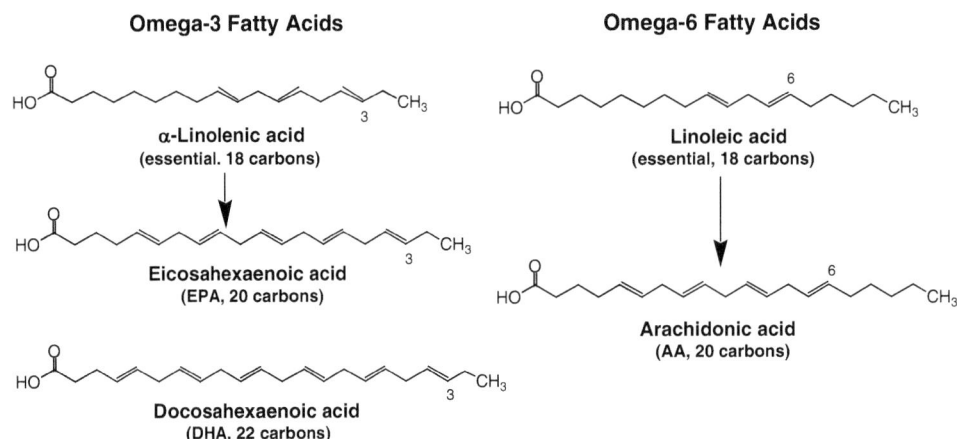

Fig. (2). Polyunsaturated fatty acids (PUFAs).

Arachidonic acid is converted to the prostaglandins and thromboxanes (prostanoids) by the "cyclo-oxygenase" isoenzymes types 1 and 2 (COX-1, COX-2), prostaglandin-endoperoxide synthase (PTGS), and a peroxidase [59]. Prostaglandins can stimulate synthesis of pro-inflammatory cytokines, such as interleukin-6 (IL-6) and TNF-α [60]. EPA is converted to leukotrienes (members of the eicosanoid family) through a lipoxygenase. All of these lipid products contribute to local regulation of inflammatory and immunological responses [61]. DHA, EPA, and arachidonic acid also are involved in the synthesis of resolvins—oxidized fatty acids with demonstrated anti-inflammatory, tissue-healing, and neuroprotective functions in addition to those of DHA and EPA themselves [58, 62, 63]. Neuroprotective effects are also mediated by the protein, brain-derived neurotrophic factor (BDNF), production of which is enhanced by ω-3 fatty acids. PUFAs of the ω-3 type have a key role in the BDNF-activated tyrosine kinase receptor-B (TrkB) signaling pathway, again contributing to neuro-protective effects [64]. The preceding chemical reactions occur primarily in the liver, but also in brain, once ω-3 and ω-6 fatty acids are transferred through the blood-brain barrier [58]. The varied effects of fatty acids include support of the structural integrity and fluidity of neuronal and other cell membranes; enzyme activities; lipid-protein interactions, and their role as precursors for eicosanoids, such as prostaglandins, leukotrienes and thromboxanes which contribute to the regulation of inflammatory responses [58, 59, 65]. Moreover, fatty acids are crucial for the transmission of nerve impulses and strongly influence brain development [65, 66].

3.2. Clinical Applications of Fatty Acids

An emerging view is that the complex group of PUFAs and other fatty acids may exert significant benefits in preventing or ameliorating several general medical illnesses [65]. In addition, their deficiency has been associated with some psychiatric disorders [65-67]. Notably, in a large prospective study, higher dietary intake of EPA and DHA was associated with a lower risk of clinical depression in a 10-year follow-up of 3317 young adults in the US, particularly in women [68]. Furthermore, growing evidence suggests

involvement of PUFAs in the pathophysiology of BD. For example, greater seafood consumption, which is a main food source of ω-3 PUFAs, predicted lower lifetime prevalence rates of postpartum depression, and BD [69, 70]. Also, fish oil as a dietary supplement may reduce the severity of manic and depressive symptoms in juvenile BD [70].

The content of EPA and DHA in erythrocyte membranes seems to represent a reliable clinical index of the status of ω-3 PUFAs [71]. Type I BD has been associated with decreased concentrations of these PUFAs and of arachidonic acid in red blood cell membranes in some studies [72-74], but not in another [75]. In contrast, plasma concentrations of fatty acids including EPA, arachidonic and α-linolenic acids were higher in BD patients than in healthy controls [76], and the severity of manic symptoms was lower with higher circulating levels of EPA and arachidonic acid, and a lower ratio of the two fatty acids [77]. Among BD patients there also is evidence of altered metabolism of α-6-linoleic acid [78, 79]. Other findings of potential interest include association of circulating concentrations of fatty acids with symptomatic expression of BD. For example, greater symptom-severity in BD patients correlated with lower plasma levels of ω-3 fatty acids including EPA, but also with higher levels of ω-6 fatty acids including arachidonic [80]. In addition, giving supplemental ethyl-EPA to BD patients led to magnetic resonance spectroscopic (MRS) evidence of increased cerebral concentrations of N-acetylaspartate (NAA), considered to be a biomarker of neuronal integrity and suggesting a neuroprotective effect of ω-3 fatty acids [81].

Mood-altering or -stabilizing medicines, including lithium and the anticonvulsants carbamazepine, lamotrigine and valproate are standard treatments for BD. Their use has been associated with evidence of decreased metabolic turnover of arachidonic acid in cerebral phospholipids, as well as decreased production of prostaglandin-E2 and of the expression of enzymes involved in the metabolism of arachidonic acid, including cytosolic phospholipase-A2, cyclo-oxygenase-2 or acyl-CoA-synthase [82, 83]. These biological effects support the hypothesis that dietary supplementation of the intake of ω-3 PUFAs may be effective in the treatment of BD, possibly through mechanisms that may parallel pharmacodynamic relationships to actions of standard mood-stabilizing agents. For instance, ω-3 fatty acids may produce a general dampening of signal transduction pathways associated with phosphatidylinositol, arachidonic acid, and other molecular systems through direct inhibition of protein kinase-C (PKC), reduced production of cytokines, blockade of calcium ion channels, and modification of the composition of cell membranes [84-87]. Some of these actions also have been associated with the effects of lithium and valproate [1].

Encouraged by these varied preliminary findings, several studies have explored the therapeutic potential of augmenting dietary intake of PUFAs for patients with BD. Reported beneficial effects include reducing the severity of mania when ω-3 fatty acids were added to standard antimanic treatments [88], beneficial effects on bipolar depression of addition of EPA [89, 90], as well as possible reduction of long-term recurrence rates in BD patients [91]. Nevertheless, despite some encouraging findings, this research has not been consistent or compelling (Table **1**) [80, 81, 88-95]. For example, there was no improvement in risk of recurrences following acute bipolar depression after addition of EPA versus placebo to standard ongoing treatment [92], or evidence of an antimanic benefit after supplementing oral intake of EPA and DHA [93, 94]. Another small study found little benefit of adding ω-3 fatty acids with or without cytidine for children with possible BD [95].

3.3. Comments about Fatty Acids

There are a series of interesting associations between clinical states in BD patients (and others) and concentrations of fatty acids in erythrocyte membranes or plasma. They have encouraged efforts to supplement intake of PUFAs including DHA and EPA for therapeutic effects in mania and perhaps in bipolar as well as unipolar major depression. However, the reported clinical effects of such interventions have been modest and inconsistent. Moreover, the expectation of highly selective effects of administering PUFAs in bipolar disorder may be unrealistic.

4. ANTI-INFLAMMATORY AGENTS AND ANTI-OXIDANTS

4.1. Introduction

Support for the hypothesis that inflammatory responses are associated with mood and other psychiatric disorders has been gathering for several decades [96-98]. Most of this evidence pertains to nonbipolar major depression. Some recent studies have considered anti-inflammatory agents as potential innovative treatments for depression, including in BD [99]. Evidence supporting an association between clinical depression and inflammatory responses includes adverse effects on mood of clinically administered cytokine peptides involved in inflammatory responses, such as interferon [100, 101]. Cytokines are small proteins with local and systemic regulatory effects on cell functions associated with inflammatory responses, as are eicosanoids derived from PUFAs [102]. Cytokines include chemokines, interferons, interleukins, lymphokines, and tumor necrosis factors. Some inflammatory cytokines, especially interleukin-4 (IL-4) or -6 (IL-6) and tumor necrosis factor-alpha (TNF-α), as well as eicosanoids and other products of arachidonic acid metabo-

lism, including prostaglandins, been found to be elevated in depressed subjects [102], as well as in mania [103-105].

Conversely, antidepressant treatment has been associated with decreased release of cytokines, including some interleukins and tumor necrosis factors [103, 107], and responses to antidepressant treatment have been associated with declining circulating concentrations of cytokines [107, 108]. Serum concentrations of some cytokines also may be reduced by mood-stabilizing and antipsychotic agents [104]. In addition, there are associations between release of cytokines and exposure to a range of environmental factors and health measures (including stress, childbirth, malnutrition, inactivity, obesity, smoking, and altered intestinal functioning), some of which have been considered risk factors for depression but also of other psychiatric and general medical disorders [107]. In sum, there is evidence of an association between abnormal mood states and inflammatory responses, but the lack selectivity for mood disorders and their relationship to causes versus effects of mood disorders is unclear, and their expression may be relatively nonspecific distress signals.

4.2. Therapeutic Experimentation with Anti-inflammatory Agents

As noted above, ω-3 PUFAs, which can exert anti-inflammatory effects, have shown benefits when added to standard antidepressants in at least 29 controlled trials in major depressive disorder. Eicosapentaenoic acid (EPA) was of particular interest, but with only moderate overall efficacy, considerable heterogeneity of outcomes, and evidence of biased reporting of positive findings [83, 109, 110]. In addition, several controlled treatment trials have considered effects of adding various exogenous anti-inflammatory agents to standard treatments, mostly in patients diagnosed with unipolar major depression or schizophrenia [109].

Such candidate treatments include cyclo-oxygenase-2 (COX-2) inhibitors, TNF-α antibodies, and the anti-inflammatory tetracycline antibiotic minocycline. These agents have somewhat inconsistent or weak evidence of effectiveness in major depressive episodes, lack diagnostic specificity in showing some benefits in schizophrenia as well as depression, have not been investigated extensively with BD patients, and have not been evaluated as monotherapies [109].

Among nonsteroidal anti-inflammatory drugs (NSAIDs), the COX-2 antagonist celecoxib (Cerebrex®) has been particularly well studied. In four of five trials of adding it or a placebo to ongoing, standard antidepressant treatment, at 200-400 mg/day for six weeks, celecoxib afforded significant antidepressive benefit, with an overall odds ratio versus placebo of 6.6 [95% CI: 2.6-17] [109, 111, 112]. Again, these effects were not diagnostically specific as three of four controlled trials in schizophrenia also showed benefit of celecoxib [109]. Moreover, the safety of long-term use of this and other COX-2 inhibitors in psychiatric patients, particularly regarding risks of adverse cardiac effects and stroke, is uncertain [109, 110].

Among tests of other candidate adjunctive, anti-inflammatory treatments, there is a placebo-controlled trial of the biological TNF-α antibody preparation infliximab (Remicade®), administered in three infusions of 5 mg/kg over

Table 1.   Clinical trials of fatty acids for bipolar disorder.

Study	Design	Sample & Intervention	Outcome Measures	Results
Stoll *et al.*, 1999 [91]	4-mo, double-blind RCT	30 BD patients given EPA (440 mg) + DHA (240 mg) or PBO daily + TAU	HDRS, CGI, GAS, YMRS	Longer remission with ω-3 fatty acids
Chiu *et al.*, 2005 [93]	4-wk, double-blind RCT	15 manic BD-I patients given EPA (440 mg) + DHA (240 mg), or PBO daily	YMRS, PANSS, HDRS, CGI	No effect
Osher *et al.*, 2005 [89]	6-mo, open trial	12 depressed BD-I outpatients given EPA (1.5-2.0 g) daily + TAU	HDRS	≥50% less depressed at ≥4 wks in 80% of cases
Frangou *et al.*, 2006 [90]	12-wk, double-blind RCT	24–26 depressed BD-I patients given ethyl-EPA (1 or 2 g) or PBO daily + TAU	HDRS, CGI	ω-3 fatty acid (both doses) effective vs. depression
Keck *et al.*, 2006 [92]	4-mo, double-blind RCT	59 depressed + 57 RC BD patients given EPA (6 mg) or PBO daily + TAU	CGI, IDS-C, YMRS	No effect
Frangou *et al.*, 2007 [81]	12-wk double-blind RCT	14 BD-I patients given ethyl-EPA (2 g) or PBO daily	cerebral NAA	ω-3 increased brain NAA
Gracious *et al.*, 2010 [80]	16-wk double-blind RCT	51 BP-I or –II juveniles (6–17 yrs) given flax-seed oil (550 mg of α-LNA/g) or olive oil as PBO daily, alone or with TAU	CDRS-R, CPRS, CGI-BP, GAF, K-SADS, SEFCA, YMRS	No effects
Murphy *et al.*, 2012 [94]	4-mo double-blind RCT	15 BD-I patients given cytidine + EPA (3 g) vs. 15 given EPA + PBO vs. 15 given PBO daily	YMRS, MADRS, GAF	No effects
Wozniak *et al.*, 2015 [95]	12-wk double-blind RCT	12 "BD spectrum" juveniles (aged 5–12 yrs) given ω-3+inositol, ω-3+ PBO, or inositol+PBO	YMRS, BPRS, CDRS, CGI, HDRS	Mania less intense with ω-3 + inositol
Shakeri *et al.*, 2016 [88]	3-mo double-blind RCT	50 BD-I patients given ω-3 fatty acids (1 g) daily vs. 50 given TAU	YMRS	Less intense mania with ω-3 fatty acids

Abbreviations: BD, bipolar disorder; *BPRS*, Brief Psychiatric Rating Scale; *CDRS*, Clinical Depression Rating Scale; *CGI-BP*, Clinical Global Impression scale for Bipolar Disorder; *CPRS*, Children's Psychiatric Rating Scale; *DHA*, docosahexaenoic acid; *EPA*, eicosapenaenoic acid; *GAF*, Global Assessment of Functioning scale; *GAS*, Global Assessment Scale; *HDRS*, Hamilton Depression Rating Scale; *IDS-C*, Inventory of Depressive Symptomatology [clinicians]; *K-SADS-PL*, Schedule for Affective Disorders and Schizophrenia for school-age Children (K), Present and Lifetime versions; *α-LNA*, alpha-linolenic acid; MADRS, Montgomery-Asberg Depression Rating Scale; *NAA*, N-acetylaspartate (estimated by magnetic resonance spectroscopy); *PANSS*, Positive and Negative Syndrome Scale; *PBO*, placebo; *RC*, rapid-cycling (≥4 episodes/year); *SEFCA*, Side Effects Form for Children and Adolescents; *TAU*, treatment as usual; *YMRS*, Young Mania Rating Scale; ω-3; omega-3 fatty acids (usually EPA or DHA).

six weeks, with follow-up to 12 weeks to a mix of 60 unipolar and bipolar depression patients. There was some decrease in depressive symptoms, but only among subjects who also had initially elevated serum concentrations of the inflammatory peptide, high-specificity C-reactive protein (hs-CRP) [113].

There have been fewer studies of anti-inflammatory agents added to standard mood-stabilizing treatments for BD patients, and specifically for bipolar depression [4, 19]. A recent comprehensive review of controlled trials of agents with anti-inflammatory effects for acute bipolar depression, identified only 8 trials involving 312 participants, in which anti-inflammatory agents were added to ongoing standard treatments [99].

The largest number of trials (n=5, with 140 subjects treated for a mean of 13 weeks) involved the ω-3 unsaturated fatty acids docosahexaenoic (DHA) or eicosapentaenoic (EPA) acids, alone or combined, and considered as anti-inflammatory agents [99]. Only two of the five trials found the PUFAs to be more effective than control treatments (placebo, or mineral or olive oils) [90, 91], and in one other there was a weak effect [89]. Risks of switching of mood into hy-

pomania or mania were minimal [114], but effects of PUFAs as a treatment for mania have been inconsistent in two trials [93, 94]. However, a pilot study in juveniles diagnosed with BD found suggestive evidence that ω-3 unsaturated fatty acids may be of benefit for manic symptoms [95].

In one placebo-controlled trial of celecoxib (400 mg/day for 6 weeks in 23 subjects), and another involving aspirin (240 mg/day in 30 subjects), neither nonsteroidal anti-inflammatory agent added to standard treatments was better than placebo for bipolar depression [99, 115].

Two controlled trials involved addition to standard treatments of N-acetylcysteine (NAC; Mucomyst® and others), 2 g/day for six months, in a total of 224 subjects. This amino acid derivative is an effective antidote for overdoses of acetaminophen (paracetamol) by acting to protect against depletion of glutathione with damage to hepatic cells; it also exerts beneficial effects in several conditions associated with inflammation, and is a mucolytic. Neither trial found significant antidepressant effects of NAC compared to a placebo [116, 117].

Among other even less well evaluated agents, a placebo-controlled, add-on trial (with 44 subjects treated for 6 weeks) of the potentially toxic, oral hypoglycemic agent pioglitazone (Actos®), with anti-inflammatory effects that include reducing output of TNF-α and modulating arachidonic acid metabolism, also found no evidence of antidepressant efficacy in BD [99, 118]. Treatment with minocycline for general medical indications has been reported to have incidental, apparent beneficial effects in case reports of various psychiatric disorders including bipolar depression, and requires study in controlled trials [109, 119]. Finally, the endogenous neurosteroid pregnenolone (a precursor of cortisol and other steroids) was tested in 80 patients diagnosed with bipolar depression, at a dose of 500 mg/day for 12 weeks [120]. The results were inconsistent, depending on the outcome measures employed. The same agent also has been reported to have beneficial effects in schizophrenia [120]. The preceding trials are summarized in Table **2** [115-118, 121-123].

4.3. Conclusions: Anti-inflammatory Agents

The overall impression arising from the information just reviewed is that the hypothesis that inflammatory changes associated with major mental illnesses, including bipolar depression, might lead to the development of novel treatments has only limited support. The relationship of inflammatory markers to particular psychiatric disorders appears to be nonspecific and may represent secondary pathophysiological responses, perhaps limiting the likelihood of leading to specific treatments. Even treatments with some promise (notably, polyunsaturated fatty acids and the COX-2 inhibitor celecoxib) have been tested only as adjuncts intended to boost responses of standard treatments, and even then, their effects have usually been modest and inconsistent in small numbers of trials for bipolar depression.

5. PROBIOTIC SUPPLEMENTS

5.1. Introduction

Probiotics are microörganisms that may provide health benefits when taken orally, supposedly by altering the balance between unfavorable bacteria in the intestines and more benign microorganisms including *Lactobacilli* and related *Bifidobacteria* which are naturally occurring gut flora [1, 124]. The concept appears to have arisen from observations of unusual longevity among certain Eastern European cultures whose diets include yoghurt. Proposed health benefits of the consumption of foods rich in milk-fermenting bacteria are suspiciously broad, and include: [a] reduced gastrointestinal discomfort, [b] strengthening of the immune system, [c] improved memory, and [d] benefits in psychiatric disorders ranging from autism and anxiety to obsessive-compulsive disorder, as well as depression [124-130]. Broad popularity of the consumption of lactobacillus-rich foods such as yoghurts has far outrun scientific evidence to support the broad and optimistic proposed health benefits of the approach.

Table 2.   **Trials of anti-inflammatory agents or antioxidants for bipolar disorder.**

Study	Design	Sample & Intervention	Outcomes	Results
Anti-Inflammatory Agents				
Nery *et al.*, 2008 [115]	6-wk double-blind RCT	28 depression of mixed BD patients given mood-stabilizer or atypical antipsychotic + celecoxib (400 mg/day) or PBO	HDRS, YMRS	Depression improved rapidly, not sustained
Saroukhani *et al.*, 2013 [121]	6-wk double-blind RCT	32 stable BD men continued lithium with aspirin (240 mg/day) or PBO	HDRS, YMRS	No significant difference in depression (erectile dysfunction improved)
Antioxidants				
Berk *et al.*, 2008 [116]	24-wk double-blind RCT	75 BD patients given NAC (1 g/day) or PBO plus treatment-as-usual	MADRAS, BDRS YMRS, GAF, CGI, *etc.*	Significantly improved depression (MADRS)
Berk *et al.*, 2011 [122]	8-wk open-label trial	149 depressed BD patients given NAC (2 g/day)	BDRS, MADRAS, CGI	Significantly improved depression (MADRS)
Berk *et al.*, 2012 [117]	24-wk double-blind RCT	93 BD patients given NAC openly (8 wks), then NAC *vs.* PBO	MADRAS, BDRS, YMRS, GAF, CGI, *etc.*	Depression not improved
Brennan *et al.*, 2013 [123]	12-wk double-blind RCT	40 depressed BD patients given ALCAR (1-3 g/day) + ALA (0.66-1.8 g/day), or PBO	HDRS, MADRS, YMRS, CGI	Depression not improved
Zeinoddini *et al.*, 2015 [118]	6-wk double-blind RCT	48 BD patients given pioglutazone (30 mg/day) or PBO, with lithium (to 0.6-0.8 mEq/L serum)	HDRS, YMRS	Significantly improved depression (HDRS)

Abbreviations: *ALA*, α-lipoic acid; *ALCAR*, acetyl-L-carnitine; *BDRS*, Bipolar Depression Rating Scale; *CGI*, Clinical Global Impression scale; *GAF*, Global Assessment of Functioning scale; HDRS, Hamilton Depression Rating Scale; *MADRS*, Montgomery-Asberg Depression Rating Scale; NAC, N-actylcysteine; PBO, placebo; *YMRS*, Young Mania Rating Scale; other abbreviations as for Table 1.

5.2. Clinical Experimentation with Probiotics

Oral administration of probiotic live microörganisms in daily doses of 108-1010 colony forming units (CFU) for 1-2 months has been a typical treatment. Favored organisms have included *Bifidobacteria* (longum, breve, and infantis) and *Lactobacilli* (casei, helveticus, plantarum, and rhaminosus). In at least 15 controlled clinical trials, such interventions have yielded suggestive evidence of possible modest impact on symptoms of depression or anxiety, but have not been studied specifically in bipolar depression [131, 132]. These findings would appear to encourage further study.

CONCLUSION

Of the wide-ranging and unusual treatment proposals considered here, the NMDA-antagonist ketamine and other agents like it are particularly interesting as innovative, rapidly acting, experimental treatments for bipolar depression with possible antisuicidal effects, but with practical limitations of short-action, unproved efficacy and safety with repeated administration, and potential for abuse. Unsaturated fatty acids (including DHA and EPA) and some anti-inflammatory agents (notably celecoxib, which may be less cardiotoxic than was initially proposed) have suggestive but inconsistent support as antidepressant, including for bipolar depression. Probiotic treatments have been claimed to exert beneficial effects across an extraordinary range of clinical conditions, but their value for bipolar depression specifically remains speculative. All of these innovative approaches require much more clinical investigation.

LIST OF ABBREVIATIONS

AChn	=	Nicotinic Acetylcholine Receptors
AMPA	=	α-amino-3-hydroxy-5-methyl-4-isoxazolepropionic acid
BD	=	Bipolar Disorder
BDNF	=	Brain-derived Neurotrophic Factor
CFU	=	Colony Forming Units
COX-1	=	Cyclo-oxygenase Isoenzymes Types 1
COX-2	=	Cyclo-oxygenase Isoenzymes Type 2
DAT	=	Dopamine Transporter
DHA	=	Docosahexaenoic Acid
ECT	=	Electroconvulsive Treatment
EPA	=	Eicosapentaenoic Acid
GABA$_A$	=	γ-aminobutyric Acid Type A Receptors
hs-CRP	=	High-specificity C-reactive Protein
IL-4	=	Interleukin-4
IL-6	=	Interleukin-6
MAO	=	Monoamine Oxidase
MRS	=	Magnetic Resonance Spectroscopic
NAA	=	N-acetylaspartate
NAC	=	N-acetylcysteine
NET	=	Norepinephrine Transporter
NIMH	=	National Institute of Mental Health
NMDA	=	N-methyl-D-aspartate
NO	=	Nitric Oxide
NSAIDS	=	Nonsteroidal Anti-inflammatory Drugs
PKC	=	Protein kinase-C
PTGS	=	Prostaglandin-endoperoxide Synthase
PUFAs	=	Polyunsaturated Fatty Acids
SERT	=	Serotonin Transporter
TNF-α	=	Tumor Necrosis Factor-alpha
TrkB	=	Tyrosine Kinase Receptor-B

CONSENT FOR PUBLICATION

Not applicable.

CONFLICT OF INTEREST

The authors and immediate family members have no financial relationships with commercial organizations that might appear to represent conflicts of interest in the work presented.

ACKNOWLEDGEMENTS

Supported in part by a grant from the Bruce J. Anderson Foundation and by the McLean Private Donors Psychopharmacology Research Fund (to RJB).

REFERENCES

[1] Baldessarini RJ. Chemotherapy in Psychiatry, third edition. New York: Springer Press, 2013.
[2] Pacchiarotti I, Bond DJ, Baldessarini RJ, *et al*. International Society for Bipolar Disorders (ISBD) Task Force report on antidepressant use in bipolar disorders. Am J Psychiatry 2013; 170(11): 1249-62.
[3] Vázquez GH, Tondo L, Undurraga J, Baldessarini RJ. Overview of antidepressant treatment of bipolar depression. Int J Neuropsychopharmacol 2013; 16(7): 1673-85.
[4] McGirr A, Vöhringer PA, Ghaemi SN, Lam RW, Yatham LN. Safety and efficacy of adjunctive second-generation antidepressant therapy with a mood-stabilizer or an atypical antipsychotic in acute bipolar depression: systematic review and meta-analysis of randomized, placebo-controlled trials. Lancet Psychiatr 2016; 3(12): 1138-46.
[5] Tondo L, Vázquez GH, Baldessarini RJ. Mania associated with antidepressant-treatment: comprehensive meta-analytic review. Acta Psychiatr Scand 2010; 121(6): 404-14.
[6] Selle V, Schalkwijk S, Vázquez GH, Baldessarini RJ. Treatments for acute bipolar depression: meta-analyses of placebo-controlled, monotherapy trials of anticonvulsants, lithium and antipsychotics. Pharmacopsychiatry 2014; 47(2): 43-52.
[7] Suttajit S, Srisurapanont M, Maneeton N, Maneeton B. Quetiapine for acute bipolar depression: a systematic review and meta-analysis. Drug Des Devel Ther 2014; 8(16): 827-38.
[8] Franklin R, Zorowitz S, Corse AK, Widge AS, Deckersbach T. Lurasidone for the treatment of bipolar depression: an evidence-based review. Neuropsychiatr Dis Treat 2015; 11(8): 2143-52.
[9] Baldessarini RJ, Vieta E, Calabrese JR, Tohen M, Bowden CL. Bipolar depression: overview and commentary. Harv Rev Psychiatry 2010; 18(3): 143-57.
[10] Caddy C, Amit BH, McCloud TL, *et. al.* Ketamine and other glutamate receptor modulators for depression in adults. Cochrane Database Syst Rev 2015; 23(9): CD011612, 183 pp.
[11] Coyle CM, Laws KR. Use of ketamine as an antidepressant: systematic review and meta-analysis. Hum Psychopharmacol Clin Exptl 2015; 30(3): 152-63.
[12] Lee EE, Della Selva MP, Liu A, Himelhoch S. Ketamine as a novel treatment for major depressive disorder and bipolar depression: systematic review and quantitative meta-analysis. Gen Hosp Psychiatry 2015; 37(2): 178-84.

[13]   McCloud TL, Caddy C, Jochim J, *et al.* Ketamine and other gluta-mate receptor modulators for depression in bipolar disorder in adults. Cochrane Database Syst Rev 2015; 9: 67.

[14]   Park M, Niciu MJ, Zarate CA Jr. Novel glutamatergic treatments for severe mood disorders. Curr Behav Neurosci Rep 2015; 2(4): 198-208.

[15]   Romeo B, Choucha W, Fossati P, Rotge J-Y. Meta-analysis of short- and mid-term efficacy of ketamine in unipolar and bipolar depression. Psychiatry Res 2015; 230(2): 682-8.

[16]   Kishimoto T, Chawla JM, Kagi K, *et al.* Single-dose infusion of ketamine and non-ketamine N-methyl-D-aspartate receptor antago-nist for unipolar and bipolar depression: meta-analysis of efficacy, safety and time trajectories. Psychol Med 2016; 46(7): 1459-72.

[17]   Kohrs R, Durieux ME. Ketamine: teaching an old drug new tricks. Anesthesia Analgesia 1998; 87(5): 1186-93.

[18]   World Health Organization (WHO). Critical review of ketamine, 2006. Accessible at http://www.who.int/medicines/areas/quality_safety/4.3 KetamineCritReview.pdf; accessed 10 Oct 2016.

[19]   Vollenweider F, Leenders K, Oye I, Hell D, Angst J. Differential psychopathology and patterns of cerebral glucose utilization pro-duced by S- and R-ketamine in healthy volunteers using positron emission tomography (PET). Eur Neuropsychopharmacol 1997; 7(1): 25-38.

[20]   Haile C, Murrough J, Isofescu D, *et al.* Plasma brain-derived neu-rotrophic factor (BDNF) and response to ketamine in treatment-resistant depression. Int J Neuropsychopharmacol 2014; 17(2): 331-6.

[21]   Abdallah CG, Adams TG, Kelmendi B, *et al.* Ketamine's mecha-nism of action: a path to rapid-acting antidepressants. Depres Anxi-ety 2016; 33(8): 689-97.

[22]   Muller J, Pentyala S, Dilger J, Pentyala S. Ketamine enantiomers in rapid and sustained antidepressant effects. Ther Adv Psychophar-macol 2016; 6(3): 185-92.

[23]   Sanacora G, Schatzberg AD. Ketamine: promising path of false prophecy in the development of novel therapeutics for mood disor-ders? Neurosychopharmacology 2015; 40(2): 259-67.

[24]   Zanos P, Moaddel R, Morris PJ, *et al.* NMDAR inhibition-dependent antidepressant actions of ketamine metabolites. Nature 2016; 533(7604): 481-6.

[25]   Bobo WV, VandeVoort JL, Croarkin PE, *et al.* Ketamine for treat-ment-resistant unipolar and bipolar major depression: critical re-view and implications for clinical practice. Depress Anxiety 2016; 33(8): 698-710.

[26]   Rot M, Collins KA, Murrough JW, *et al.* Safety and efficacy of repeated-dose intravenous ketamine for treatment-resistant depres-sion. Biol Psychiatry 2010; 67(2): 139-45.

[27]   Rasmussen KG, Lineberry TW, Galardy CW, *et al.* Serial infusions of low-dose ketamine for major depression. J Psychopharmacol 2013; 27(5): 444-50.

[28]   Singh JB, Fedgchin M, Daly E, *et al.* Intravenous esketamine in adult treatment-resistant depression: double-blind, double-randomization, placebo-controlled study. Biol Psychiatry 2016; 80(6): 424-31.

[29]   Pharmabiz.com. US FDA grants breakthrough therapy status to Janssen's antidepressant medicine, esketamine. 2016; Aug. Acces-sible at www.pharmabiz.com/NewsDetails.Aspx?aid=96950& sid=2; accessed 18 Aug 2016.

[30]   Salat K, Siwek A, Starowicz G, *et al.* Antidepressant-like effects of ketamine, norketamine and dehydronorketamine in forced swim test: role of activity at NMDA receptor. Neuropharmacology 2015; 99: 301-7.

[31]   Rasmussen K, Jarvis M, Zorumski C. Ketamine anesthesia in ECT. Convuls Ther 1996; 12(4): 217-23.

[32]   Okamoto N, Nakai T, Sakamoto K, *et al.* Rapid antidepressant effect of ketamine anesthesia during electroconvulsive therapy of treatment-resistant depression: comparing ketamine with propofol anesthesia. J ECT 2010; 26(3): 223-7.

[33]   Ghasemi M, Kasemi M, Yoosefi A, *et al.* Rapid antidepressant effects of repeated doses of ketamine compared with electroconvul-sive therapy in hospitalized patients with major depressive disor-der. Psychiatry Res 2014; 215(2): 355-61.

[34]   Dang Y-H, Ma X-C, Zhang J-C, *et al.* Targeting NMDA receptors in the treatment of major depression. Curr Pharmaceut Design 2014; 20(32): 5151-9.

[35]   Zarate CA Jr, Mathews D, Ibrahim L, *et al.* Randomized trial of a low trapping non-selective N-methyl-D-aspartate (NMDA) channel blocker in major depression. Biol Psychiatry 2013; 74(4): 257-64.

[36]   Serra G, Koukopoulos A, De Chiara L, *et al.* Three-year, naturalis-tic, mirror-image assessment of adding memantine to the treatment of 30 treatment-resistant patients with bipolar disorder. J Clin Psy-chiatry 2015; 76(1): e91-7.

[37]   Domino EF. Taming the ketamine tiger 1965. Anesthesiology 2010; 113(3): 678-84.

[38]   Berman RM, Cappiello A, Anand A, *et al.* Antidepressant effects of ketamine in depressed patients. Biol Psychiatry 2000; 47(4): 351-4.

[39]   Skolnick P. Antidepressants for the new millennium. Eur J Phar-macol 1999; 375(1-3): 31-40.

[40]   Pennybaker SJ, Niciu MJ, Luckenbaugh DA, Zarate CA. Sympto-matology and predictors of antidepressant efficacy in extended re-sponders to a single ketamine infusion. J Affect Disord 2016; 0165-0327(16): 31206.

[41]   Xu Y, Hackett M, Carter G, *et al.* Effects of low-dose and very low-dose ketamine among patients with major depression: system-atic review and meta-analysis. Int J Neuropsychopharmacol 2016; 19(4).

[42]   Fond G, Loundou A, Rabu C, *et al.* Ketamine administration in depressive disorders: systematic review and meta-analysis. Psy-chopharmacology 2014; 231(8): 3663-76.

[43]   McGirr A, Berlim MT, Bond DJ, *et al.* Systematic review and meta-analysis of randomized, double-blind, placebo-controlled tri-als of ketamine in the rapid treatment of major depressive episodes. Psychol Med 2015; 45(4): 693-704.

[44]   Parsaik AK, Singh B, Khosh-Chashm D, Mascarenhas SS. Efficacy of ketamine in bipolar depression: systematic review and meta-analysis. J Psychiatr Pract 2015; 21(6): 427-35.

[45]   Alberich S, Martínez-Cengotitabengoa M, López P, *et al.* Efficacy and safety of ketamine in bipolar depression: systematic review. Rev Psiquiatria Salud Ment 2016; 10(2): 104-112.

[46]   Van de Voort JL, Morgan RJ, Kung S, *et al.* Continuation phase intravenous ketamine in adults with treatment-resistant depression. J Affect Disord 2016; 206(12): 300-4.

[47]   Lara DR, Bisol LW, Munari LR. Antidepressant, mood-stabilizing and procognitive effects of very low dose sublingual ketamine in refractory unipolar and bipolar depression. Int J Neuropsycho-pharmaol 2013; 16(9): 2111-7.

[48]   Permoda-Osip A, Skibinska M, Bartowska-Sniatkowka A, *et al.* Factors connected with efficacy of single ketamine infusion in bi-polar depression. Psychiatria Polska 2014; 48(1): 35-47.

[49]   Diazgranados N, Ibrahim L, Brutsche NE, *et al.* Randomized, add-on trial of an N-methyl-D-aspartate antagonist in treatment-resistant bi-polar depression. Arch Gen Psychiatry 2010; 67(8): 793-802.

[50]   Zarate CA Jr, Brutsche NE, Ibrahim L, *et al.* Replication of keta-mine's antidepressant activity in bipolar depression: randomized, controlled add-on trial. Biol Psychiatry 2012; 71(11): 939-46.

[51]   Ionescu DF, Luckenbaugh DA, Niciu MJ, Richards EM, Zarate CA Jr. Single infusion of ketamine improves depression scores in pa-tients with anxious bipolar depression. Bipolar Disord 2015; 17(4): 438-43.

[52]   Rush AJ. Ketamine for treatment-resistant depression: ready or not for clinical use? Am J Psychiatry 2013; 170(10): 1079-81.

[53]   Schatzberg AJ. A word to the wise about ketamine. Am J Psychia-try 2014; 171(3): 262-4.

[54]   Malhi GS, Byrow Y, Cassidy F, *et al.* Ketamine: stimulating anti-depressant treatment? Br J Psychiatry Open 2016; 2(3): e5-9.

[55]   Newport DJ, Schatzberg AF, Nemeroff CB. Whither ketamine as an antidepressant: panacea or toxin? Depres Anxiety 2016; 33(8): 685-8.

[56]   Zhang MW, Harris KM, Ho RC. Is off-label repeat prescription of ketamine as a rapid antidepressant safe? Controversies, ethical con-cerns, and legal implications. BMC Med Ethics 2016; 17(1): 4-12.

[57]   Bozzatello P, Brignolo E, De Grandi E, Bellino S. Supplementation with omega-3 fatty acids in psychiatric disorders: review of litera-ture data. J Clin Med 2016; 5(8): 1-26.

[58]   Scorletti F, Byrne CD. Omega-3 fatty acids, hepatic lipid metabo-lism and nonalcoholic fatty liver disease. Ann Rev Nutrition 2013; 33(1): 231-48.

[59]   Powell WS, Rokach K. Biosynthesis, biological effects, and recep-tors of hydroxyeicosatetraenoic(HETEs) and oxyeicosatetraenoic

acids (oxo-ETEs) derived from arachidonic acid. Biochim Biophys Acta 2015; 1851(4): 340-55.

[60] Anderson GD, Hauser SD, McGarity KL, *et al.* Selective inhibition of cyclo-oxygenase-2 (COX-2) reverses inflammation and expression of COX-2 and interleukin-6 in rat adjuvant arthritis. J Clin Invest 1996; 97(11): 2672-9.

[61] Salmon JA, Higgs GA. Prostaglandins and leukotrienes as inflammatory mediators. Br Med Bull 1987; 43(2): 285-96.

[62] Bagga D, Wang L, Farias-Eisner R, Glaspy JA, Reddy ST. Differential effects of prostaglandin derived from omega-6 and omega-3 polyunsaturated fatty acids on COX-2 expression and IL-6 secretion. Proc Natl Acad Sci 2003; 100(4): 1751-6.

[63] Ji RR, Xu ZZ, Strichartz G, Serhan CN. Emerging roles of resolvins in the resolution of inflammation and pain. Trends Neurosci 2011; 34(11): 599-609.

[64] Rao JS, Ertley RN, Lee HJ, *et al.* Omega-3 polyunsaturated fatty acid deprivation in rats decreases frontal cortex BDNF *via* a p38 MAPK-dependent mechanism. Mol Psychiatry 2007; 12(1): 36-46.

[65] Watson RR, DeMeester D (Eds). Omega-3 Fatty Acids in Brain and Neurological Health. New York: Academic Press, 2014.

[66] Youdim KA, Martin A, Joseph JA. Essential fatty acids and the brain: possible health implications. Int J Dev Neurosci 2000; 18(4-5): 383-99.

[67] Balanzá-Martínez V, Fries GR, Colpo GD, *et al.* Therapeutic use of omega-3 fatty acids in bipolar disorder. Expert Rev Neurother 2011; 11(7): 1029-47.

[68] Colangelo LA, He K, Whooley MA, Daviglus ML, Liu K. Higher dietary intake of long-chain omega-3 polyunsaturated fatty acids is inversely associated with depressive symptoms in women. Nutrition 2009; 25(10): 1011-9.

[69] Hibbeln JR. Seafood consumption, DHA content of mothers' milk and prevalence rates of postpartum depression: a cross-national, ecological analysis. J Affect Disord 2002; 69(1-3): 15-29.

[70] Clayton EH, Hanstock TL, Hirneth SJ, *et al.* Reduced mania and depression in juvenile bipolar disorder associated with long-chain omega-3 polyunsaturated fatty acid supplementation. Eur J Clin Nutr 2009; 63(8): 1037-40.

[71] Harris WS, von Schacky C, Park Y. Standardizing methods for assessing omega-3 fatty acid biostatus. Chapt 19 in: McNamara RK (Ed). The Omega-3 Fatty Acid Deficiency Syndrome: Opportunities for Disease Prevention. Hauppauge, NY: Nova Science Publishers 2013; pp 385-98.

[72] Chiu CC, Huang SY, Su KP, *et al.* Polyunsaturated fatty acid deficit in patients with bipolar mania. Eur Neuropsychopharmacol 2003; 13(2): 99-103.

[73] McNamara RK, Jandacek R, Rider T, Tso P, Pandey GN. Selective deficits in erythrocyte docosahexaenoic acid composition in adult patients with bipolar disorder and major depressive disorder. J Affect Disord 2010; 126(1-2): 303-11.

[74] McNamara RK, Nandagopal JJ, Strakowski SM, DelBello MP. Preventative strategies for early-onset bipolar disorder: towards a clinical staging model. CNS Drugs 2010; 24(12): 983-6.

[75] Clayton EH, Hanstock TL, Hirneth SJ, Kable CJ, Garg ML, Hazell PL. Long-chain omega-3 polyunsaturated fatty acids in the blood of children and adolescents with juvenile bipolar disorder. Lipids 2008; 43(11): 1031-8.

[76] Pomponi M, Janiri L, La Torre G, *et al.* Plasma levels of omega-3 fatty acids in bipolar patients: deficit restricted to DHA. J Psychiatr Res 2013; 47(3): 337-42.

[77] Sublette ME, Bosetti F, DeMar JC, *et al.* Plasma free polyunsaturated fatty acid levels are associated with symptom severity in acute mania. Bipolar Disord 2007; 9(7): 759-65.

[78] Evans, SJ, Kamali M, Prossin AR, *et al.* Association of plasma omega-3 and omega-6 lipids with burden-of-disease measures in bipolar subjects. J Psychiatr Res 2012; 46(11): 1435-41.

[79] Evans SJ, Ringrose RN, Harrington GJ, *et al.* Dietary intake and plasma metabolomic analysis of polyunsaturated fatty acids in bipolar subjects reveal dysregulation of linoleic acid metabolism. J Psychiatr Res 2014; 57(10): 58-64.

[80] Gracious BL, Chirieac, MC, Costescua S, *et al.* Randomized, placebo-controlled trial of flax oil in pediatric bipolar disorder. Bipolar Disord 2010; 12(2): 142-54.

[81] Frangou S, Lewis M, Wollard J, Simmons A. Preliminary *in vivo* evidence of increased N-acetyl-aspartate following eicosapentanoic acid treatment in patients with bipolar disorder. J Psychopharmacol 2007; 21(4): 435-9.

[82] Hibbeln JR, Palmer JW, Davis JM. Are disturbances in lipid-protein interactions by phospholipase-A2 a predisposing factor in affective illness? Biol Psychiatry 1989; 25(7): 945-61.

[83] Appleton KM, Rogers PJ, Ness AR. Updated systematic review and meta-analysis of the effects of omega-3 long-chain polyunsaturated fatty acids on depressed mood. Am J Clin Nutrition 2010; 91(3): 757-70.

[84] Sperling RI, Benincaso AI, Knoell CT, Larkin JK, Austen KF, Robinson RD. Dietary omega-3 polyunsaturated fatty acids inhibit phosphoinositide formation and chemotaxis in neutrophils. J Clin Invest 1993; 91(2): 651-60.

[85] Holian, Nelson R. Action of long chain fatty acids on protein kinase C activity: comparison of omega-6 and omega-3 fatty acids. Anticancer Res 1992; 12(3): 975-80.

[86] Pepe S, Bogdanov K, Hallaq H, Spurgeon H, Leaf A, Lakatta E. Omega-3 polyunsaturated fatty acid modulates dihydropyridine, effects on L-type Ca^{2+} channels, cytosolic $Ca^{2+,}$ and contraction in adult rat cardiac myocytes. Proc Natl Acad Sci USA 1994; 91(19): 8832-6.

[87] Maes M, Smith R. Fatty acids, cytokines, and major depression. Biol Psychiatry 1998; 43(5): 313-4.

[88] Shakeri J, Khanegi M, Golshani S, *et al.* Effects of omega-3 supplement in the treatment of patients with bipolar I disorder. Int J Prev Med 2016; 7(5): 77-85.

[89] Osher Y, Bersudsky Y, Belmarker RH. Omega-3 eicosapentaenoic acid in bipolar depression: report of a small open-label study. J Clin Psychiatry 2005; 66(6): 726-9.

[90] Frangou S, Lewis M, McCrone P. Efficacy of ethyl-eicosapentaenoic acid in bipolar depression: randomized double-blind placebo-controlled study. Br J Psychiatry 2006; 188: 46-50.

[91] Stoll AL, Severus WE, Freeman MP, *et al.* Omega-3 fatty acids in bipolar disorder. Arch Gen Psychiatry 1999; 56(5): 407-12.

[92] Keck PE, Mintz J, McElroy SL, *et al.* Double-blind, randomized, placebo-controlled trials of ethyl-eicosapentanoate in the treatment of bipolar depression and rapid cycling bipolar disorder. Biol Psychiatry 2006; 60(9): 1020-2.

[93] Chiu CC, Huang SY, Chen CC, Su SK. Omega-3 fatty acids are more beneficial in the depressive phase than in the manic phase in patients with bipolar I disorder. J Clin Psychiatry 2005; 66(12): 1613-4.

[94] Murphy BL, Stoll, AL, Harris PQ, *et al.* Omega-3 fatty acid treatment with or without cytidine fails to show therapeutic properties in bipolar disorder. J Clin Psychopharmacol 2012; 32(5): 699-703.

[95] Wozniak J, Faraone SM, Chan J, *et al.* Randomized clinical trial of high eiscosapentaenoic acid omega-3 fatty acids and inositol as monotherapy and in combination in the treatment of pediatric bipolar spectrum disorders: pilot study. J Clin Psychiatry 2015; 76(11): 1548-55.

[96] Maes M. Evidence for an immune response in major depression: review and hypothesis. Prog Neuro-psychopharmacol Biol Psychiatry 1995; 19(1): 11-38.

[97] Leonard B, Maes M. Mechanistic explanations how cell-mediated immune activation, inflammation and oxidative and nitrosative stress pathways and their sequels and concomitants play a role in the pathophysiology of unipolar depression. Neurosci Behav Rev 2012; 36(2): 764-85.

[98] Leboyer M, Berk M, Yolken RH, *et al.* Immuno-psychiatry: agenda for clinical practice and innovative research. BMC Med 2016; 14(1): 173.

[99] Rosenblat JD, Kakar R, Berk M, *et al.* Anti-inflammatory agents in the treatment of bipolar depression: systematic review and meta-analysis. Bipolar Disord 2016; 18(2): 89-101.

[100] Reichenberg A, Yirmiya R, Schuld A, *et al.* Cytokine-associated emotional and cognitive disturbances in humans. Arch Gen Psychiatry 2001; 58(5): 445-52.

[101] Udina M, Castellvi P, Moreno-Espana J, *et al.* Interferon-induced depression in chronic hepatitis C: systematic review and meta-analysis. J Clin Psychiatry 2012; 73(8): 1128-38.

[102] Dowlati Y, Herrmann N, Swardfager W, *et al.* Meta-analysis of cytokines in major depression. Biol Psychiatry 2010; 67(5): 446-57.

[103] Xia Z, DePierre JW, Nässberger L. Tricyclic antidepressants inhibit IL-6, IL-1-beta and TNF-alpha release in human blood monocytes and IL-2 and interferon-gamma in T cells. Immunopharmacology 1996; 34(1): 27-37.

[104] McNamara RK, Lotrich FE. Elevated immune-inflammatory signaling in mood disorder: a new therapeutic target? Expert Rev Neurother 2012; 12(9): 1143-61.

[105] Modabbernia A, Taslimi S, Brietzke E, Ashrafi M. Cytokine alterations in bipolar disorder: meta-analysis of 30 studies. Biol Psychiatry 2013; 74(1): 15-25.

[106] Hannestad J, DellaBioia N, Bloch M. Effect of antidepressant medication treatment on serum levels of inflammatory cytokines: meta-analysis. Neuropsychopharmacology 2011; 36(12): 2452-9.

[107] Berk M, Williams LJ, Jacka FN, et al. So depression is an inflammatory disease, but where does the inflammation come from? BMC Med 2013; 11(9): 200-16.

[108] Eller T, Vasar V, Shlik J, Maron E. Pro-inflammatory cytokines and treatment response to escitalopram in major depressive disorder. Prog Neuro-psychopharmacol Biol Psychiatry 2008; 32(2): 445-50.

[109] Fond G, Hamdani N, Kapczinski F, et al. Effectiveness and tolerance of anti-inflammatory drugs add-on therapy in major mental disorders: systematic qualitative review. Acta Psychiatr Scand 2014; 129(3): 163-79.

[110] Nissen SE, Yeomans ND, Solomon DH, et al. Cardiovascular safety of celecoxib, naproxen, or ibuprofen for arthritis. N Engl J Med 2016; 375(26): 2519-29.

[111] Na KS, Lee KJ, Lee JS, Cho YS, Jung HY. Efficacy of adjunctive celecoxib treatment for patient with major depressive disorder: a meta-analysis. Prog Neuro-Psychopharmacol Biol Psychiatry 2014; 48(1): 79-85.

[112] Faridhosseini F, Sadeghi R, Farid L, Pourgholami M. Celecoxib: new augmentation strategy for depressive mood episodes: systematic review and meta-analysis of randomized placebo-controlled trials. Hum Psychopharmacol Clin Exp 2014; 29(3): 216-23.

[113] Raison VL, Rutherford RE, Woolwine BJ, et al. Randomized controlled trial of t18he tumor necrosis factor antagonist infliximab for treatment-resistant depression: role of baseline inflammatory biomarkers. JAMA Psychiatry 2013; 70(1): 31-41.

[114] Sarris J, Mischoulon D, Schweitzer I. Omega-3 for bipolar disorder: meta-analyses of use in mania and bipolar depression. J Clin Psychiatry 2012; 73(1): 81-6.

[115] Nery FG, Monkul AES, Hatch JP, et al. Celecoxib as an adjunct in the treatment of depressive or mixed episodes of bipolar disorder: double-blind, randomized, placebo-controlled study. Hum Psychopharmacol Clin Exp 2008; 23(2): 87-94.

[116] Berk M, Copolov DL, Dean OM, et al. N-acetylcysteine for depressive symptoms in bipolar disorder: double-blind randomized placebo-controlled trials. Biol Psychiatry 2008; 64(6): 468-75.

[117] Berk M, Dean OM, Cotton SM, et al. Maintenance N-actylcysteine treatment for bipolar disorder; double-blind randomized placebo-controlled trial. BMC Med 2012; 10(8): 91-102.

[118] Zeinoddini A, Sorayani M, Hassanzadeh E, et al. Pioglitazone adjunctive therapy for depressive episode of bipolar disorder; randomized, double-blind, placebo-controlled trial. Depress Anxiety 2015; 32(3): 167-73.

[119] Dean OM, Data-Franco J, Giorlando F, Berk M. Minocycline: therapeutic potential in psychiatry. CNS Drugs 2012; 26(5): 391-401.

[120] Brown ES, Park J, Marx CE, et al. Randomized, double-blind, placebo-controlled trial of pregnenolone for bipolar depression. Neuropsychopharmacology 2014; 39(12): 2867-73.

[121] Saroukhani S, Emami-Parsa M, Modabbernia A, et al. Aspirin for treatment of lithium-associated sexual dysfunction in men: randomized double-blind placebo-controlled study. Bipolar Disord 2013; 15(6): 650-6.

[122] Berk M, Dean O, Cotton SM, et al. Efficacy of N-acetylcysteine as an adjunctive treatment in bipolar depression: open label trial. J Affect Disord 2011; 135(1-3): 389-94.

[123] Brennan BP, Jensen JE, Hudson JI, et al. A placebo-controlled trial of acetyl-L-carnitine and α-lipoic acid in the treatment of bipolar depression. J Clin Psychopharmacol 2013; 33(5): 627-35.

[124] Hill C, Guarner F, Reid G, et al. International Scientific Association for Probiotics and Prebiotics consensus statement on the scope and appropriate use of the term probiotic. Nature Rev Gastroenterol Hepatol 2014; 11(8): 506-14.

[125] Rijkers GT, de Vos WM, Brummer RJ, et al. Health benefits and health claims of probiotics: bridging science and marketing. Br J Nutrition 2011; 106(9): 1291-6.

[126] Maynard CL, Elson CO, Hatton RD, Weaver CT. Reciprocal interactions of the intestinal microbiota and immune system. Nature 2012; 489(7145): 231-41.

[127] Foster JA, McVey-Neufeld KA. Gut-brain axis: how the microbiome influences anxiety and depression. Trends Neurosci 2013; 36(5): 305-12.

[128] Bustos Fernandez LM, Lasa JS, Man F. Intestinal microbiota: its role in digestive diseases. J Clin Gastroenterol 2014; 48(8): 657-66.

[129] Louis P, Hold GL, Flint HJ. The gut microbiota, bacterial metabolites and colorectal cancer. Nature Rev Microbiol 2014; 12(10): 661-72.

[130] Akkasheh G, Kashani-Poor Z, Tajabadi-Ebrahimi M, et al. Clinical and metabolic response to probiotic administration in patients with major depressive disorder: randomized, double-blind, placebo-controlled trial. Nutrition 2016; 32(3): 315-20.

[131] Pirbaglou M, Katz J, de Souza RJ, et al. Probiotic supplementation can positively affect anxiety and depressive symptoms: systematic review of randomized controlled trials. Nutr Res 2016; 36(9): 889-98.

[132] Wang H, Lee IS, Braun C, Enck P. Effect of probiotics on central nervous system functions in animals and humans: systematic review. J Neurogastroenterol Motil 2016; 22(4): 589-60.

Send Orders for Reprints to reprints@benthamscience.ae

REVIEW ARTICLE

Unmet Needs in Schizophrenia

Maurizio Pompili[1,*], Gloria Giordano[1], Mario Luciano[2], Dorian A. Lamis[3], Valeria Del Vecchio[2], Gianluca Serafini[4], Gaia Sampogna[2], Denise Erbuto[1], Peter Falkai[5] and Andrea Fiorillo[2]

[1]*Department of Neurosciences, Mental Health and Sensory Organs, Suicide Prevention Center, Sant'Andrea Hospital, Sapienza University of Rome, Rome, Italy;* [2]*Department of Psychiatry, University of Campania "L. Vanvitelli", Naples, Italy;* [3]*Department of Psychiatry and Behavioral Sciences, Emory University School of Medicine, Atlanta, GA, USA;* [4]*Department of Neuroscience, Rehabilitation, Ophthalmology, Genetics, Maternal and Child Health, Section of Psychiatry, University of Genoa, Genoa, Italy;* [5]*Department of Psychiatry and Psychotherapy, Ludwig-Maximilians-University Munich, Munich, Germany*

Abstract: ***Background:*** Schizophrenia is a complex psychiatric disorder that represents a challenge for all clinicians. Although treatment must address both positive and negative symptoms, several authors have reported the importance of managing unmet needs among patients with schizophrenia. Unmet needs in schizophrenia include difficulties at various clinical, psychosocial, relational, economic, and occupational levels. An important unmet need is represented by insight into the illness that is associated with treatment adherence and compliance with medical prescriptions.

Conclusion: In order to improve our understanding and management of schizophrenia, it is critically important to address the complexity of needs among patients with schizophrenia.

ARTICLE HISTORY

Received: March 01, 2017
Revised: July 11, 2017
Accepted: July 11, 2017

DOI:
10.2174/1871527316666170803143927

Keywords: Cognitive, emotional, psychosocial, psychiatric disorder, symptoms, schizophrenia.

1. INTRODUCTION

Schizophrenia is the most severe psychiatric condition affecting around 24 million people worldwide [1], and causes approximately 1% of disability-adjusted life years (DALYs) [2]. In 2013, schizophrenia was among the top 25 leading causes of disability worldwide, with a high health, social, and economic burden not only for patients, but also for caregivers and society as a whole [3]. Recent evidence has suggested that individuals with schizophrenia have an excess mortality which is mainly attributable to physical illnesses [4], with an overall mortality being twice than that of the general population [5, 6].

Social disability is largely due to impairments in cognitive, emotional, and psychological functions, that cause difficulties in social relationships, a reduced ability to find and/or to maintain a job as well as to have a satisfactory quality of life [7]. From a public health perspective, patients with schizophrenia have reduced accessibility to health services and appropriate treatments [8], and decreased productivity is

associated with a significant economic burden for both society and public health system [3]. The annual costs of schizophrenia have been estimated to be approximately 60 billion dollars, including direct medical costs, non-health care costs, and lost productivity. This is mainly due to the fact that individuals become ill early in life and have high rates of unemployment and medical comorbidities [9].

The current management of schizophrenia focuses on the treatment of acute symptoms as well as on long-term treatment aimed at preventing relapses after patients have experienced an improvement in acute symptoms [10]. Refinement of schizophrenia management has been stimulated and supported by the development of empirically validated measures for the assessment of needs together with the elaboration and diffusion of clinical practice guidelines (CPGs). Management has become more specific through the administration of questionnaires, clinical rating scales, and diagnostic interviews, developed for describing and quantifying psychopathological symptoms and signs, particularly in clinical research. The routine use of these instruments has been shown to improve decision-making and patient care [11]. In the last 20 years, there has been a growing interest in recognizing patients' psychosocial functioning and quality of life as essential parts of treatment aims, with a subsequent need for specific tools created to measure them. As a result of the

*Address correspondence to this author at the Department of Neurosciences, Mental Health and Sensory Organs, Sant'Andrea Hospital, Sapienza University of Rome, Via di Grottarossa 1035, 00189 Rome, Italy; Tel: +39-06-3377-5675; Fax: +39-06-3377-5342; E-mail: maurizio.pompili@uniroma1.it

improved understanding of patients' psychosocial unmet needs, several interventions have been developed and tested to promote the recovery and empowerment of individuals with schizophrenia. These strategies include cognitive-behavioral therapy, cognitive remediation (CR), and family psychoeducation being the most effective non-pharmacological treatment to improve the quality of life of patients with schizophrenia and reduce their psychosocial unmet needs [12].

The World Health Organization estimated that the treatment gap for schizophrenia across the world, including other non-affective psychoses, may be as high as 32.2%. Thus, it is clear that the management of schizophrenia represents a challenge for clinicians: a complex process of interactions among research, clinical practice, service provision, users' experiences, and mental health advocacy is recommended. Consequently, the aim of our review is to examine the myriad of complex problems experienced by patients diagnosed with schizophrenia in order to better understand their needs and improve their quality of psychiatric care.

2. MATERIALS AND METHOD

To provide a review about the importance of unmet needs in the management of schizophrenia, we performed a Pub-Med/MEDLINE, Scopus, PsycLIT, and PsycINFO search to identify all articles and book chapters on the topic up to 2016. For this aim, we used the following search terms: "unmet needs AND schizophrenia", "unmet needs AND management of schizophrenia" or "psychotic disorder" or "schizoaffective disorder" or "psychosis". Later, in a second step, we searched the same terms specifying (title and abstract) as electronic search strategy in Medline to adequately focus on the specific field of interest. The reference lists of articles included in the review were also manually checked for relevant studies. All English full-text articles reporting original data about the main topic were included. The reference lists of the articles included in the review were manually checked for relevant studies.

3. MANAGEMENT OF SCHIZOPHRENIA

The management of patients with schizophrenia is very complex: the reduction of positive and negative symptoms of this condition represents the first goal of treatment, but importantly this is not enough. During the middle of the last century, management of symptoms with the recently discovered neuroleptics represented the core of the therapeutic process: the needs of patients with schizophrenia have been mainly defined by medical staff and they were principally of a clinical nature. Subsequently, with the deinstitutionalization and the development of community-based mental health services, patients encountered the difficulties of living in the community. In addition to symptoms' reduction, clinicians had to consider patients' social relationships, housing, and working among the main goals of treatment. In the last twenty years, with the rising awareness of human rights, the empowerment of mentally ill patients, and the increasing social sensibility, the existential needs of psychiatric patients, such as freedom, respect, and spirituality, has become essential in order to obtain a meaningful life [13]. Therefore, the primary treatment goal for patients with schizophrenia

changed from the management of positive and negative symptoms to the promotion of well-being and recovery [14]. All available guidelines for the treatment of schizophrenia suggest the need for an integrated treatment approach, given that pharmacological treatment alone is not enough to improve quality of life and promote recovery of patients with schizophrenia [15, 16]. Thus, it is important that psychosocial interventions be utilized in addition to medication to address the symptoms experienced by patients with schizophrenia. Illness Management and Recovery (IMR) is one such an approach, which is designed to help people with severe mental illness manage their symptoms and achieve personal recovery goals [17]. In a recent review of the literature [18], the authors concluded that IMR shows promise for improving patient-level outcomes and suggested that IMR should continue to be implemented and tested in RCTs.

4. MEDICAL UNMET NEEDS

4.1. Comorbidity, Complications and Lifestyle

Schizophrenia presents many comorbidities and complications that quite often contribute to poor health outcomes. Substance abuse is one of the most frequent comorbidities in schizophrenia (about 37-53%) that may negatively affect diagnosis, symptoms, treatment, and prognosis [11]. The Substance Abuse and Mental Health Services Administration [19] found that only 12.4% of the American adults that receive a dual diagnosis have access to both mental health and substance abuse services. Also anxiety and depression are other frequent comorbidities in schizophrenia, both during and after the onset of psychotic symptoms; the prevalence rates are about 15% for panic disorder, 29% for post-traumatic stress disorder, 23% for obsessive-compulsive disorder, and 50% for depression [20]. The presence of a comorbidity has a negative impact on patients' outcome and quality of life [21]; therefore, clinicians should pay attention to medical severity and environmental risk factors.

Many patients with schizophrenia are inactive and present with disorganized patterns of nutrition and hygiene: these altered lifestyle behaviours are often associated with an higher incidence of several physical diseases, such as metabolic, cardiovascular, and sexual dysfunctions, with a consequent reduction of life expectancy of approximately 20 years [22].

A study conducted by Daumit and colleagues [23] clearly demonstrated that obesity, diabetes and smoking are two times more frequent in schizophrenia than in the general population. Schizophrenia is associated with a higher risk of metabolic syndrome (MS), characterized by obesity, insulin resistance, hypertension and elevated triglycerides, with a consequent higher mortality risk [24]. Several studies have demonstrated that patients with schizophrenia are at a greater risk of heart diseases such as coronary heart diseases, stroke, and arrhythmias [25-27]. Recent studies have indicated that certain metabolic abnormalities may significantly contribute to cardiovascular diseases, a leading cause of death among patients with schizophrenia [28]. When compared to approximately one-half in the general population, more than two-thirds of schizophrenia patients, die from coronary heart diseases [29], and they have a 2.5 fold greater risk of death than the general population [30]. In patients with schizophrenia, type 2 diabetes is often considered as having a 5-time higher prevalence compared to the general population (especially in patients receiving clozapine and olanzapine) [31]. Several studies have reported that about 40% of patients who suffer from both schizophrenia and diabetes do not receive any treatment for the latter [24]. A genetic influence for explaining the higher prevalence of metabolic disorders in patients with schizophrenia, even in those who are drug-naïve, has been hypothesized [32]. This hypothesis is further supported by the higher frequency of metabolic problems including diabetes, in first-degree relatives of patients with schizophrenia [33, 34]. Moreover, they have a 2-fold greater standardized mortality ratio for cardiovascular disease [35]. Increased adiposity is associated with decreases in insulin sensitivity leading to an increased risk of hyperglycemia and hyperlipidemia. Second generation antipsychotics (SGAs) may largely contribute to the increased metabolic dysregulation [36-38], and some of the current available SGAs may have substantially more metabolic side-effects than others [39].

Patients with schizophrenia also have a substantial risk of comorbid respiratory disorders. Heavy smoking is particularly frequent in this patient population and it contributes to the occurrence of several respiratory disorders, such as chronic obstructive pulmonary diseases and pneumonia (80% versus 20% of the general population) [40]. In addition, patients with schizophrenia present with a higher occurrence of viral infections, such as HIV and hepatitis B and C, often related to substances abuse and/or unprotected sexual activity [41]. All of these conditions may significantly compromise patients' compliance to treatments and quality of life.

Despite this excess of mortality due to comorbid physical illnesses, the somatic well-being of individuals with schizophrenia has been neglected for decades, which may be attributable to several factors [6]. The first factor is related to patients' behaviors. In fact, patients with schizophrenia are usually more worried by their psychotic symptoms and may fail to seek the appropriate treatment for physical diseases. Moreover, they have a reduced number of physical checkups and poor communication skills to report their problems and manage their medication [41].

A second factor is related to the use of antipsychotic treatment for the management of schizophrenia. Antipsychotic drugs and other medications that are prescribed to patients with schizophrenia are associated with a number of side effects such as weight gain, abnormal prolactin increase, cardiac effects, motor side-effects, blood dyscrasias, and may have many interactions with other psychotropic and non-psychotropic drugs [6]. Table 1 summarizes the main pharmacological unmet needs (adverse effects) for newer available SGAs in patients with schizophrenia.

System-related factors may also explain the reduced life expectancy of individuals with schizophrenia. Indeed, they have less access to health care, more often psychiatric units are not integrated with the general hospital, and medical interventions occur more frequently than in individuals without schizophrenia [42].

Lastly, attitudes of clinicians may also contribute to higher mortality rates. On one hand, psychiatrists often neglect their skills in recognizing and treating physical illnesses, and consider patients' complaints as expressions of the mental illness rather than of a physical disorder; on the other hand, clinicians from other medical specialties often feel uncomfortable in treating patients with schizophrenia [8].

Table 1. **Pharmacological unmet needs (adverse effects) for newer available SGAs in patients with schizophrenia.**

	Risperidone 4-8 mg/day	Paliperidone 9-12 mg/day	Quetiapine 300-800 mg/day	Olanzapine 10-20 mg/day	Clozapine 300-800 mg/day	Aripiprazole 10-30 mg/day	Amisulpride 400-800 mg/day	Ziprasidone 120-160 mg/day	Asenapine 5-20 mg/day	Zotepine 100-300 mg/day	Lurasidone 40-160 mg/die	Sertindole 12-24 mg/day
Extrapyramidal side effects	++	+	+/-	+/−	-	+/-	+/−	+/−	+	+	++	+/−
Akathisia	+	+	+/−	+/−	-	+	+/−	+/−	+	+/−	++	+/−
QTc prolongation	+/-	+/−	+	-	+	+/-	++	++	+	+	+/−	+/−
Weight gain	+	++	+/-	++	++	+/-	+/−	+/-	+/−	+	+	+
Cholesterol increase	+	+	+	++	++	+/−	+/−	+/−	+/−	+/−	+/−	+
Glucose increase	+	+		++	++	+/−	-	+/−	+/−	+/−	+/−	+
Diabetes mellitus	+	+	+/-	++	++	+/-	-	+/−	+/−	+/−	+/−	+/−
Dyslipidemia	+	+	+/-	++	+	+/-	+/−	+/−	+/−	+/−	+/−	+/−
Prolactin increase	++	++	-	+	-	-	++	+	+	+	+	++
Sonnolence and sedation	+	+	++	++	++	-	-	+/−	++	++	++	+

Note: ++ Greater propensity to induce the specified adverse event; + propensity to induce the specified adverse event; +/− smaller propensity to induce the specified adverse event or inconsistent data according to the current literature; − no effects regarding the specified adverse event.

Some of the determinants of a poor physical health in this psychiatric population are represented by lifestyle modifiable risk factors, adverse effects of antipsychotics and poor access to mental health services. Overall, it is clear that psychiatrists should include the physical assessment in their clinical examination, improve the access of patients to primary care facilities, and evaluate their metabolic parameters.

4.2. Pharmacotherapy and Attitudes Towards Drugs

Compliance may be defined as "the extent to which a person's behaviour coincides with the medical advices he/she received" [43]. It is difficult to obtain complete compliance in several chronic disorders. Patients with schizophrenia often refuse to take medications, spontaneously interrupt pharmacotherapy or diverge from the clinicians' prescriptions [44]. Studies have demonstrated that a third of patients are fully compliant with pharmacotherapy, another third is partially compliant, and the last third does not follow prescription indications at all [45]. The rates of partial compliance with antipsychotic medications tend to increase over time with discharge from a psychiatric ward: at least 50% of patients will be partially or not compliant within one year after discharge, and 75% within 2 years [46]. Adherence to treatment is not always an all-or-nothing phenomenon (*i.e.*, the subject is compliant or not): often we may identify a "partial compliance" in which the patients do not follow entirely the specialist's prescriptions. In particular, patients may take a medication dose that is less than the registered one, may take the correct dose at a wrong time, or may have an irregular (on/off) dosing behavior and premature interruption [43]. Compliance may be also considered as an indicator of quality and efficiency of the physician-patient relationship that may be seen as a result of various factors influencing the patient's tendency to follow medical indications. These factors include patient's attitudes towards drugs and illness, the presence of adverse effects and the involvement of caregivers in motivating the subject to take medications. In addition, the presence of some psychotic symptoms such as delusions may reduce patients' compliance: individuals who feel persecuted, at risk of poisoning or grandiose for manic symptoms are often reluctant to take medications [47]. Similarly, negative symptoms such as apathy may decrease patient's motivation to adhere to treatment [48]. Moreover, cognitive symptoms may prevent patients from effectively adhering to their medication regimen, with consequences of forgotten doses or mistaken medications [49]. Insight and compliance are interconnected: poor or lack of insight may lead to a complete denial of illness, with consequent rejecting or interruption of all forms of treatment when they feel better [50]. This may determine a destabilization of patients and a more severe prognosis [50]. Several studies reported the strong association between insight and adherence to treatment. In 2002, Novak-Grubic and Tavcar [51] demonstrated that poor insight in psychotic patients increases the risk of non-compliance with medications two fold compared with patients with a better insight. A partial compliance may subsequently implicate an uncompleted control of symptoms, relapses and rehospitalization, with possible long-term functional disabilities, such as reduction in autonomy or employment, homelessness, and even suicide [52].

A cross-sectional study conducted in 2011 by Beck and colleagues [53] revealed that awareness into the illness contributes to therapy adherence through patient's perception of needing antipsychotics. Moreover, the same study showed a direct negative association between concerns regarding antipsychotics and adherence to treatment as well as an indirect negative consequence of a distrust about medications and compliance *via* antipsychotic specific attitudes. Psychiatrists should not only improve the patient's perceived necessity of pharmacological treatment, but also try to investigate the patient's distrust in pharmacotherapy in a more personalized manner. A study conducted by Miner and colleagues [54] showed that patients with more negative symptoms have a better compliance, whereas, those with mixed syndrome are more often non-adherent. Schennach-Wolff *et al.* [55] showed that the most important predictable factors for a positive attitude towards adherence were reduction in PANSS general psychopathology sub-score, employment status, greater illness insight and treatment with SGAs. The authors also highlighted the importance of providing adherence-focused psychotherapy and psychoeducation into daily clinical practice [55]. Rocca *et al.* [56] analyzed a sample of 50 patients with schizophrenia and concluded that lack of insight; more severe PANSS scores and later onset of schizophrenia were correlated with a worse global medication attitude. Further, the unawareness into treatment need predicted a poorer medication global attitude. Individuals taking SGAs reported lower negative attitudes and better global medication attitude than patients treated with first generation antipsychotics (FGAs). Higher rates of antipsychotic non-adherence, one of the most significant unmet needs related to treatment, are responsible for many social negative consequences. Medication non-adherence plays an important role in relapse rates, poor outcome, and high costs [57]. Several previous studies have reported that patients discontinuing antipsychotics may be two to five times as likely to relapse as other patients, leading to unnecessary suffering and increased costs [58-60]. Adherence to treatment still remains an important goal in the management of schizophrenia. A more complex and articulated view of the patients is warranted to better understand their real needs in order to achieve an improved quality of life and reduce their psychosocial impairment.

5. PHARMACOLOGICAL UNMET NEEDS

Several studies have demonstrated that negative symptoms of schizophrenia are more difficult to treat, contribute to a poorer functional outcome and quality of life, tend to persist longer, and often cause a higher burden for caregivers than positive symptoms [61-63]. Many SGAs and FGAs are currently available for the management of both positive and negative symptoms: while FGAs (*e.g.*, haloperidol, fluphenazine, and chlorpromazine) are more effective in treating positive symptoms, new SGAs (*e.g.*, aripiprazole, risperidone, quetiapine, olanzapine, clozapine, and paliperidone) are more efficient in addressing negative symptoms. Both SGA and FGA medications may cause several adverse effects. FGAs more frequently cause sedation, anticholinergic effects, extrapiramidal symptoms, cardiac arrhythmias, seizure, hyperprolactinemia, and sexual dysfunction, whereas, SGAs may induce agranulocytosis, hypotension, sedation, and metabolic syndrome. The occurrence of relevant adverse effects often significantly reduces treatment compliance [64].

The metabolic syndrome has been mainly associated with the use of SGAs. It has been defined by the National Cholesterol Education Program (NCEP) [65] Expert Panel as an interrelated constellation of cardiovascular risk factors linked to insulin resistance and including obesity, dyslipidemia, impaired glucose tolerance, and hypertension [33, 65, 66] and it has been related to an increased cardiovascular mortality of 2.6 times and in all-cause mortality of approximately 2 [67]. In the Clinical Antipsychotic Trails for Intervention Effectiveness (CATIE) study, McEvoy *et al.* [68] showed that patients with schizophrenia who were taking antipsychotics had metabolic syndrome of 42.7% at baseline, which is approximately twice the prevalence of the general population. Specifically, studies confirmed that the prevalence and incidence of the metabolic syndrome was two to three times higher in patients with schizophrenia [69] and bipolar disorders [70] compared to the general population. De Hert *et al.* [71] compared the prevalence of metabolic syndrome in patients who were treated for their first-episode of psychosis with FGAs and SGAs, and found that patients treated with SGAs had three times the incidence of the metabolic syndrome and twice the incidence of weight gain as compared to those who were treated with FGAs, but these differences disappeared when clozapine and olanzapine were excluded from the analyses.

Treatment with SGAs may cause alterations in serum lipid such as elevated levels of cholesterol, triglycerides, alterations of levels of low (LDL) and high-density lipoprotein (HDL), and hyperinsulinemia [72-74]. Antipsychotic treatment is often associated with an increase in body weight and adiposity, ranging from modest effects reported with amisulpride, ziprasidone, and aripiprazole to clinically significant increases with olanzapine (4-10 kg). It is still unclear if the side effects and weight gain induced by metabolic changes are dose-dependent. Several studies demonstrated that weight gain liability differs significantly among SGAs. Clozapine and olanzapine seem to be associated with the greatest risk of weight gain and a higher risk of hyperlipidemia [73]. Over 10 mg daily of olanzapine determine weight gain, but often with a significant dose-response induction [75, 76]. Risperidone, quetiapine, amisulpride, and zotepine frequently show low to moderate levels of weight gain; conversely, minimal mean weight gain and the lowest risk of hyperlidemia are reported with ziprasidone and aripiprazole [73]. Studies highlighted that SGAs interfere with insulin metabolism by inducing insulin resistance and reducing its release from the pancreatic beta cells by blocking their M3 receptors. Several studies have demonstrated that different SGAs are associated with disparate effects on glucose and lipid metabolism: clozapine and olanzapine are more often associated with an increased risk of diabetes mellitus and dyslipidaemia [73]. Scarce data are available about the risk for treatment-induced diabetes mellitus and dyslipidaemia with risperidone and quetiapine [33]. The metabolic syndrome should represent a prime target for therapeutic intervention, since it significantly increases the risk of cardiovascular diseases at any level of LDL cholesterol [33].

Cardiac event risk is a prominent safety concern with antipsychotic utilization since patients with schizophrenia have a greater risk of cardiac events than the general population [77]. QTc, the measure of time between the beginning of the Q wave and the end of the T wave corrected for heart rate in the electrocardiogram, is important have under control since an interval prolongation may result in fatal arrhythmias, torsade de pointes, and sudden deaths [78]. These cardiac adverse effects are dose-dependent [79]. Recent evidence indicates that the greatest prolongation from baseline QTc is observed with thioridazine (mean: 30.1 milliseconds), especially in combination with a tryciclic antidepressant therapy [80]; the second longest QTc prolongation (mean: 15.9 milliseconds) is associated with ziprasidone [81]; whereas, the lowest prolongation is found with olanzapine (mean: 1.7 milliseconds) [81]. The cardiovascular risk is often increased only if the patient has pre-existing cardiac disease or an autonomic nervous system dysfunction [82, 83]. It is still a matter of debate whether SGAs are associated with major cardiac safety when compared to FGAS. Many investigators have suggested that SGAs should be preferred in clinical practice because they do not increase cardiac risk [84-90]. Conversely, Ray and colleagues [77] found that SGAS determine similar dose-related increased risk of sudden cardiac death (twice) in comparison with FGAS. Several studies [80, 91-98] confirmed that SGAs increase the cardiac risk to the same extent as FGAs.

The most important factors implicated in the onset of cardiovascular disorder include cigarette smoking and obesity with its consequences, such as dyslipidemia, hypertension, and insulin resistance leading to diabetes. It has been demonstrated that cardiovascular disorders are the leading cause of death in individuals with serious mental illness [99]. It is possible that an increased risk of cardiovascular events may be due both to the schizophrenia itself, given that this condition is often associated with unhealthy lifestyles including poor nutrition, substance abuse, smoking, lack of exercise, poverty and stress, and medications' side effects [99].

6. PSYCHOSOCIAL UNMET NEEDS

6.1. Unsufficient Treatment Options of Cognitive Impairment: Pharmacological and Non-pharmacological Options

Pharmacological treatment is likely to not be enough to manage the multiple impairments of schizophrenia. Cognitive impairment represents one of these unregulated aspects. It is now considered one of the most disabling dimensions of schizophrenia, and in many cases it persists during pharmacological treatment [14]. Cognition is a complex collection of different mental processes including the capacity to perceive, learn, think, memorize, study, analyze information, and program adaptive behaviours. Frequently, antecedents of this impairment are already evident during childhood, resulting in a more disabled occupational and social functioning as well as reduced capacity for independent living [14]. Cognitive symptoms are commonly associated with functional outcome: executive functions, verbal memory and vigilance have been reported to be the most important predictors of functional outcome [100]. In recent years, several studies have focused on the prominence of cognitive deficits of patients with schizophrenia. Individuals experiencing psychosis often present with several impairments in many neurocognitive domains, such as executive functioning, memory, attention, semantic memory, motor processing, vigilance, verbal learning, verbal and spatial working memory [101]. Cognitive impairment is included in the group of negative symptoms of schizophrenia. The expression "deficit symptoms" is in reference to negative symptoms that are present as enduring symptoms and during and/or between episodes of positive symptom exacerbation, and observable regardless of the patient's medication status. The negative symptoms of schizophrenia may be described as an impairment of normal emotional responses, behaviors and thought processes, resulting in blunting or flattening affect, alogia/aprosody, avolition/apathy, anhedonia, and asociality. Negative symptoms contribute to most of the long-term morbidity and poor functional outcomes in patients diagnosed with schizophrenia, which reduces quality of life and increases functional disability and burden of illness [63]. Primary negative symptoms are prominent and persistent in up to 26% of patients with schizophrenia, and they are estimated to occur in up to 58% of outpatients at any given time. Several studies have demonstrated the almost inefficacy of antipsychotics in managing negative symptoms [102]. Buchanan and colleagues [103] compared the efficacy of clozapine (200-600 mg/day) and haloperidol (10-30 mg/day) in partially responsive outpatients with a diagnosis of schizophrenia and found that clozapine was superior to haloperidol in treating positive symptoms, but there was no evidence for clozapine being efficacious or having significant long-term effects for primary or secondary negative symptoms.

Kopelowicz *et al.* [104] investigated a sample of 39 outpatients with schizophrenia, and severe negative symptoms and deficit symptoms. The patients were treated for 12 weeks with 5-30 mg/day of olanzapine. Overall, 13 patients had deficit negative symptoms and 26 had non-deficit negative symptoms. The authors showed that patients who had non-deficit negative symptoms had an improvement in positive and negative symptoms, level of functioning, and extrapiramidal side effects. In contrast, patients meeting criteria for the deficit syndrome improved significantly over baseline only in extrapiramidal side effects. In a recent review, Chue and Lalonde [105] outlined the lack of evidence for the use of antipsychotics in the treatment of negative symptoms of schizophrenia. Similarly, a meta-analysis of five double blind placebo-controlled studies demonstrated that only amisulpiride showed a mild improvement in the Schedule for the Assessment of Negative Symptoms (SANS) score at endpoint in patients with schizophrenia who have predominant negative symptoms [106]. More recent studies demonstrated that FGAs may determine, in addition to producing adverse motor system effects, higher-level cognitive adverse effects. Such adverse effects on working memory are well established in animal models [107-109]. Similar effects have been reported in both psychiatrically healthy human subjects [110] and schizophrenia patients regarding working memory, processing speed, motor skills, and other higher-order cognitive abilities [111-114].

6.2. Intervention Studies

Clinical studies with SGAs have revealed that they have pro-cognitive benefits. An initial study conducted by Kane *et al.* [115] showed that clozapine reduces negative symptoms and improves cognitive deficits. In addition to comparable, if not superior, control of positive symptoms with fewer extrapyramidal symptoms and less risk for tardive dyskinesia, SGAs have demonstrated meaningful benefits for schizophrenia patients in terms of quality of life and daily function *via* cognitive improvements [116]. Among SGAs, asenapine represents a new molecule with few side effects. Asenapine has demonstrated its effectiveness in improving different cognitive domains although potential negative and/or cognitive symptoms effects of asenapine need to be more closely investigated in long-term prospective studies. Cognitive functioning in patients with acute exacerbation of schizophrenia symptoms was assessed in a 6-week, randomized, double-blind, placebo- and risperidone-controlled study [117]. Patients were randomly assigned to fixed doses of asenapine (5 mg BID), risperidone (3 mg BID), or placebo. A battery of neurocognitive tests, administered at baseline, week 3, and week 6 or last visit, assessed the speed of processing, working memory, verbal learning and memory visual learning and memory, and reasoning and problem solving. Dunlap's D >0.25 was used to indicate a moderate or greater effect size. The researchers examined 180 patients with schizophrenia and found that those treated with 5 mg twice daily of asenapine demonstrated improvements on all cognitive tests related to verbal learning and memory compared to those receiving risperidone 6 mg daily or placebo. On most measures of cognitive functions, the effect size for active treatment *vs.* placebo was greater with asenapine than that with risperidone [118]. Among the new drugs, lurasidone plays an important role in the management of schizophrenia. Lurasidone is a new benzisothiazol derivative with potent binding affinity for D2, 5-HT2A, and 5HT7 receptors (antagonist), moderate affinity for 5HT1A (partial agonist) and α2C receptors (antagonist), and no appreciable affinity for H1 and M1 receptors [119]. Several studies have supported the hypothesis that lurasidone may have a precognitive effect [120-122] as confirmed by Harvey *et al.* [123] in a 3-week, double blind, active controlled study including lurasidone and ziprasidone. In a follow-up study, the authors showed the superiority of lurasidone 160 mg/die compared to placebo (Cohen's d = 0.37) and quetiapine 600 mg/die (d = 0.41), while lurasidone 80 mg/d, quetiapine XR 600 mg/d, and placebo did not significantly differ [124]. In a recent 6-week randomized trial, Harvey and colleagues [125] described improved cognitive performance in schizophrenia patients treated with each of the flexible doses of lurasidone 40-160 mg/d, compared to quetiapine XR 200-800 mg/d. All doses of lurasidone were superior to all doses of quetiapine for cognitive performance.

In summary, it is clear how important elucidating the biological and neurological mechanisms underlying negative symptoms in schizophrenia. In fact, the development of a negative symptom treatment is still considered a major unmet need in this disabling condition. Further studies and rigorous pharmacological research are needed in order to develop more effective and better tolerated treatments.

7. COGNITIVE REMEDIATION

In addition to pharmacotherapy, another intervention strategy for neurocognition in schizophrenia is represented by cognitive remediation (CR). Fig. (1) depicts the key assumptions and rationale underlying CR in schizophrenia.

From the 1980s to 1990s, studies on CR consisted of experimental manipulations on a particular task or in broad rehabilitation programs which were very similar to those applied to brain-injured patients [126]. During that period, researchers studied the modifiability of performance on cognitive tasks, such as problem solving, reaction time, vigilance and verbal memory, employing several approaches including coaching, monetary reinforcement, and performance strategies [127]. Later, more comprehensive and longer lasting cognitive programs were used in patients with schizophrenia, including cognitive exercise conducted in group [128]. Indeed, CR now includes interventions encompassing environmental aids, compensation strategies and techniques that enhance executive functions and social cognition, repetitive drill-like exercises that challenge sensory information processing, attention and memory [127].

Although it remains unclear what form of repetitive challenge is required to stimulate neuroplasticity, CR training may induce structural and functional brain changes, being able to reverse neurocognitive deficits through neural plasticity [129]. Cognitive enhancement has been found to be asso-

ciated with gray matter preservation in several brain regions as well as an increase in gray matter volume in the left amygdala [129]. One of the several approaches of this kind of rehabilitation is based on the theory of neuroplasticity, using the auditory discrimination. Specifically, three studies [130-132] with samples of 29, 55, and 56 patients with schizophrenia, respectively, demonstrated that 50 hours of CR improved peripheral blood levels of the neurotrophin, BDNF, compared to an active control condition. Eack and colleagues [133], in a two-year intervention combining CR and social skills training during the onset of schizophrenia, demonstrated an improvement of cognitive performance.

Recent studies have also reported the possible benefits associated with CR in schizophrenia patients. Cella *et al.* [134] found that participants in a CR group reported significant improvements in recall memory, reduced negative symptoms as well as lower cognitive complains. Similarly, Au *et al.* [135] demonstrated improvements in vocational, clinical, psychological, and neurocognitive outcomes at the short-term period and after 7 and 11 months of follow-up in a sample of ninety patients with schizophrenia or schizoaffective disorders. Significant improvements on the training tasks have been also observed with computerized CR among 130 chronic schizophrenic patients by Gomar and colleagues [136]. Furthermore, although no differences emerged between groups on specific skills or psychosocial functioning,

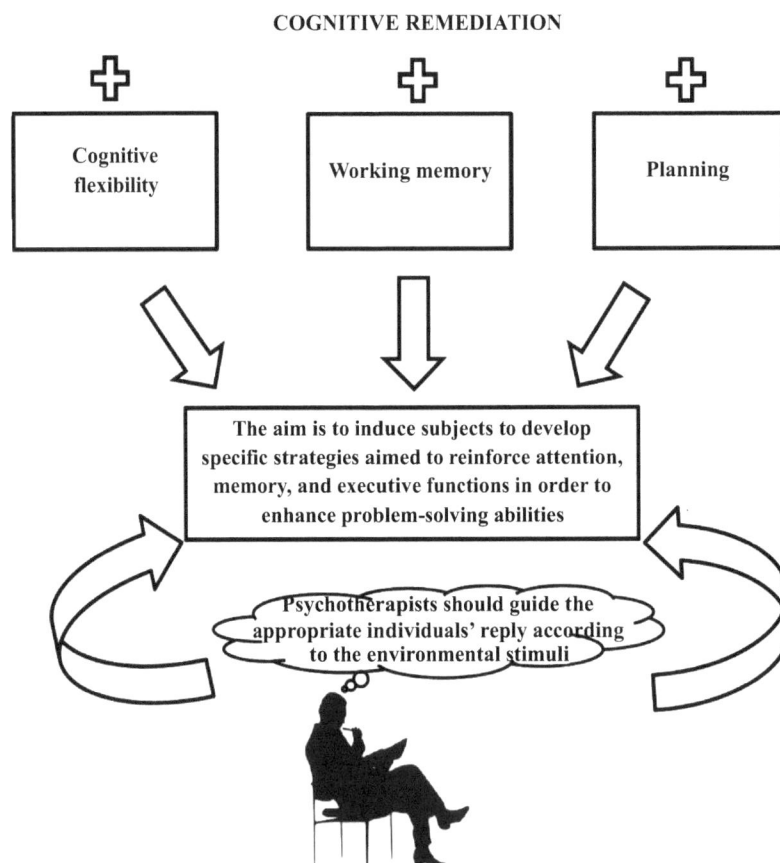

Fig. (1). Key assumptions and rationale underlying cognitive remediation in schizophrenia.
Source: Wykes T, Reeder C (eds) (2005). Cognitive remediation therapy for schizophrenia. Theory and Practice. Routledge, London.

subjects who underwent CR improved more significantly in attention, working memory and empathy than those treated with computer skills [137]. Interestingly, Puig *et al.* [138] demonstrated significant improvements in verbal memory and executive functions, with medium-to-large effect sizes in a sample of fifty adolescents diagnosed with early-onset schizophrenia. Moreover, CR integrated within a supported education setting demonstrated interesting outcomes in specific areas of functioning and mental health [139] and CR was also shown to exert a significant effect on both disorganization and negative symptoms [140].

Computer-assisted CR therapy has been associated with improvements in speed of processing, working memory and reasoning, and problem-solving cognitive domains with significant benefits over time regarding patients' quality of life and self-esteem [141]. Problem solving, memory and attention were also significantly improved with large effect sizes based on a study conducted Trapp and colleagues [142]. According to Tan and King [143], CR subjects also obtained greater attainment of vocational or independent living skills and improved functional outcomes both at post-intervention and 1-year follow-up; however, other studies [144] did not show any significant differences between CR and an individualized therapy in a sample of 138 participants. Finally, other additional evidence [145-147] has supported the assumption that remediation programs are promising with regard to social functioning and that CR may significantly improve cognitive performance providing neurobiological protective effects in patients with schizophrenia. Table **2** summarizes the most relevant CR studies in patients with schizophrenia.

In sum, CR may significantly ameliorate neurocognitive deficits in schizophrenia improving quality of life and psychosocial functioning among schizophrenia patients.

8. UNMET NEEDS IN THE PSYCHOSOCIAL PERSPECTIVE

Patients with schizophrenia are frequently unemployed, single, less educated, and have poor or no social contacts, which reflect several difficulties in various areas of daily life [148]. These patients are often at a high risk of isolation, have problems with housing, and their incomes depend on community aids [149]. In a recent observational descriptive cross-sectional study in Chile, Jorquera and colleagues [150] examined data from a sample of 29 young subjects with first episode schizophrenia. They found that the areas with more reported needs were; psychotic symptoms with 65.5% of the sample, 21.1% of which reported it unmet; and daytime activities, where 44.8% of patients reported a need, 61.54% of them as unmet. Moreover, Gaite and colleagues [151] showed that social contacts were strongly associated with patient's quality of life, with stigmatization and social exclusion being the strongest predictors [152]. Unfortunately, even family members are often stigmatized for their association with schizophrenia [153]: family members are looked on with suspicion for dealing with their sick relative and may be subjected to lack of socialization and reduced job opportunities.

Quality of life among patients with schizophrenia is worse than that of general population and other physically ill patients [154, 155]. It has been consistently found that the longer the length of the illness, the worse quality of life. Negative and depressive symptoms are also associated with a poorer quality of life. On the contrary, a better quality of life is related to being young, female, married with a low educational level. Having few side effects of drugs, being integrated into community support programs and receiving psychotherapy are also associated with an enhanced quality of life.

Impairment in social skills is an important deficit in psychosocial functioning among patients with schizophrenia: often stressful interactions with the social environment leads to social isolation [156]. Robert Liberman proposed a model of social skills training in order to enhance patients' interpersonal and communication skills, illness management, community reintegration, workplace social skills, and instrumental activities of daily life [157]. Training in social abilities is composed of three main settings: receiving skills (social perception), processing skills (social cognition) and sending information skills (behavioral responding or expression) [157]. This training teaches patients to better deal with stressful life events and solve problems of everyday life, reduce negative symptoms and hospitalizations, improve insight levels, manage pharmacotherapy ingestion, and increase the general quality of life [158, 159].

CONCLUSION

Several studies have confirmed that a needs' assessment in schizophrenia should be considered as one of the most important aspects in the management and recovery of this complex psychiatric condition. Defining the main needs of patients with schizophrenia will advance treatment strategies in order to reach better therapeutic results and recovery. To date, various unmet needs are known among schizophrenic patients regarding efficacy, particularly negative symptoms and cognitive deficits, together with treatment resistance, safety and tolerability concerns for currently available antipsychotics, reduced adherence to treatment and stigmatizing behaviours.

The introduction of SGAs has, at least partially, helped clinicians address the most relevant unmet needs for schizophrenia patients according to their enhanced effectiveness. These new medications have significantly improved the quality of daily life as well as the general outcomes for these patients by reducing the occurrence of extrapyramidal side effects, excessive sedation, and prolactin dysfunction; however, the challenge remains for other relevant adverse effects, such as weight gain and metabolic syndrome. Thus, focusing on specific non-pharmacological interventions addressing healthy eating, supporting the active engagement in physical activities as well as the need to have blood tests performed at regular intervals may be very important. Unfortunately, monotherapy is an exception among these patients and is clearly related to an increased risk of treatment adverse effects [160].

Table 2.   Most relevant studies about cognitive remediation in patients with schizophrenia.

	Study Type	Sample	Main Results	Conclusions	Limitations/Shortcomings
Cella *et al.*, 2016	Cross-sectional case-control study	Twenty-five service of which ten received group CR and 15 individual CR	Participants assessed positively group CR and judged it helpful while therapists rated it feasible. The two methods exert similar effects on cognition. After CR, participants reported improvements in recall memory, reduced negative symptoms, as well as lower cognitive complains.	Take part in small CR therapy groups may be useful for schizophrenia patients	1) The small sample size; 2) The study did not measure functioning; 3) Therapeutic alliance has been not measured.
Au *et al.*, 2015	Prospective follow-up case-control study	Ninety schizophrenia or schizoaffective disorders participants of which 45 randomly assigned into the ISE+CR and 45 to ISE alone	Similar improvements were reported immediately and after 7 and 11month follow-ups while no significant group differences emerged. Significant positive trends over time in vocational, clinical and cognitive outcomes consistently have been observed for the ISE+CR group.	Both the ISE+CR and ISE groups showed improvements in vocational, clinical, psychological, and neurocognitive outcomes	1) The non-significant results might have been attributed to the plateau effect induced by the Wisconsin Card Sorting Test component; 2) The non-significant findings might be due to the small sample size;
Gomar *et al.*, 2015	6-month follow up case-control study	130 chronic schizophrenic patients randomly assigned to computerized CR, an active computerized CC or TAU	Iimprovements on the training tasks have been observed with computerized CR, although this did not reflect gains on the primary outcome measures and most other neuropsychological tests relative to CC or TAU conditions.	Computerized CR is not effective in schizophrenia	1) Dropout resulted in 17% of patients 2) Results did not imply the possibility that CR combined with other cognitive interventions, and detailed rehabilitation programs may be efficacious.
Kurtz *et al.*, 2015	Cross-sectional case-control study	Sixty-four schizophrenia or schizoaffective disorder outpatients assigned to a standardized program of SST, and SST+Computer Skills	The CR group improved more significantly in attention, working memory, and empathy than the Computer Skills group. However, no differences emerged between groups on other skills or in terms of psychosocial functioning.	CR ameliorates working memory and consequently empathy in schizophrenia.	1) Participants in the CR and Computer Skills groups received lower hours of training compared to previous studies; 2) The type of CR did not test the link between targeted cognitive skills and learning of social skills; 3) The administration of both CR and SST may have impacted the influence of acquired cognitive skills on acquisition of specific social skills.
Puig *et al.*, 2014	Randomized, controlled trial	Fifty adolescents with early-onset schizophrenia, of which 25 were randomly assigned to receive CR and 25 TAU	After CR, significant improvements were reported in verbal memory and executive functions, with medium-to-large effect sizes. Medium-sized effect size emerged for improvements after CR in daily living and adaptive functioning, whereas large effect size were observed for improvements in family burden. These changes were maintained after 3 months (except for functional gains).	Adolescents with early-onset schizophrenia may significantly benefit from CR	1) The small sample size; 2) Findings may be not generalized to adult patients with chronic schizophrenia
Kidd *et al.*, 2014	8-month randomized controlled trial	Thirty-seven psychotic students	The treatment group showed better retention in the academic program and a trend of improvement in a range of academic functional domains. However, the outcomes were not improved with CR which resulted associated with significant and sustained improvements in self-esteem.	CR integrated within a supported education setting showed enhanced outcomes in some areas of functioning and mental health, with no effect on long-term cognitive functioning.	1) The relatively small sample size; 2) The degree to which assessor blinding was sustained is questionable; 2) Teacher ratings were less standardized than other measures.
Cella *et al.*, 2014	Randomized controlled trial	85 schizophrenia patients of which 43 participating in a CR training plus treatment as usual and 42 to TAU	After CR, the therapy group had a significant reduction in disorganized and negative symptom dimensions compared to the TAU group. No effect of CR has been observed on symptoms.	CR may exert a significant effect on both disorganization and negative symptoms.	1) The small sample size; 2) Results are limited by the type of CR and may not extend to other programmes with reduced therapist contact.
Vianin *et al.*, 2014	14-week prospective follow-up study	16 right-handed schizophrenia patients who underwent CR training	Increased activation in Broca's area together with improvements in performance of executive/frontal tasks, was observed after CR training.	Metacognitive techniques of verbalization have been supposed as the main factor underlying the specified brain changes	1) The exploratory nature of this study; 2) The small sample size; 3) The possible contribution of antipsychotic drug to the cognitive improvement is unclear; 3) The number of female participants was very low
Garrido *et al.*, 2013	Cross-sectional study	Sixty-seven schizophrenia subjects randomly assigned to computer-assisted CR or an active control condition	Improvements in speed of processing, working memory and reasoning and problem-solving cognitive domains have been reported with computer-assisted CR therapy. Significant improvements over time concerning QoL and self-esteem were also reported in this group.	Computer-assisted CR is associated with improvements in neuropsychological performance, QoL and self-esteem in schizophrenia.	1) The relatively small sample size that may limit the power to detect subtle differences in cognitive change between groups.

(Table 2) Contd....

	Study Type	Sample	Main Results	Conclusions	Limitations/Shortcomings
Trapp *et al.*, 2013	Cross-sectional study	Sixty schizophrenia patients, of which thirty received computer-assisted CR training, and thirty occupational therapy	Problem solving, memory and attention were significantly improved with high effect sizes. Employment status, a post test verbal memory performance measure and a measure of executive functioning outperformed all other measures in the prediction of time to relapse.	CR may strengthen cognition directly and positively acts on clinical course indirectly through improved neurocognition.	1) The relatively small sample size; 2) It is possible that changes in employment level may have occurred and interacted with clinical outcome; 3) Milder forms of relapse before re-hospitalisation presumably remained undetected
Tan and King, 2013	One-year follow-up study	70 schizophrenia participants were randomized to receive a 60-hour programme of either CR or physical exercise	Participants who received CR had significantly greater improvement in all neurocognitive domains. Also, the CR group obtained greater attainment of vocational or independent living skills and better functional outcomes at post-intervention and 1-year follow-up.	CR was able to show significant positive effects on both neurocognition and functional outcomes	1) The small sample size; 2) The main results may be not generalized to other populations.
Franck *et al.*, 2013	Cross-sectional case-control study	138 participants of which 65 randomized to CR and 73 to an individualized therapy	No difference was demonstrated for the main outcome. Significant improvements were reported in most of outcomes including cognition (executive functions, selective attention, verbal memory, and visuospatial abilities) and clinician measures (symptoms and awareness to be hampered by cognitive deficits in everyday) in both treatment arms after treatment. Self-esteem improved only after an individualized therapy, and working memory improved only after CR a, but there were no differences in changes between groups.	A similar efficacy has been observed for both CR and an individualized therapy	1) Potential medication effects on outcome may be not excluded; 2) The level of medication and changes of treatments have not been considered; 3) The absence of evaluation of the impact of CR on daily functioning or an assessment of social cognition are other additional limitations.
Keefe *et al.*, 2012	Cross-sectional case-control study	53 adult schizophrenia patients randomized to a CR condition including the Posit Science Brain Fitness auditory training program with weekly Neuropsychological and Educational Approach to Remediation "bridging groups" or a control condition of computer games	After 20 sessions, patients in the CR condition showed mean MATRICS Consensus Cognitive Battery composite score improvements that were 3.7 T-score points greater than in patients in the computer-games control group. At the end of treatment, a trend in favor of CR resulted not statistically significant	CR interventions improve cognitive performance in patients with schizophrenia	1) The small sample size; 2) The ideal or minimal dose, frequency, and time course of CR treatment response remains unclear
Farreny *et al.*, 2012	6-month case-control follow-up study	62 schizophrenia or schizoaffective disorder participants were randomized to 32 group sessions of Problem Solving and Cognitive Flexibility training or 32 group sessions of activities focused on leisure	Patients in the CR group showed significant improvements in executive function, negative symptoms and functioning at post-treatment compared with controls. Significant improvements in executive function and functioning were maintained after 6-month of follow-up.	Problem Solving and Cognitive Flexibility training may improve executive thinking and functioning outcomes	1) Metacognition has not been appropriately investigated; 2) The small sample size.
Wölwer and Frommann, 2011	6-month case-control study	Thirty-eight schizophrenia or schizoaffective disorder inpatients randomly assigned to 6 weeks of treatment with the TAR targeted at facial affect recognition or CR Training primarily targeted at neurocognition	The effects on theory of mind and social competence were no longer significant in the smaller group of patients who completed treatment. TAR effects may be generalized to other social cognitive domains not primarily addressed. TAR may also enhance social skills and social functioning.	Remediation programs targeting social cognition seem to be more promising with regard to social functioning than programs targeting neurocognition.	1) The smaller sample size; 2) The larger variance of the completer sample; 3) The differential improvement in social competence under TAR as compared to CRT is smaller in effect size
Eack *et al.*, 2010	2-year randomized controlled trial	53 stable but cognitively disabled schizophrenia or schizoaffective disorder outpatients	Patients who received CET showed significantly greater preservation of gray matter volume over 2 years in the left hippocampus, parahippocampal gyrus, and fusiform gyrus, and significantly greater gray matter increases in the left amygdala compared with those who received enriched supportive therapy. Less gray matter loss in the left parahippocampal and fusiform gyrus and greater gray matter increases in the left amygdala were significantly related to improved neurocognition and mediated the beneficial cognitive effects of CET.	CET can provide neurobiologic protective and enhancing effects.	1) The absence of an appropriately matched group of healthy subjects; 2) The absence of functional neuroimaging data limits the pathophysiological significance of the main results; 3) Overall structural changes in regional brain volumes were not large; 4) No effects were observed in the dorsolateral prefrontal cortex, and only modest effects in the anterior cingulate and hippocampus

(Table 2) Contd....

	Study Type	Sample	Main Results	Conclusions	Limitations/Shortcomings
Adcock *et al.,* 2009	Cross-sectional case-control study	Auditory training group (N = 29) and control group (N = 26)	Active cognitive training was associated with improvements not only in the trained functions of verbal working memory and immediate verbal learning but also improved verbal memory performance. Active cognitive training exercises are associated with increases in peripheral BDNF and to NMDA receptor activity.	The program of training may be of functional benefit and may open a critical window for successful psychosocial rehabilitation	1) The preliminary nature of the main findings; 2) It is unclear what specific components of the exercises are the active ingredients; 3) Whether benefits may be attributable to the exercises' sensory component is a matter of debate;
Fisher *et al.,* 2009		Fifty-five clinically stable schizophrenia subjects randomized to 50 hours of computerized auditory training or a control condition with computer games	Individuals receiving active training demonstrated significant effects in global cognition, verbal working memory, verbal learning, and memory. Auditory psychophysical performance was also improved according to gains in global cognition and verbal working memory.	Intensive training in early auditory processes and auditory-verbal learning is associated with substantial gains in verbal cognitive processes linked to psychosocial functioning in schizophrenia	1) The small sample size; 2) The relatively high level of education of participants; 3) The recruitment through self-referral or clinician referral; 4) No intent-to-treat analysis has been conducted; 5) Whether this intervention may be successfully adapted to real-world treatment settings is unclear
Eack *et al.,* 2009	2-year follow-up study	Early-course schizophrenia or schizoaffective disorder outpatients randomized to CET (N=31) or EST (N=27)	Of the 58 subjects who were randomly assigned and treated, 84.5% and 79.3% completed one- and two-years of treatment, respectively. Significant differential effects in favour of CET on social cognition, cognitive style, social adjustment, and symptomatology composites have been observed during the first year of treatment. After two years, moderate effects were observed in favour of CET for enhancing neurocognitive function. These differential effects on social cognition, cognitive style, and social adjustment composites were maintained at year 2 and even extended to negative symptoms.	CET appears to be an effective approach to the remediation of cognitive deficits in early schizophrenia and can significantly help in reducing disability.	1) Patients studied were mostly male and Caucasian; 2) Treatment groups were not matched for the number of hours of clinician contact; 3) Rater bias cannot be ruled out (assessing clinicians were not blind to the treatments); 4) Within-composite analyses need to be interpreted with caution; 5) The small sample size

Note: Cognitive remediation (CR); Cognitive enhancement treatment (CET); Computer skills training program (Computer Skills); control condition (CC); Enriched supportive therapy (EST); Integrated Supported Employment (ISE); Quality of life (QoL); Social skills-training (SST); Training of Affect Recognition (TAR); Treatment as usual (TAU).

In addition, patient adherence to treatment which is impaired due to the lack of insight into the illness, cognitive deficits, negative symptoms, and alcohol/substance abuse plays a fundamental role in the long-term outcomes of schizophrenia patients; therefore, the utilization of long-acting antipsychotics for this unmet treatment need in schizophrenia should be considered. Although many schizophrenia patients are referred to psychopharmacological treatment, a significant percentage may be considered treatment resistant. Conversely, according to existing evidence [10], patients treated with non-pharmacological approaches show more rapid remission and minor relapses when compared to those who have only been treated with pharmacological agents. Specifically, given the relevance of cognitive impairments in determining negative outcomes in schizophrenia patients, CR has been reported to significantly improve neurocognitive deficits, ameliorating psychosocial functioning and quality of life. CR may significantly improve the course of the illness enhancing patients' coping strategies and indirectly increased social functioning with the final result of reducing illness relapses and hospital admissions. It has been widely accepted that the course of schizophrenia may be affected by life stressors, psychological environment, patients' competence, and specific coping strategies [161, 162]. Learning how to cope with impairments is crucial for schizophrenia patients and has been increasingly identified as a fundamental aim for the management of schizophrenia symptoms [162].

In summary, given the complexity of schizophrenia as a chronic and disabling illness affecting patients' social functioning and the persistence of various unmet needs, there is the absolute need to consider novel treatment (both pharmacological and non-pharmacological) strategies and/or combined therapeutic approaches for schizophrenic patients.

CONSENT FOR PUBLICATION

Not applicable.

CONFLICT OF INTEREST

The authors declare no conflict of interest, financial or otherwise.

ACKNOWLEDGEMENTS

Declared none.

REFERENCES

[1]   World Health Organization (WHO). 2011. Schizophrenia. Retrieved February 27, 2011.

[2]   Picchioni MM, Murray RM. Schizophrenia. BMJ 2007; 335(7610): 91-5.

[3]   Chong HY, Teoh SL, Wu DB, Kotirum S, Chiou CF, Chaiya-kunapruk N. Global economic burden of schizophrenia: a systematic review. Neuropsychiatr Dis Treat 2016; 12: 357-73.

[4]   Correll CU, Detraux J, De Lepeleire J, De Hert M. Effects of antipsychotics, antidepressants and mood stabilizers on risk for physical diseases in people with schizophrenia, depression and bipolar disorder. World Psychiatry 2015; 14: 119-36.

[5]   Vancampfort D, Stubbs B, Mitchell AJ, et al. Risk of metabolic syndrome and its components in people with schizophrenia and related psychotic disorders, bipolar disorder and major depressive disorder: a systematic review and meta-analysis. World Psychiatry 2015; 14: 339-47.

[6]   Leucht S, Burkard T, Henderson J, Maj M, Sartorius N. Physical illness and schizophrenia: a review of the literature. Acta Psychiatr Scand 2007; 116: 317-33.

[7]   Bottlender R, Strauß A, Möller H. Social disability in schizophrenic, schizoaffective and affective disorders 15 years after first admission. Schizophr Res 2010; 116: 9-15.

[8]   Del Vecchio V, Luciano M, Sampogna G, et al. The role of relatives in pathways to care of patients with a first episode of psychosis. Int J Soc Psychiatry 2015; 61: 631-17.

[9]   Lieberman JA, Dixon LB, Goldman HH. Early detection and intervention in schizophrenia: a new therapeutic model. JAMA 2013; 310: 689-90.

[10] Pompili M, Montebovi F, Forte A, et al. Support management in schizophrenia: a systematic review of current literature. Patient Intellig 2012; 4: 79-101.

[11] Torres-González F, Ibanez-Casas I, Saldivia S, et al. Unmet needs in the management of schizophrenia. Neuropsychiatr Dis Treat 2014; 10: 97-110.

[12] Dixon LB, Dickerson F, Bellack AS, et al. The 2009 schizophrenia PORT psychosocial treatment recommendations and summary statements. Schizophr Bull 2010; 36: 48-70

[13] Galderisi S, Heinz A, Kastrup M, Beezhold J, Sartorius N. Toward a new definition of mental health. World Psychiatry 2015; 14: 231-3.

[14] Green MF. Impact of cognitive and social cognitive impairment on functional outcomes in patients with schizophrenia. J Clin Psychiatry 2016; 77(2): 8-11.

[15] NICE. National Institute for Health and Care Excellence. Psychosis and schizophrenia in adults: prevention and management. 2014. Available at: https: //www.nice.org.uk/guidance/cg178.

[16] Kreyenbuhl J, Buchanan RW, Dickerson FB, Dixon LB. Schizophrenia patient outcomes research team (port). the schizophrenia patient outcomes research team (PORT): updated treatment recommendations 2009. Schizophr Bull 2010; 36(1): 94-103.

[17] Mueser KT, Meyer PS, Penn DL, Clancy R, Clancy DM, Salyers MP. The illness management and recovery program: rationale, development, and preliminary findings. Schizophr Bull 2006; 32(Suppl1): S32-S43.

[18] McGuire AB, Kukla M, Green A, Gilbride D, Mueser KT, Salyers MP. Illness management and recovery: a review of the literature. Psychiatric Serv 2014; 65(2): 171-9.

[19] Substance abuse and mental health services administration. Results from the 2011 national survey on drug use and health: summary of national findings. rockville, MD: substance abuse and mental health services administration; 2012.

[20] Siris SG. Depression in schizophrenia: perspective in the era of "Atypical" antipsychotic agents. Am J Psychiatry 2000; 157(9): 1379-89.

[21] Cohen CI, Vahia I, Reyes P, et al. Focus on geriatric psychiatry: schizophrenia in later life: clinical symptoms and social well-being. Psychiatr Serv 2008; 59(3): 232-4.

[22] Biddle S. Physical activity and mental health: evidence is growing. World Psychiatry 2016; 15: 176-8.

[23] Daumit GL, Pratt LA, Crum RM, Powe NR, Ford DE. Characteristics of primary care visits for individuals with severe mental illness in a national sample. Gen Hosp Psychiatry 2002; 24(6): 391-5.

[24] Meyer JM, Nasrallah HA. Medical illness and schizophrenia. Arlington, VA: American Psychiatric Publishing, Inc; 2009.

[25] Appleby L, Thomas S, Ferrier N, Lewis G, Shaw J, Amos T. Sudden unexplained death in psychiatric in-patients. Br J Psychiatry 2000; 176: 405-6.

[26] Glassman AH, Bigger JT Jr. Antipsychotic drugs: prolonged QTc interval, torsade de pointes, and sudden death. Am J Psychiatry 2001; 158(11): 1774-82.

[27] Lin HC, Hsiao FH, Pfeiffer S, Hwang YT, Lee HC. An increased risk of stroke among young schizophrenia patients. Schizophr Res 2008; 101(1-3): 234-41.

[28] Newcomer JW. Antipsychotic medications: metabolic and cardiovascular risk. J Clin Psychiatry 2007; 68 Suppl 4: 8-13.

[29] Hennekens CH. Increasing global burden of cardiovascular disease in general populations and patients with schizophrenia. J Clin Psychiatry 2007; 68 Suppl 4: 4-7.

[30] Saha S, Chant D, McGrath J. A systematic review of mortality in schizophrenia: is the differential mortality gap worsening over time? Arch Gen Psychiatry 2007; 64(10): 1123-31.

[31] McBain H, Mulligan K, Haddad M, Flood C, Jones J, Simpson A. Self management interventions for type 2 diabetes in adult people with severe mental illness. Cochrane Database Syst Rev 2016; 4: CD011361.

[32] Gough SC, O'Donovan MC. Clustering of metabolic comorbidity in schizophrenia: a genetic contribution? J Psychopharmacol 2005; 19(6 Suppl): 47-55.

[33] Newcomer JW. Second-generation (atypical) antipsychotics and metabolic effects: a comprehensive literature review. CNS Drugs 2005; 19 Suppl 1: 1-93.

[34] Spelman LM, Walsh PI, Sharifi N, Collins P, Thakore JH. Impaired glucose tolerance in first-episode drug-naive patients with schizophrenia. Diabet Med 2007; 24(5): 481-5.

[35] Osby U, Correia N, Brandt L, Ekbom A, Sparen P. Mortality and causes of death in schizophrenia in Stockholm county, Sweden. Schizophr Res 2000; 45(1-2): 21-8.

[36] Johnsen E. Review: metabolic side effects of second-generation antipsychotics. Evid Based Ment Health 2011; 14(2): 47.

[37] De Hert M, Dobbelaere M, Sheridan EM, Cohen D, Correll CU. Metabolic and endocrine adverse effects of second-generation antipsychotics in children and adolescents: a systematic review of randomized, placebo controlled trials and guidelines for clinical practice. Eur Psychiatry 2011; 6(3): 144-58.

[38] DeBattista C, DeBattista K. Safety considerations of the use of second generation antipsychotics in the treatment of major depression: extrapyramidal and metabolic side effects. Curr Drug Saf 2010; 5(3): 263-6.

[39] Rummel-Kluge C, Komossa K, Schwarz S, et al. Head-to-head comparisons of metabolic side effects of second generation antipsychotics in the treatment of schizophrenia: a systematic review and meta-analysis. Schizophr Res 2010; 123(2-3): 225-33.

[40] Winterer G. Why do patients with schizophrenia smoke? Curr Opin Psychiatry 2010; 23(2): 112-9.

[41] Bowie CR, Harvey PD. Cognition in schizophrenia: impairments, determinants, and functional importance. Psychiatr Clin North Am 2005; 28: 613-33.

[42] Jones LE, Clarke W, Carney CP. Receipt of diabetes services by insured adults with and without claims for mental disorders. Med Care 2004; 42: 1167-75.

[43] Kampman O, Lehtinen K. Compliance in psychoses. Acta Psychiatrica Scandinavica 1999; 100: 167-75.

[44] Valenstein M, Copeland LA, Blow FC, et al. Pharmacy data identify poorly adherent patients with schizophrenia at increased risk for admission. Med Care 2002; 40: 630-9.

[45] Llorca PM. Partial compliance in schizophrenia and theimpact on patient outcomes. Psychiatry Res 2008; 161: 235-47.

[46] Weiden P, Zygmunt A. Medication noncompliance in schizophrenia. Part I. Assessment. J Pract Psychiatry Behav 2016; 3: 106-10.

[47] Fleischhacker W, Oehl MA, Hummer M. Factors influencing compliance in schizophrenia patients. J Clin Psychiatry 2003; 64(suppl 16): 10-3.

[48] Oehl M, Hummer M, Fleischhacker WW. Compliance with antipsychotic treatment. Acta Psychiatrica Scandinavica 2000; 102: 83-6.

[49] ProuteauA, Verdoux H, Briand C, et al. 2005. Cognitive predictors of psychosocial functioning outcome in schizophrenia: a follow-up study of subjects participating in a rehabilitation program. Schizophrenia Res 2000; 77: 343-53.

[50] Dam J. Insight in schizophrenia: a review. Nordic J Psychiatry 2006; 60: 114-20.

[51] Novak-Grubic, V, Tavcar R. Predictors of noncompliance in males with first-episode schizophrenia, schizophreniform and schizoaffective disorder. Eur Psychiatry 2002; 17: 148-54.

[52] Herings RM, Erkens JA. Increased suicide attempt rate among patients interrupting use of atypical antipsychotics. Pharmacoepidemiol Drug Saf 2000; 12: 423-4.

[53] Beck EM, Cavelti M, Kvrgic S, Kleim B, Vauth R. Are we addressing the 'right stuff' to enhance adherence in schizophrenia? Understanding the role of insight and attitudes towards medication. Schizophr Res 2011; 132(2011): 42-9.

[54] Miner CR, Rosenthal RN, Hellerstein DJ, Muenz LR. Prediction of compliance with outpatient referral in patients with schizophrenia and psychoactive substance use disorders. Arch Gen Psychiatry 1997; 54(8): 706-12.

[55] Schennach-Wolff R, Jäger M, Seemüller F, et al. Attitude towards adherence in patients with schizophrenia at discharge. J Psychiatr Res 2009; 43(16): 1294-301.

[56] Rocca P, Crivelli B, Marino F, Mongini T, Portaleone F, Bogetto F. Correlations of attitudes toward antipsychotic drugs with insight and objective psychopathology in schizophrenia. Comprehensive Psychiatry 2008; 49: 170-6.

[57] Perkins DO. Predictors of noncompliance in patients with schizophrenia. J Clin Psychiatry 2002; 63(12): 1121-8

[58] Davis JM, Kane JM, Marder SR, et al. Dose response of prophylactic antipsychotics. J Clin Psychiatry 1993; 54 Suppl: 24-30

[59] Fenton WS, Blyler CR, Heinssen RK. Determinants of medication compliance in schizophrenia: empirical and clinical findings. Schizophr Bull 1997; 23(4): 637-51

[60] Robinson D, Woerner MG, Alvir JM, et al. Predictors of relapse following response from a first episode of schizophrenia or schizoaffective disorder. Arch Gen Psychiatry 1999; 56(3): 241-7.

[61] Hunter R, Barry S. Negative symptoms and psychosocial functioning in schizophrenia: neglected but important targets for treatment. Eur Psychiatry 2012; 27: 432-6.

[62] Kirkpatrick B, Fenton WS, Carpenter WT Jr, Marder SR. The NIMH-MATRICS consensus statement on negative symptoms. Schizophrenia Bull 2006; 32: 214-19.

[63] Milev P, Ho BC, Arndt S, Andreasen NC. Predictive values of neurocognition and negative symptoms on functional outcome in schizophrenia: a longitudinal first-episode study with 7-year follow-up. Am J Psychiatry 2005; 162: 495-506.

[64] Ames D, Carr-Lopez SM, Gutierrez MA, et al. Detecting and managing adverse effects of antipsychotic medications: current state of play. Psychiatr Clin North Am 2016; 39(2): 275-311.

[65] Third Report of the National Cholesterol Education Program (NCEP) Expert Panel on Detection, Evaluation, and Treatment of High Blood Cholesterol in Adults (Adult Treatment Panel III) final report. Circulation 2002; 106(25): 3143-421.

[66] Gilmer TP, Dolder CR, Lacro JP, et al. Adherence to treatment with antipsychotic medication and health care costs among Medicaid beneficiaries with schizophrenia. Am J Psychiatry 2004; 161(4): 692-99.

[67] Lakka HM, Laaksonen DE, Lakka TA, et al. The metabolic syndrome and total and cardiovascular disease mortality in middle-aged men. JAMA 2002; 288(21), 2709-16 (2002).

[68] McEvoy JP, Meyer JM, Goff DC, et al. Prevalence of the metabolic syndrome in patients with schizophrenia: baseline results from the clinical antipsychotic trials of intervention effectiveness (CATIE) schizophrenia trial and comparison with national estimates from NHANES III. Schizophr Res 2005; 80(1): 19-32

[69] Meyer JM, Stahl SM. The metabolic syndrome and schizophrenia. Acta Psychiatr Scand 2009; 119(1): 4-14.

[70] De Hert M, Schreurs V, Vancampfort D, Van Winkel R. Metabolic syndrome in people with schizophrenia: a review. World Psychiatry 2009; 8(1): 15-22.

[71] De Hert M, Schreurs V, Sweers K, et al. Typical and atypical antipsychotics differentially affect long-term incidence rates of the metabolic syndrome in first-episode patients with schizophrenia: a retrospective chart review. Schizophr Res 2008; 101(1-3): 295-303.

[72] Hasnain M, Vieweg WV, Fredrickson SK, et al. Clinical monitoring and management of the metabolic syndrome in patients receiving atypical antipsychotic medications. Prim Care Diabetes 2009; 3(1): 5-15.

[73] Meyer JM, Koro CE. The effects of antipsychotic therapy on serum lipids: a comprehensive review. Schizophr Res 2004; 70(1): 1-17.

[74] Stahl SM, Mignon L, Meyer JM. Which comes first: atypical antipsychotic treatment or cardiometabolic risk? Acta Psychiatr Scand 2009; 119(3): 171-9.

[75] Kinon BJ, Volavka J, Stauffer V, et al. Standard and higher dose of olanzapine in patients with schizophrenia or schizoaffective disorder: a randomized, double-blind, fixed-dose study. J Clin Psychopharmacol 2008; 28(4): 392-400.

[76] Rondanelli M, Sarra S, Antoniello N, et al. No effect of atypical antipsychotic drugs on weight gain and risk of developing type II diabetes or lipid abnormalities among nursing home elderly patients with Alzheimer's disease. Minerva Med 2006; 97(2): 147-51.

[77] Brown S, Inskip H, Barraclough B. Causes of the excess mortality of schizophrenia. Br J Psychiatry 2000; 177: 212-7.

[78] Ray WA, Chung CP, Murray KT, Hall K, Stein CM. Atypical antipsychotic drugs and the risk of sudden cardiac death. N Engl J Med 2009; 360(3): 225-35.

[79] Correll CU, Frederickson AM, Figen V, et al. The QTc interval and its dispersion in patients receiving two atypical antipsychotics. Eur Arch Psychiatry Clin Neurosci 2009; 259(1): 23-7.

[80] Fenton M, Rathbone J, Reilly J, Sultana A. Thioridazine for schizophrenia. Cochrane Database Syst Rev (3), CD001944 (2007).

[81] Harrigan EP, Miceli JJ, Anziano R, et al. A randomized evaluation of the effects of six antipsychotic agents on QTc, in the absence and presence of metabolic inhibition. J Clin Psychopharmacol 2004; 24(1): 62-9.

[82] Jolly K, Gammage MD, Cheng KK, Bradburn P, Banting MV, Langman MJ. Sudden death in patients receiving drugs tending to prolong the QT interval. Br J Clin Pharmacol 2009; 68(5): 743-51.

[83] Mackin P. Cardiac side effects of psychiatric drugs. Hum Psychopharmacol 2008; 23(1): 3-14.

[84] Barnett AH, Millar HL, Loze JY, L'Italien GJ, van Baardewijk M, Knapp M. UK cost-consequence analysis of aripiprazole in schizophrenia: diabetes and coronary heart disease risk projections (STAR study). Eur Arch Psychiatry Clin Neurosci 2009; 259(4): 239-47.

[85] Herrmann N, Lanctot KL. Atypical antipsychotics for neuropsychiatric symptoms of dementia: malignant or maligned? Drug Saf 2006; 29(10): 833-43.

[86] Jerrell JM, McIntyre RS. Cerebro- and cardiovascular conditions in adults with schizophrenia treated with antipsychotic medications. Hum Psychopharmacol 2007; 22(6): 361-4.

[87] Greenberg WM, Citrome L. Ziprasidone for schizophrenia and bipolar disorder: a review of the clinical trials. CNS Drug Rev 2007; 13(2): 137-77.

[88] Nakagawa S, Pedersen L, Olsen ML, Mortensen PB, Sorensen HT, Johnsen SP. Antipsychotics and risk of first-time hospitalization for myocardial infarction: a population-based case-control study. J Intern Med 2006; 260(5): 451-8.

[89] Riedel M, Eich FX, Moller HJ. A pilot study of the safety and efficacy of amisulpride and risperidone in elderly psychotic patients. Eur Psychiatry 2009; 24(3): 149-53.

[90] Takeuchi H, Uchida H, Suzuki T, Watanabe K, Kashima H. Changes in metabolic parameters following a switch to aripiprazole in Japanese patients with schizophrenia: one-year follow-up study. Psychiatry Clin Neurosci 2010; 64(1): 104-6.

[91] Correll CU, Harris JL, Pantaleon Moya RA, Frederickson AM, Kane JM, Manu P. Low-density lipoprotein cholesterol in patients treated with atypical antipsychotics: missed targets and lost opportunities. Schizophr Res 2007; 92(1-3): 103-7.

[92] Elbe D, Carandang CG. Focus on ziprasidone: a review of its use in child and adolescent psychiatry. J Can Acad Child Adolesc Psychiatry 2008; 17(4): 220-9.

[93] Cysneiros RM, Terra VC, Machado HR, et al. May the best friend be an enemy if not recognized early: possible role of omega-3 against cardiovascular abnormalities due to antipsychotics in the treatment of autism. Arq Neuropsiquiatr 2009; 67(3B): 922-6.

[94] Roh S, Ahn DH, Nam JH, Yang BH, Lee BH, Kim YS. Cardiomyopathy associated with clozapine. Exp Clin Psychopharmacol 2006; 14(1): 94-8.

[95] Haddad PM, Sharma SG. Adverse effects of atypical antipsychotics: differential risk and clinical implications. CNS Drugs 2007; 21(11): 911-36.

[96] Dodd ML, Dolenc TJ, Karpyak VM, Rasmussen KG. QTc dispersion in patients referred for electroconvulsive therapy. J Ect 2008; 24(2): 131-3.

[97]   Schneider RA, Lizer MH. Apparent seizure and atrial fibrillation associated with paliperidone. Am J Health Syst Pharm 2008; 65(22): 2122-5.

[98]   Wang JF, Min JY, Hampton TG, et al. Clozapine-induced myocarditis: role of catecholamines in a murine model. Eur J Pharmacol 2008; 592(1-3): 123-7.

[99]   Baldessarini RJ. Atypical antipsychotic drugs and the risk of sudden cardiac death. N Engl J Med 2009; 360(20): 2136-7.

[100]   Green MF, Kern RS, Braff DL, Mintz J. Neurocognitive deficits and functional outcome in schizophrenia: are we measuring the 'right stuff'? Schizophr Bull 2000; 26(1): 119-36.

[101]   Saykin, AJ, Shtasel DL, Gur RE, et al. Neuropsychological deficits in neuroleptic naive patients with first-episode schizophrenia. Arch Gen Psychiatry 1994; 51(2): 124-31.

[102]   Hovington CL, Bodnar M, Joober R, Malla AK, Lepage M. Identifying persistent negative symptoms in first episode psychosis. BMC Psychiatry 2012; 12: 224.

[103]   Buchanan RW, Breier A, Kirkpatrick B, Ball P, Carpenter WT Jr. Positive and negative symptom response to clozapine in schizophrenic patients with and without the deficit syndrome. Am J Psychiatry 1998; 155: 751-60.

[104]   Kopelowicz A, Zarate R, Tripodis K, Gonzalez V, Mintz J. Differential efficacy of olanzapine for deficit and nondeficit negative symptoms in schizophrenia. Am J Psychiatry 2000; 157: 987-93.

[105]   Chue P, Lalonde JK. Addressing the unmet needs of patients with persistent negative symptoms of schizophrenia: emerging pharmacological treatment options. Neuropsychiatr Dis Treat 2014; 10: 777-89.

[106]   Levine SZ, Leucht S. Treatment response heterogeneity in the predominant negative symptoms of schizophrenia: analysis of amisulpride vs placebo in three clinical trials. Schizophr Res 2014; 156(1): 107-14.

[107]   Arnsten AF, Cai JX, Steere JC, Goldman-Rakic PS. Dopamine D2 receptor mechanisms contribute to age-related cognitive decline: the effects of quinpirole on memory and motor performance in monkeys. J Neurosci 1995; 15: 3429-39.

[108]   Castner SA, Williams GV, Goldman-Rakic PS. Reversal of antipsychotic-induced working memory deficits by short-term dopamine D1 receptor stimulation. Science 2000; 287: 2020-2.

[109]   Sawaguchi T, Goldman-Rakic PS. The role of D1-dopamine receptor in working memory: local injections of dopamine antagonists into the prefrontal cortex of rhesus monkeys performing an oculomotor delayed-response task. J Neurophysiol 1994; 71: 515-28.

[110]   Ramaekers JG, Louwerens JW, Muntjewerff ND, et al. Psychomotor, cognitive, extrapyramidal, and affective functions of healthy volunteers during treatment with an atypical (amisulpride) and a classic (haloperidol) antipsychotic. J Clin Psychopharmacol 1999; 19: 209-21.

[111]   Bedard MA, Scherer H, Stip E, Cohen H, Rodriguez JP, Richer F. Procedural learning in schizophrenia: further consideration on the deleterious effect of neuroleptics. Brain Cogn 2000; 43: 31-9.

[112]   Kapur S, Zipursky R, Jones C, Remington G, Houle S. Relationship between dopamine D(2) occupancy, clinical response, and side effects: a double-blind PET study of first-episode schizophrenia. Am J Psychiatry 2000; 157(4): 514-20.

[113]   Purdon SE, Woodward N, Lindborg SR, Stip E. Procedural learning in schizophrenia after 6 months of double-blind treatment with olanzapine, risperidone, and haloperidol. Psychopharmacology 2003; 169(3-4): 390-7.

[114]   Reilly JL, Harris MS, Keshavan MS, Sweeney JA. Adverse effects of risperidone on spatial working memory in first-episode schizophrenia. Arch Gen Psychiatry 2006; 63(11): 1189-97.

[115]   Kane J, Honigfeld G, Singer J, Meltzer H. Clozapine for the treatment-resistant schizophrenic. A double-blind comparison with chlorpromazine. Arch Gen Psychiatry 1988; 45(9): 789-96.

[116]   Gründer G, Heinze M, Cordes J, et al. Effects of first-generation antipsychotics vs second-generation antipsychotics on quality of life in schizophrenia: a double-blind, randomised study. Lancet Psychiatry 2016; 3(8): 717-29.

[117]   Fleming K, Potkin SG, Binneman B, Keller DS, Alphs L, Panagides J. Asenapine improves cognitive function in acute schizophrenia: a placebo- and risperidone-controlled trial. J Clin Psychiatry 2007; 68(10): 1492-500.

[118]   Potkin SG, Fleming K, Binneman B, Keller DS, Alphs L, Panagides J. Asenapine cognitive function effects in acute schizo-

phrenia: a placebo- and risperidone-controlled trial. Am J Psychiatry 2007; 18: 176-82.

[119]   Ishibashi T, Horisawa T, Tokuda K, et al. Pharmacological profile of lurasidone, a novel antipsychotic agent with potent 5-HT7 and 5-HT1A receptor activity. J Pharmacol Exp Ther 2010; 334: 171-81.

[120]   Ishiyama T, Tokuda K, Ishibashi T, et al. Lurasidone (SM-13496), a novel atypical antipsychotic drug, reversesMK-801-induced impairment of learning andmemory in the rat passive-avoidance test. Eur J Pharmacol 2007; 572: 160-70.

[121]   Enomoto T, Ishibashi T, Tokuda K, et al. Lurasidone reverses MK-801-induced impairment of learning and memory in the Morris water maze and radial-arm maze tests in rats. Behav Brain Res 2008; 186: 197-207.

[122]   Horisawa T, Ishibashi T, Nishikawa H, et al. The effects of selective antagonists of serotonin 5-HT7 and 5-HT1A receptors on MK-801-induced impairment of learning andmemory in the passive avoidance and Morriswatermaze tests in rats: mechanistic implications for the beneficial effects of the novel atypical antipsychotic lurasidone. Behav Brain Res 2011; 220: 83-90.

[123]   Harvey PD, Ogasa M, Cucchiaro J, et al. Performance and interview-based assessments of cognitive change in a randomized, double-blind comparison of lurasidone vs. ziprasidone. Schizophr Res 2011; 127: 188-94.

[124]   Harvey PD, Siu CO, Hsu J, Cucchiaro J, Maruff P, Loebel A. Effect of lurasidone on neurocognitive performance in patients with schizophrenia: a short-term placebo- and active-controlled study followed by a 6-month double-blind extension. Eur Neuropsychopharmacol 2013; 23: 1373-82.

[125]   Harvey PD, Siu CO, Ogasa M, Loebel A. Effect of lurasidone dose on cognition in patients with schizophrenia: Post-hoc analysis of a long-term, double-blind continuation study. Schizophr Res 2015; 166: 334-8.

[126]   Ben-Yishay Y, Rattok J, Lakin P, et al. Neuropsychological rehabilitation: quest for a holistic approach. Semin Neurol 1985; 5: 252-9.

[127]   Hogarty GE, Flesher S, Ulrich R, et al. Cognitive enhancement therapy for schizophrenia. Arch Gen Psychiatry 2004; 61: 866-76.

[128]   Eack SM, Hogarty GE, Cho RY, et al. Neuroprotective effects of cognitive enhancement therapy against gray matter loss in early-schizophrenia: results from a 2-year randomized controlled trial. Arch Gen Psychiatry 2010; 67(7): 674-82.

[129]   Adcock RA, Dale C, Fisher M, et al. When top-down meets bottom-up: auditory training enhances verbal memory inschizophrenia. Schizophr Bull 2009; 35(6): 1132-41.

[130]   Fisher M, Holland C, Subramaniam K, Vinogradov S. Neuroplasticity-based cognitive training in schizophrenia: an interim report on the effects 6 months later. Schizophr Bull 2009; 36(4): 869-79.

[131]   Vinogradov S, Fisher M, Holland C, Shelly W, Wolkowitz O, Mellon SH. Is serum brain-derived neurotrophic factor a biomarker for cognitive enhancement inschizophrenia? Biol Psychiatry 2009; 66(6): 549-53.

[132]   Eack SM, Greenwald DP, Hogarty SS. Cognitive enhancement therapy for early-courseschizophrenia: effects of a two-year randomized controlled trial. Psychiatr Serv 2009; 60(11): 1468-76.

[133]   Cella M, Reeder C, Wykes T. Group cognitive remediation for schizophrenia: exploring the role of therapist support and metacognition. Psychol Psychother 2016; 89(1): 1-14.

[134]   Au DW, Tsang HW, So WW, et al. Effects of integrated supported employment plus cognitive remediation training for people with schizophrenia and schizoaffective disorders. Schizophr Res 2015; 166(1-3): 297-303.

[135]   Gomar JJ, Valls E, Radua J, et al. Cognitive rehabilitation study group. a multisite, randomized controlled clinical trial of computerized cognitive remediation therapy for schizophrenia. Schizophr Bull 2015; 41(6): 1387-96.

[136]   Kurtz MM, Mueser KT, Thime WR, Corbera S, Wexler BE. Social skills training and computer-assisted cognitive remediation in schizophrenia. Schizophr Res 2015; 162(1-3): 35-41.

[137]   Puig O, Penadés R, Baeza I. Cognitive remediation therapy in adolescents with early-onset schizophrenia: a randomized controlled trial. J Am Acad Child Adolesc Psychiatry 2014; 53(8): 859-68.

[138]   Kidd SA, Kaur J, Virdee G, George TP, McKenzie K, Herman Y. Cognitive remediation for individuals with psychosis in a supported education setting: a randomized controlled trial. Schizophr Res 2014; 157(1-3): 90-8.

[139]   Cella M, Reeder C, Wykes T. It is all in the factors: effects of cognitive remediation on symptom dimensions. Schizophr Res 2014; 156(1): 60-2.

[140]   Garrido G, Barrios M, Penadés R. Computer-assisted cognitive remediation therapy: cognition, self-esteem and quality of life in schizophrenia. Schizophr Res 2013; 150(2-3): 563-9.

[141]   Trapp W, Landgrebe M, Hoesl K, *et al.* Cognitive remediation improves cognition and good cognitive performance increases time to relapse--results of a 5 year catamnestic study in schizophrenia patients. BMC Psychiatry 2013; 13: 184.

[142]   Tan BL, King R. The effects of cognitive remediation on functional outcomes among people with schizophrenia: a randomised controlled study. Aust NZJ Psychiatry 2013; 47(11): 1068-80.

[143]   Franck N, Duboc C, Sundby C. Specific *vs* general cognitive remediation for executive functioning in schizophrenia: a multicenter randomized trial. Schizophr Res 2013; 147(1): 68-74.

[144]   Keefe RS, Vinogradov S, Medalia A, *et al.* feasibility and pilot efficacy results from the multisite cognitive remediation in the schizophrenia trials network (crstn) randomized controlled trial. J Clin Psychiatry 2012; 73(7): 1016-22.

[145]   Farreny A, Aguado J, Ochoa S, *et al.* REPYFLEC cognitive remediation group training in schizophrenia: looking for an integrative approach. Schizophr Res 2012; 142(1-3): 137-44.

[146]   Wölwer W, Frommann N. Social-cognitive remediation in schizophrenia: generalization of effects of the training of affect recognition (TAR). Schizophr Bull 2011; 37(2): S63-70.

[147]   Moreno-Küstner B, Mayoral F, Rivas F, *et al.* Factors associated with use of community mental health services by schizophrenia patients using multilevel analysis. BMC Health Serv Res 2011; 11: 257.

[148]   Schennach R, Riedel M, Obermeier M, *et al.* Remission and recovery and their predictors in schizophrenia spectrum disorder: results from a 1-year follow-up naturalistic trial. Psychiatr Q 2012; 83(2): 187-207.

[149]   Jorquera N, Alvarado R, Libuy N, de Angel V. Association between Unmet Needs and Clinical Status in Patients with First Episode of Schizophrenia in Chile. Front Psychiat 2015; 6: 57.

[150]   Gaite L, Vázquez-Barquero JL, Borra C, *et al.* EPSILON study group. Quality of life in patients with schizophrenia in five european countries: the EPSILON study. Acta Psychiatr Scand 2002; 105(4): 283-92.

[151]   van der Plas AG, Hoek HW, van Hoeken D, Valencia E, van Hemert AM. Perceptions of quality of life and disability in homeless persons with schizophrenia and persons with schizophrenia living in non-institutional housing. Int J Soc Psychiatry 2012; 58: 629-34.

[152]   Phelan JC, Bromet EJ, Link BG. Psychiatric illness and family stigma. Schizophr Bull 1998; 24(1): 115-26.

[153]   Awad AG, Voruganti LNP, Heslegrave RJ. A conceptual model of quality of life in schizophrenia: description and preliminary clinical validation. Qual Life Res 1997; 6: 21-6.

[154]   Bobes J, Garcia-Portilla MP. Quality of life in schizophrenia. In: Katschnig H, Freeman H, Sartorius N, eds. *Quality of Life in Mental Disorders*. Chichester, UK: John Wiley & Sons Ltd; 2005: 153-68.

[155]   Chien WT, Leung SF, Yeung FKK, Wong WK. Current approaches to treatments for schizophrenia spectrum disorders, part II: psychosocial interventions and patient-focused perspectives in psychiatric care. Neuropsych Dis Treat 2013; 9: 1463-81.

[156]   Liberman RP, Wallace CJ, Blackwell G, Kopelowicz A, Vaccaro JV, Mintz J. Skills training versus psychosocial occupational therapy for persons with persistent schizophrenia. Am J Psychiatry 1998; 155(8): 1087-91.

[157]   Kopelowicz A, Liberman RP, Zarate R. Recent advances in social skills training for schizophrenia. Schizophr Bull 2006; 32(Suppl 1): S12-S23.

[158]   Pilling S, Bebbington P, Kuipers E, *et al.* Psychological treatments in schizophrenia: II. Meta-analyses of randomized controlled trials of social skills training and cognitive remediation. Psychol Med 2002; 32(5): 783-91.

[159]   Pompili M, Serafini G, Innamorati M, *et al.* Unmet treatment needs in schizophrenia patients: is asenapine a potential therapeutic option? Expert Rev Neurother 2011; 11: 989-1006.

[160]   Zubin J, Spring B. Vulnerability - a new view of schizophrenia. J Abnorm Psychol 1977; 86: 103-26.

[161]   Nuechterlein KH, Dawson ME. A heuristic vulnerability/stress model of schizophrenic episodes. Schizophr Bull 1984; 10: 300-12.

[162]   Anthony WA, Liberman RP. The practice of psychiatric rehabilitation: historical, conceptual, and research base. Schizophr Bull 1986; 12: 542-59.

Send Orders for Reprints to reprints@benthamscience.ae

REVIEW ARTICLE

Older and Newer Strategies for the Pharmacological Management of Agitation in Patients with Bipolar Disorder or Schizophrenia

Giovanni Amodeo[1,*], Andrea Fagiolini[1], Gabriele Sachs[2] and Andreas Erfurth[3]

[1]*Department of Molecular Medicine, University of Siena School of Medicine, Viale Bracci 1, Siena 53100, Italy;* [2]*Department of Psychiatry and Psychotherapy, Medical University of Vienna, Waehringer Guertel 18-20, 1090 Vienna, Austria;* [3]*6th Psychiatric Department, Otto-Wagner-Spital, Baumgartner Hoehe 1, 1140 Vienna, Austria*

Abstract: ***Background***: The management of acute agitation in patients with bipolar disorder or schizophrenia is a multifaceted and dynamic task, which presents unique and complex challenges to healthcare providers.

Objective: To ascertain and describe which medications are best to use in patients with agitation, affected by bipolar disorder or schizophrenia.

Method: Selective review of current literature and guidelines referred to the treatment of agitation in individuals affected with bipolar disorder or schizophrenia

Results: When possible, the pharmacologic management of agitation should be preceded by a in-depth evaluation of the possible causes of the agitation. The use for of first and second-generation antipsychotic medications, of benzodiazepines and of the newer inhaled antipsychotic loxapine, is reviewed and commented.

Conclusion: The mainstay of medication treatment of acute agitation should be based on a thotough assessment cause. If agitation is due to delirium or to another physial condition, an attempt to address the underlying causes should be always considered. When agitation is primarily due to schizophrenia or bipolar disorder, antipsychotics and/or benzodiazepines are usually the mainstay of treatment. Newer inhaled formulation of loxapine has shown ability to rapidly reduce the agitation in mild to moderate patients with schizophrenia or bipolar disorder, with a decrease in agitation that was evident since the first assessment, 10 minutes after the first dose.

ARTICLE HISTORY

Received: January 03, 2017
Revised: July 11, 2017
Accepted: July 11, 2017

DOI:
10.2174/1871527316666170919115507

Keywords: Agitation, bipolar, schizophrenia, antipsychotics, benzodiazepines, loxapine, intramuscular, oral, inhaled.

1. INTRODUCTION

Treatment of agitation represents a major clinical challenge [1]. In many circumstances, behavior control methods such as de-escalation, verbal intervention, offering food and/or beverages, letting patients smoke or offering nicotine substitutes (*e.g.* nicotine patches or gums), may be useful to begin with the initial management of agitation and to prevent its escalation into aggression or violence [2, 3]. However, when the above mentionated attempts fail to control agitation, the use of specific psychotropic drugs becomes crucial. Before starting medications, an attempt should be made to establish the cause for agitation, which can inform treatment choice. However, acute agitation is common and may occur across a range of somatic, psychiatric, and substance abuse disorders, and a diagnosis is often still unclear when rapid intervention is necessary.

Nonetheless, the choice of medication for an agitated patient should be informed at least by a provisional diagnosis and by the presumed etiology underlying the observed symptoms. For instance, agitation that is deemed as likely to stem from organic causes (*e.g.* hypoglycemia, hypoxia, thyroid storm) should not be treated with an antipsychotic, whereby the prescription of an antipsychotic and/or benzodiazepine is appropriate for agitation that has a psychiatric etiology. It is believed that abnormalities in the biogenic amines - dopamine, norepinephrine, and serotonin - as well as adenosine [4], glutamate [5] and the inhibitory neurotransmitter ã-aminobutyric acid (GABA) are involved in the etiology of agitation due to psychiatric reasons [6-8]. Specifically, it is hypothesized that agitation associated with psychosis, mania,

*Address correspondence to this author at the Department of Molecular Medicine, Division of Psychiatry, University of Siena School of Medicine, Viale Bracci 1, Siena 53100, Italy; Tel: +39-0577-586275; E-mail: giovanniamodeo86@gmail.com

and substance abuse is mainly correlated with elevated dopaminergic neurotransmission, whereby decreased GABAergic transmission is the primary characteristic of agitation associated with dementia, depression, and anxiety [9].

In agitated patients affected by bipolar disorder or schizophrenia, benzodiazepines or second-generation antipsychotics (SGA) are usually preferred over first-generation antipsychotics (FGA) but there are instances in which older antipsychotics or newer medications represent a valid alternative.

2. TYPES OF MEDICATION

There is no medication or class of medications that has proven to be the "best" in all cases of patients with bipolar disorder or schizophrenia that present with agitation. However, the choice usually falls on antipsychotics (first or second generation) and benzodiazepines, which may be administered in oral, intramuscular or intravenous formulations. A recent addition to the armamentarium for the treatment of agitation is inhaled loxapine, which is approved by the FDA for the acute treatment of agitation in individuals with bipolar disorder or schizophrenia [10] and by the EMA for the quick control of mild to moderate agitation in adult patients with bipolar disorder or schizophrenia [11].

2.1. First Generation Antipsychotics

First Generation Antipsychotics (FGA) have been widely used for management of agitation in bipolar disorder and schizophrenia. The mechanism of action that is involved in FGA ability to control agitation is not know, but is likely related to their ability to antagonize dopamine receptors, which leads to a reduction of activation and psychomotor agitation while addressing the underlying psychotic symptoms. Also, some FGAs are structurally similar to gamma-amino-butyric acid (GABA) - an inhibitory neurotransmitter - and are hence able to directly act on the GABA receptor [12].

Compared to haloperidol, chlorpromazine, a low-potency phenothiazine, has a higer propensity to cause hypotension, particularly in the elderly, causes more pain at the site of injection, has more anticholinergic side effects, and a higher likelihood to lower the seizure threshold [13-15]. Also, when used intravenously chlorpromazine may cause prolonged unconsciousness [16]. Moreover the use at high doses may be associated with sudden death [17]. As a result, intramuscular chlorpromazine is not recommended [18] and the phenothiazines in general are seldom considered as a first choice for the management of agitation.

Haloperidol is a highly potent and selective dopamine-2 (D2) receptor antagonist and has a long track record of effective usege for the management of acute agitation [19, 20]. For a relatively long time, haloperidol used to be considered as a safe and effective medication when administered intramuscularly or intravenously. However, serious adverse events have been described, including neuroleptic malignant syndrome [21], dystonia and other extrapyramidal side-effects, which may even worsen agitation [18]. In addition, it has been reported that FGAs sometimes cause dysphoria after use [22, 23].

Although the exact incidence of EPS adverse events is unclear, one study reported that EPS symptoms were observed in up to 20% of agitated individuals that received haloperidol monotherapy versus a percentage of only 6% of subjects that were treated with haloperidol combined with lorazepam [24]. Also, the combination of haloperidol-lorazepam was related to a faster reduction in agitation [25]. Other studies have reported that a combination of haloperidol with promethazine or diphenhydramine may lower EPS incidence [26, 27].

For these reasons, haloperidol is often administered together with other medications, such as lorazepam, promethazine, or diphenhydramine [19]. Yet, the use of multiple medications to control agitation may rise the risks of cardiovascular side effects, excessive sedation and pharmacokinetic or pharmacodynamics interactions.

Other worrisome adverse events that have been described for haloperidol, include torsade de pointes [28, 29], cardiac arrest and sudden death [30, 17].

For the reasons above, haloperidol carries a label warning that specifies that "higher doses and intravenous administration of haloperidol appear to be associated with a higher risk of QT prolongation and TdP". [31]. The updated FDA warning notes that high doses and intravenous use of haloperidol increase the risk of QT prolongation and TdP and that particular caution necessary when treating patients with any dose or formulation of haloperidol have other conditions that have been correlated to higher risk to prolong QT trait, such as electrolyte imbalance (*i.e.*, hypokalemia and hypomagnesemia). Also, particular caution is warranted when patients are affected by cardiac abnormalities, low thyroid function, familial long QT syndrome, or are receiving medications that are able to increase the QT interval.

Because of the risk of QT increase and TdP, ECG monitoring is necessary if haloperidol is administered intravenously. However, haloperidol intravenous administration is not endorsed by any regulatory agency, including the USA Food and Drug Administration [31].

Of interest, agitation itself may prolong QTc trait. For instance, compared to psychiatric out-patients, acutely agitated patients have been described to have a 50 ms longer QTc trait [32].

Also, patients with agitation may be at higher risk of death when QTc prolongation occurs, given that adrenalin may sensitize the heart and increase the risk of arrhythmias [18, 29].

The short-acting depot medication zuclopenthixol acetate has been longly used for rapid tranquillization [33]. However, injecting patient that has never been treated before with a long half-life drug may be dangerous and the Royal College of Psychiatrists' consensus advocates that such use in naïve patients only in 'exceptional circumstances'. Also, zuclopenthixol use in agitated patients is discouraged because of the delayed onset (about 8 hours) of its benefits [34] limited and by the fact that the highest plasma concentrations are reached after a relatively long period of time of 36 hours [35]. Also, fatal cardiac events and sudden deaths have been reported [18].

2.2. Second Generation Antipsychotics

Second-generation antipsychotics (SGA), also called typical antipsychotics, are frequently used for the pharmacological management of acute agitation. Aripiprazole, olanzapine and ziprasidone, come in both intramuscular and oral formulations.

Compared with FGA, SGAs carry a lower risk of side effects such as dystonia or akathisia, with rates that have usually reported as lower than 1% [36-38]. Most studies in bipolar disorder or schizophrenia have indicated that SGA are more effective than placebo, and similar to haloperidol, in reducing agitation [39-45].

Oral olanzapine is one of the best-studied SGAs for psychiatric agitation. Yet, a number of studies have also demonstrated that medications such as aripiprazole, quetiapine, risperidone, or ziprasidone are efficacious as well [46, 47]. Usually, oral medicines should be preferred over intramuscular agents when a patient is cooperative and has no contraindications to oral use. However, many agitated patients are not cooperative and oral medication may have too slow an onset in patients with severe agitation.

Intramuscular preparations of the SGA ziprasidone [48], olanzapine [49] and aripiprazole [50] show a better extrapyramidal side-effect profiles than intramuscular haloperidol, while providing similar effect sizes in terms of controlling agitation [41, 25].

These intramuscular medications are indicated by the FDA for treatment of acute agitation associated with schizophrenia [48-50] and - limited to olanzapine and aripiprazole - bipolar mania. Also, these medications have been recommended over the first-generation antipsychotics [25].

However, since the approval of intramuscular olanzapine, several adverse events have been decribed, some of which were fatal [51]. Hypotension, bradycardia and cardiorespiratory depression were noted and excessively high doses and/or concomitant prescription of benzodiazepines and/or of other antipsychotics seemed a likely contributor to death [46]. Hence, intramuscular olanzapine should not be administered together with other medications, such as benzodiazepines, antipsychotics or other CNS depressants. Careful post-injection monitoring of the patient is recommended. In the case of a severe adverse event an intensive care unit should be easily accessible.

An open-label study that compared ziprasidone with haloperidol in a sample of 132 individuals reported that intramuscular ziprasidone prescribed at 5-20 mg was equivalent or better than haloperidol prescribed at 2.5-10 mg in reducing agitation [40]. Compared with haloperidol, ziprasidone was associated with significantly less extrapyramidal side-effects. The efficacy of intramuscular ziprasidone was tested in subjects with acute psychotic agitation in two similarly designed 24-hour, multisite, randomized, double-blind trials [52, 53], which both demonstrated significant superiority to placebo.

Intramuscular aripiprazole has been approved in the EU and US for the mnagement of agitation in subjects with schizophrenia or bipolar I disorder. In several trials, intramuscular aripiprazole has proven better than placebo and well tolerated in the control of agitation in individuals with bipolar I disorder, schizophrenia and schizoaffective disorder [54-58]. Aripiprazole carries a relatively low risk of extrapyramidal symptoms, *e.g.* akathisia [59], cardiovascular effects, weight gain, hyperprolactinaemia and other metabolic issues [60-62].

Orally disintegrating formulations of aripiprazole, olanzapine, and risperidone, and have been developed but this method of administration does not improve time to onset and these medications are bioequivalent to the regular oral tablets and provide similar efficacy and safety at the same dose [49, 50, 63, 64].

Sublingual asenapine, is approved by the FDA for the treatment of patients with schizophrenia or patients with bipolar disorder and a manic or mixed episode. Differently from the orally disintegrating tablets of aripiprazole, olanzapine, and risperidone sublingual asenapine might partially be absorbed in the oral mucosa and peak plasma concentration is reached in 30-60 minutes [65]. Hence, this medication might have the advantage of at least partially avoiding first-pass metabolism; however, even more than with all oral medications, treatment requires patient cooperation [66].

In a double-blind, randomized, placebo-controlled trial for acute agitation, sublingual asenapine showed an effect size comparable to that observed for intramuscular SGA [67]. However, sublingual asenapine is not approved for acute agitation. Hence, its use for this condition would be considered off label.

2.3. Benzodiazepines and Other Anticonvulsants

Benzodiazepines (BDZ) are frequently prescribed for rapid control of agitation owing to their anxiolytic and sedative effects. Also, BDZ enhance gamma-amino-butyric acid activity, which may provide an direct antipsychotic effect *via* inhibition of dopamine mediated transmission [68]. However, the main effects of benzodiazepines for the treatment of agitation is mainly linked with their capacity to decrease arousal [69].

A relatively large number of studies have evaluated benzodiazepines and typical antipsychotics in the treatment of acute agitation. Most studies found similar efficacy, less EPS and increased sedation [69]. The most serious risks of benzodiazepines include respiratory depression,which is more frequent when high doses are prescribed. However, this adverse event can be quickly reversed with the partial agonist flumazenil. Also, case reports of behavioral disinhibition with benzodiazepines have been reported [70].

This risk seems heightened when high dses of benzodiazepines are prescribed [71] and in patients showing symptoms such as hostility or difficulty controlling impulse [70, 72].

Lorazepam is the only benzodiazepine with complete, rapid and consistent intramuscular absorption. Peak plasma concentrations are reached 60-90 minutes after dose when Intramuscular or sublingual lorazepam are administered The elimination half-life is 12-15 hours and duration of effect is at least 8-10 hours [73, 74].

Drug interactions are limited given that lorazepam is quickly metabolized *via* a conjugationn to an inactive glucuronide, with no involvement of the oxidative cytochrome P450 system. Several studies have demonstrated that lorazepam has comparable efficacy to haloperidol in the management of psychotic or manic agitation, and some trials have even indicated superiority [75-78]. Lorazepam can be administered intravenously, which may be helpful for the rapid control of severe agitation [61, 62].

Diazepam is effective when administered intravenously [79], but is not recommended for intramuscular administration due to of its erratic absorption [80]. As a result, intramuscular lorazepam, which is better and more reliably absorbed [73], is the BDZ of choice [81, 82].

Several reports, including one placebo-controlled double-blind trial involving patients with chronic schizophrenia, have suggested that clonazepam may escalate psychosis or agitation in some individuals [83-85]. Hence, clonazepam has a very limited, if any, role for the treatment of acute agitation.

Midazolam -a fast-acting benzodiazepine- is not FDA approved for acute agitation. Yet, there has been interest in the potential use of this formulation for this indication [86]. Intranasal midazolam avoids first-pass metabolism since it is absorbed by the nasal mucosa. Intranasal midazolam induced calming within 15 to 20 minutes in children [87]. The use of intravenous midazolam is limited because of the risk of respiratory depression and respiratory arrest. Hence, it should be used only in settings where a continuous monitoring of respiratory and cardiac functions is possible. Speciafically, an immediate availability of equipment for ventilation, intubation and resuscitative drugs should be present [61].

In some cases other anticonvulsive agents have been associated with the successful control of agitation particularly in manic episodes [88]. Oral gabapentin [89] and intravenous valproate [90, 61] might be interesting off-label alternatives to the use of benzodiazepines.

2.4. Newer Tratments for Agitation

Loxapine has been available for many years as an oral formulation of a FGA and has shown an established safety and efficacy profile [91]. Recently, loxapine was reformulated as an inhaled powder that can be directly administered to the lungs, at a lower dose. This results in a quick dissemination into the systemic circulation with peak plasma levels that are reached within two minutes of administration [10]. The safety and efficacy of inhaled loxapine for acute agitation have been demonstrated in two Phase III clinical trials, in schizophrenia and bipolar disorder [92, 93]. The effect sizes were comparable to those observed in similar studies of antipsychotics or lorazepam administered intramuscularly [94]. However, clinical effects were observed as early as 10 minutes after inhalation, which was the first time point that this was measured [92, 93]. Loxapine resulted superior to placebo throughout the remaining periods of the study, at all-time points that were measured. In the schizophrenia trial, the effect size (ES) difference from placebo on the Positive and Negative Syndrome Scale Excited Component (PEC) at the 2 h assessment point resulted 0.45 for loxapine 5 mg and 0.60 for loxapine 10 mg (Cohen's d) [95].

Inhaled loxapine was generally well tolerated. Extrapyramidal adverse events and akathisia were relatively uncommon and the most frequently reported adverse effect was dysgeusia. However, spirometry studies suggested risk of bronchospasm, with the potential to lead to respiratory distress and respiratory arrest. For this reason, the use of inhaled loxapine is restricted to the hospital setting [66]. Rapid treatment of bronchospasms can be achieved with bronchodilators such as short-acting β-agonists (*e.g.* inhalatory salbutamol).

Interestingly, inhalatory loxapine has been approved by the EMA for the control of agitation in adult patients with schizophrenia or bipolar disorder, these last, both during manic and depressive episodes with or without mixed features. In clinical practice the successful use of inhalatory loxapine in agitated depression has been reported [96].

CONCLUSION

The most common strategies for the pharmacological treatment of acute agitation in schizophrenia and bipolar disorder include FGA, SGA and benzodiazepines.

Given the concerns over tolerability and risks of FGA, SGA medications are usually preferred. However, SGA are not void of risks, such as hypotension and bradycardia. Cardiorespiratory depression has been observed in patients treated with intramuscular olanzapine, especially when this medication is associated with parenteral benzodiazepines. Benzodiazepines, particularly intravenous lorazepam, are a valid alternative. However, caution needs to be exercised with these drugs as well, owing to the presence of risks of severe adverse events such as respiratory depression, which however can usually be readily reversed with appropriate treatment (*e.g.* flumazenil). Hence, flumazenil and resuscitation equipment should be readily accessible, especially when benzodiazepines are used at high doses and in the intravenous route. Recently developed inhaled formulation of loxapine has shown the ability to rapidly reduce the agitation in individuals with schizophrenia or bipolar disorder, with a decrease in symptoms that was evident since the first assessment, 10 minutes after the first dose. Inhaled loxapine may be an important new tool for the treatment of mild to moderate agitation.

CONSENT FOR PUBLICATION

Not applicable.

CONFLICT OF INTEREST

The authors declare no conflict of interest, financial or otherwise.

ACKNOWLEDGEMENTS

Declared none.

REFERENCES

[1]   Erfurth A. Agitation: a central challenge in psychiatry. The World Journal of Biological Psychiatry 2016. Published ahead of print. Available at: http: //dx.doi.org/10.1080/15622975.2016.1237043
[2]   Hill S, Petit J. The violent patient. Emerg Med Clin North Am 2000; 18: 301-15.
[3]   Marder SR. A review of agitation in mental illness: treatment guidelines and current therapies. J Clin Psychiatry 2006; 67(suppl 10): 13-21.

[4]	Erfurth A. Adenosine and neuropsychiatric disorders: implications for treatment. CNS Drugs 1994; 2: 184-90.

[5]	Michael N, Erfurth A, Ohrmann P, et al. Acute mania is accompanied by elevated glutamate/glutamine levels within the left dorsolateral prefrontal cortex. Psychopharmacology (Berl) 2003; 168(3): 344-6.

[6]	Miczek KA, Fish EW, De Bold HF, et al. Social and neural determinants of aggressive behavior: pharmacotherapeutic targets at serotonin, dopamine and gamma-aminobutyric acid systems. Psychopharmacology (Berl) 2002; 163(3-4): 434-58.

[7]	Kavoussi R, Armstead P, Coccaro E. The neurobiology of impulsive aggression. Psychiatr Clin North Am 1997; 20(2): 395-403.

[8]	Van Winkle E. The toxic mind: the biology of mental illness and violence. Med Hypotheses 2000; 55(4): 356-68.

[9]	Lindenmayer JP. The pathophysiology of agitation. J Clin Psychiatry 2000; 61(suppl 14): 5-10.

[10]	Teva Pharmaceuticals USA I. Adasuve Prescribing Information. 2015. [Accessed Jul 24, 2016]. Available at: www.adasuve.com/PDF/AdasuvePI.pdf.

[11]	European Medicines Agency, http: //www.ema.europa.eu/ema/index.jsp?curl=pages/medicines/human/medicines/002400/human_med_001618.jsp&mid=WC0b01ac058001d124

[12]	Richards JR, Schneir AB. Droperidol in the emergency department: is it safe? J Emerg Med 2003; 24: 441-7.

[13]	Citrome L, Volavka J. Violent patients in the emergency setting. Psychiatr Clin North Am 1999; 22: 789-800.

[14]	Swett C, Cole JO, Hartz SC, et al. Hypotension due to chlorpromazine. Relation to cigarette smoking, blood pressure, and dosage. Arch Gen Psychiatry 1977; 34: 661-3.

[15]	Musey VC, Preedy JR, Musey PI, et al. Prolactin and blood pressure responses to perphenazine in human subjects: comparison of the oral and intramuscular routes. Am J Med Sci 1986; 291: 380-5.

[16]	Quenstedt M, Ramsay R, Bernadt M. Rapid tranquillisation. Br J Psychiatry 1992; 161: 573.

[17]	Jusic N, Lader M. Post-mortem antipsychotic drug concentrations and unexplained deaths. Br J Psychiatry 1994; 165: 787-91.

[18]	Royal College of Psychiatrists Psychopharmacology Sub-Group. The Association Between Antipsychotic Drugs and Sudden Death. Council Report CR57. London: Royal College of Psychiatrists, 1997.

[19]	MacDonald K, Wilson MP, Minassian A, et al. A retrospective analysis of intramuscular haloperidol and olanzapine in the treatment of agitation in drug- and alcohol-using patients. Gen Hosp Psychiatry 2010; 32: 443-5.

[20]	Clinton JE, Sterner S, Stelmachers Z, et al. Haloperidol for sedation of disruptive emergency patients. Ann Emerg Med 1987; 16: 319-22.

[21]	Konikoff F, Kuritzky A, Jerushalmi Y et al. Neuroleptic malignant syndrome induced by a single injection of haloperidol. BMJ 1984; 289: 1228-9.

[22]	Lambert M, Schimmelmann BG, Karow A, et al. Subjective well-being and initial dysphoric reaction under antipsychotic drugs—concepts, measurement and clinical relevance. Pharmacopsychiatry 2003; 36(suppl 3): 181-90.

[23]	Karow A, Schnedler D, Naber D. What would the patient choose: subjective comparison of atypical and typical neuroleptics. Pharmacopsychiatry 2006; 39: 47-51.

[24]	Battaglia J, Moss S, Rush J, et al. Haloperidol, lorazepam, or both for psychotic agitation: a multicenter, prospective, double-blind, emergency department study. Am J Emerg Med 1997; 15: 335-40.

[25]	Wilson MP, Pepper D, Currier GW, et al. The psychopharmacology of agitation: Consensus statement of the American Association for Emergency Psychiatry Project Beta Psychopharmacology Workgroup. West J Emerg Med 2012; 13(1): 26-34.

[26]	Raveendran NS, Tharyan P, Alexander J, et al. TREC-India II Collaborative Group. Rapid tranquillisation in psychiatric emergency settings in India: pragmatic randomized controlled trial of intramuscular olanzapine versus intramuscular haloperidol plus promethazine. BMJ 2007; 335: 865-73.

[27]	Huf G, Alexander J, Allen MH, et al. Haloperidol plus promethazine for psychosis-induced aggression. Cochrane Database Syst Rev 2009; 3: 102.

[28]	Zee-Cheng CS, Mueller CE, Seifert CF, et al. Haloperidol and torsades de pointes. Ann Int Med 1985; 12: 102.

[29]	Haverkamp W, Breithardt G, Camm AJ, et al. The potential for QT prolongation and pro-arrhythmia by non-anti-arrhythmic drugs: clinical and regulatory implications. Report on a Policy Conference of the European Society of Cardiology. Cardiovasc Res 2000; 47: 219-33.

[30]	Goldney RD, Spence ND, Bowes JA. The safe use of high dose neuroleptics in a psychiatric intensive care unit. Aust N Z J Psychiatry 1986; 20: 370-5.

[31]	US Food and Drug Administration. Information for healthcare professionals: haloperidol (marketed as Haldol, Haldol Decanoate and Haldol Lactate). [Accessed Jul 24, 2016] Available at: http://www.fda.gov/Drugs/DrugSafety/PostmarketDrugSafetyInformationforPatientsandProviders/DrugSafetyInformationforHealthcareProfessionals/ucm085203.htm

[32]	Hatta K, Takahashi T, Nakamura H, et al. Prolonged QT interval in acute psychotic patients. Psychiatry Res 2000; 94: 279-85.

[33]	Simpson D, Anderson I. Rapid tranquillisation: a questionnaire survey of practice. Psychiatric Bulletin 1996; 20: 149-52.

[34]	Chakravarti SK, Muthu A, Muthu PK, et al. Zuclopenthixol acetate (5% in'Viscoleo'): singledose treatment for acutely disturbed psychotic patients. Curr Med Res Opin 1990; 12: 58-65.

[35]	Clopixol Acuphase prescribing information. [Accessed Jul 24, 2016], available at https: //www.lundbeck.com/upload/ca/en/files/pdf/product_monograph/Clopixol_PM_MKT_ctrl_148975_13SEPT2011_CLN_eng.pdf

[36]	Correll CU, Schenk EM. Tardive dyskinesia and new antipsychotics. Curr Opin Psychiatry 2008; 21: 151-6.

[37]	Dolder CR, Jeste DV. Incidence of tardive dyskinesia with typical versus atypical antipsychotics in very high risk patients. Biol Psychiatry 2003; 53: 1142-5.

[38]	Kane JM. Tardive dyskinesia rates with atypical antipsychotics in adults: prevalence and incidence. J Clin Psychiatry 2004; 65(suppl 9): 16-20.

[39]	Breier A, Meehan K, Birkett M, et al. A double-blind, placebo-controlled dose-response comparison of intramuscular olanzapine and haloperidol in the treatment of acute agitation in schizophrenia. Arch Gen Psychiatry 2002; 59: 441-8.

[40]	Brook S, Lucey JV, Gunn KP. Intramuscular ziprasidone compared with intramuscular haloperidol in the treatment of acute psychosis: ziprasidone IM Study Group. J Clin Psychiatry 2000; 61: 933-41.

[41]	Citrome L. Comparison of intramuscular ziprasidone, olanzapine, or aripiprazole for agitation: a quantitative review of efficacy and safety. J Clin Psychiatry 2007; 68: 1876-85.

[42]	Currier GW, Simpson GM. Risperidone liquid concentrate and oral lorazepam versus intramuscular haloperidol and intramuscular lorazepam for treatment of psychotic agitation. J Clin Psychiatry 2001; 62: 153-7.

[43]	Currier GW, Chou JCY, Feifel D, et al. Acute treatment of psychotic agitation: a randomized comparison of oral treatment with risperidone and lorazepam versus intramuscular treatment with haloperidol and lorazepam. J Clin Psychiatry 2004; 65: 386-94.

[44]	Hsu W-Y, Huang S-S, Lee B-S, et al. Comparison of intramuscular olanzapine, orally disintegrating olanzapine tablets, oral risperidone solution, and intramuscular haloperidol in the management of acuteagitation in an acute care psychiatric ward in Taiwan. J Clin Psychopharmacol 2010; 30: 230-4.

[45]	Lim HK, Kim JJ, Pae CU, et al. Comparison of risperidone orodispersible tablet and intramuscular haloperidol in the treatment of acute psychotic agitation: a randomized open, prospective study. Neuropsychobiology 2010; 62: 81-6.

[46]	Battaglia J. Pharmacological management of acute agitation. Drugs 2005; 65(9): 1207-22.

[47]	Garriga M, Pacchiarotti I, Kasper S, et al. Assesment and management of agitation in psychiatry: expert consensus. World J Biol Psychiatry 2016; 17(2): 86-128.

[48]	Pfizer Inc. Geodon Prescribing Information. [Accessed Jul 24, 2016]. Available at: http: //labeling.pfizer.com/ShowLabeling.aspx?format=PDF&id=584.

[49]	Eli Lilly and Company. Zyprexa Prescribing Information. [Accessed Jul 24, 2016]. Available at: pi.lilly.com/us/zyprexa-pi.pdf.

[50]	Otsuka Pharmaceutical Company. Abilify Prescribing Information. 2012. [Accessed Jul 24, 2016]. Available at: packageinserts.bms.com/pi/pi_abilify.pdf.

[51]	Eli Lilly and Company Limited. Letter to healthcare professionals. Basingstoke, Hampshire, UK: Eli Lilly and Company Limited, 2004.

[52]	Lesem MD, Zajecka JM, Swift RH, et al. Intramuscular ziprasidone, 2 mg versus 10 mg, in the short-term management of agitated psychotic patients. J Clin Psychiatry 200; 62: 12-8.

[53]   Daniel DG, Potkin SG, Reeves KR, *et al.* Intramuscular (IM) ziprasidone 20 mg is effective in reducing acute agitation associated with psychosis: a double-blind, randomized trial. Psychopharmacology (Berl) 155; 11: 128-34.

[54]   Andrezina R, Josiassen RC, Marcus RN, *et al.* Intramuscular aripiprazole for the treatment of acute agitation in patients with schizophrenia or schizoaffective disorder: a double-blind, placebo-controlled comparison with intramuscular haloperidol. Psychopharmacology (Berl) 2006; 188(3): 281-92.

[55]   Currier GW, Citrome LL, Zimbroff DL, *et al.* Intramuscular aripiprazole in the control of agitation. J Psychiatr Pract 2007; 13(3): 159-69.

[56]   Tran-Johnson TK, Sack DA, Marcus RN, *et al.* Efficacy and safety of intramuscular aripiprazole in patients with acute agitation: a randomized, double-blind, placebo-controlled trial. J Clin Psychiatry 2007; 68(1): 111-9.

[57]   Zimbroff DL, Marcus RN, Manos G, *et al.* Management of acute agitation in patients with bipolar disorder: efficacy and safety of intramuscular aripiprazole. J Clin Psychopharmacol 2007; 27(2): 171-6.

[58]   De Filippis S, Cuomo I, Lionetto L, *et al.* Intramuscular aripiprazole in the acute management of psychomotor agitation. Pharmacotherapy 2013; 33(6): 603-14.

[59]   Kane JM, Barnes TR, Correll CU, *et al.* Evaluation of akathisia in patients with schizophrenia, schizoaffective disorder, or bipolar I disorder: a post hoc analysis of pooled data from short- and long-term aripiprazole trials. J Psychopharmacol 2010; 24(7): 1019-29.

[60]   Sanford M, Scott LJ. Intramuscular aripiprazole : a review of its use in the management of agitation in schizophrenia and bipolar I disorder. CNS Drugs 2008; 22(4): 335-52.

[61]   Kasper S, Baranyi A, Eisenburger P, *et al.* Konsensus-Statement: die Behandlung der Agitation beim psychiatrischen Notfall. CliniCum neuropsy Sonderausgabe 2013; 2013: 3-15.

[62]   Kasper S, Sachs GM, Bach M, *et al.* Schizophrenie Medikamentöse Therapie. Konsensus-Statement - State of the art 2016. Clin Cum Neuropsy 2016: 3-30.

[63]   Van Schaick EA, Lechat P, Remmerie BM, *et al.* Pharmacokinetic comparison of fast-disintegrating and conventional tablet formulations of risperidone in healthy volunteers. Clin Ther 2003; 25: 1687-99.

[64]   Thyssen A, Remmerie B, D'Hoore P, *et al.* Rapidly disintegrating risperidone in subjects with schizophrenia or schizoaffective disorder: a summary of ten phase I clinical trials assessing taste, tablet disintegration time, bioequivalence, and tolerability. Clin Ther 2007; 29(2): 290-304.

[65]   Allergan Saphris Prescribing Information. 2015. [Accessed Jul 24, 2016]. Available at: http: //www.allergan.com/assets/pdf/saphris_pi

[66]   66 Zeller L & Citrome L. Managing Agitation Associated with Schizophrenia and Bipolar Disorder in the Emergency Setting. West J Emerg Med 2016; 17(2): 165-72.

[67]   Pratts M, Citrome L, Grant W, *et al.* A single-dose, randomized, double-blind, placebo-controlled trial of sublingual asenapine for acute agitation. Acta Psychiatr Scand 2014; 130(1): 61-8.

[68]   Stimmel L. Benzodiazepines in schizophrenia. Pharmacotherapy 1996; 16(6 Pt 2): 148-51.

[69]   Allen MH. Managing the agitated psychotic patient: a reappraisal of the evidence. J Clin Psychiatry 2000; 14: 11-20.

[70]   Bond AJ. Drug-induced behavioural disinhibition: incidence, mechanisms and therapeutic implications. CNS Drugs 1998; 9: 41-57.

[71]   Rothschild AJ. Disinhibition, amnestic reactions, and other adverse reactions secondary to triazolam: a review of the literature. J Clin Psychiatry 1992; 53: 69-79.

[72]   Van der Bijl, Roelofse JA. Disinhibitory reactions to benzodiazepines: a review. J Oral Maxillofac Surg 1991; 49: 519-23.

[73]   Greenblatt DJ, Shader RI, Franke K, *et al.* Pharmacokinetics and bioavailability of intravenous, intramuscular, and oral lorazepam in humans. J Pharm Sci 1979; 68: 57-63.

[74]   Greenblatt DJ, Divoll M, Harmatz JS, *et al.* Pharmacokinetic comparison of sublingual lorazepam with intravenous, intramuscular, and oral lorazepam. J Pharm Sci 1982; 71: 248-52.

[75]   Cohen S, Khan A, Johnson S. Pharmacological management of manic psychosis in an unlocked setting. J Clin Psychopharmacol 1987; 7: 261-4.

[76]   Foster S, Kessel J, Berman ME, *et al.* Efficacy of lorazepam and haloperidol for rapid tranquilization in a psychiatric emergency room setting. Int Clin Psychopharmacol 1997; 12: 175-9.

[77]   Lenox RH, Newhouse PA, Creelman WL, *et al.* Adjunctive treatment of manic agitation with lorazepam versus haloperidol: a double-blind study. J Clin Psychiatry 1992; 53: 47-52.

[78]   Salzman C, Solomon D, Miyawaki E, *et al.* Parenteral lorazepam versus parenteral haloperidol for the control of psychotic disruptive behavior. J Clin Psychiatry 1991; 52: 177-80.

[79]   Lerner Y, Lwow E, Levitin A, *et al.* Acute high-dose parenteral haloperidol treatment of psychosis. Am J Psychiatry 1979; 136: 1061-4.

[80]   Gamble JA, Dundee JW, Assaf RA. Plasma diazepam levels after single dose oral and intramuscular administration. Anaesthesia 1975; 30: 164-9.

[81]   Atakan Z, Davies T. ABC of mental health. Mental health emergencies. BMJ 1997; 314: 1740-2.

[82]   Kerr IB, Taylor D. Acute disturbed or violent behaviour: principles of treatment. J Psychopharmacol 1997; 11: 271-77.

[83]   Binder RL. Three case reports of behavioral disinhibition with clonazepam. Gen Hosp Psychiatry 1987; 9: 151-3.

[84]   Karson CN, Weinberger DR, Bigelow L, *et al.* Clonazepam treatment of chronic schizophrenia: negative results in a double-blind, placebo-controlled trial. Am J Psychiatry 1982; 139(12): 1627-8.

[85]   Greenblatt DJ, Raskin A. Benzodiazepines: new indications. Psychopharmacol Bull 1986; 22: 77-87.

[86]   Nordstrom K, Allen MH. Alternative delivery systems for agents to treat acute agitation: progress to date. Drugs 2013; 73(16): 1783-92.

[87]   Zedie N, Amory DW, Wagner BK, *et al.* Comparison of intranasal midazolam and sufentanil premedication in pediatric outpatients. Clin Pharmacol Ther 1996; 59(3): 341-8.

[88]   Rosa AR, Fountoulakis K, Siamouli, *et al.* Is Anticonvulsant Treatment of Mania a Class Effect? Data from Randomized Clinical Trials. CNS Neurosci Ther 2011; 17: 167-177.

[89]   Erfurth A, Kammerer C, Grunze H, *et al.* An open label study of gabapentin in the treatment of acute mania. J Psychiatr Res 1998; 32(5): 261-4.

[90]   Grunze H, Erfurth A, Amann B, *et al.* Intravenous valproate loading in acutely manic and depressed bipolar I patients. J Clin Psychopharmacol 1999; 19(4): 303-9.

[91]   Zisook S, Click MA. Evaluations of loxapine succinate in the ambulatory treatment of acute schizophrenic episodes. Int Pharmacopsychiatry 1980; 15(6): 365-78.

[92]   Lesem MD, Tran-Johnson TK, Riesenberg RA, *et al.* Rapid acute treatment of agitation in individuals with schizophrenia: multicentre, randomised, placebo-controlled study of inhaled loxapine. Br J Psychiatry 2011; 198(1): 51-8.

[93]   Kwentus J, Riesenberg RA, Marandi M, *et al.* Rapid acute treatment of agitation in patients with bipolar I disorder: a multicenter, randomized, placebo-controlled clinical trial with inhaled loxapine. Bipolar Disord 2012; 14(1): 31-40.

[94]   Citrome L. Addressing the need for rapid treatment of agitation in schizophrenia and bipolar disorder: focus on inhaled loxapine as an alternative to injectable agents. Ther Clin Risk Manag 2013; 9: 235-45.

[95]   Citrome L. Inhaled loxapine for agitation revisited: focus on effect sizes from 2 Phase III randomised controlled trials in persons with schizophrenia or bipolar disorder. Int J Clin Pract 2012; 66(3): 318-25.

[96]   Kasper S, Di Pauli J, Erfurth A, *et al.* Inhalatives Loxapin - Praxiserfahrungen nach dem ersten Anwendungsjahr. Clini Cum Neuropsy 2015; 11: 1-8.

REVIEW ARTICLE

Pharmacological Treatment of Cognitive Symptoms in Major Depressive Disorder

Zihang Pan[1,2], Radu C. Grovu[1,3], Danielle S. Cha[1], Nicole E. Carmona[1], Mehala Subramaniapillai[1], Margarita Shekotikhina[1], Carola Rong[1], Yena Lee[1,2] and Roger S. McIntyre[1,2,4,5,6,*]

[1]Mood Disorders Psychopharmacology Unit, University Health Network, Toronto, ON, Canada; [2]Institute of Medical Science, University of Toronto, Toronto, ON, Canada; [3]The Centre for Addiction and Mental Health (CAMH), Toronto, ON, Canada; [4]Department of Pharmacology, University of Toronto, Toronto, ON, Canada; [5]Department of Psychiatry, University of Toronto, Toronto, ON, Canada; [6]Brain and Cognition Discovery Foundation, Toronto, ON, Canada

Abstract: *Background*: Cognitive dysfunction is a core transdiagnostic domain of Major Depressive Disorder (MDD) and is a principal determinant of functional recovery. However, it has been insufficiently targeted within the current therapeutic framework for MDD.

Objective: To highlight these unmet cognitive needs in MDD.

Method: An article search was conducted using PubMed from inception to November 2016: *Major Depressive Disorder* (and/or variant) was cross-referenced with the following terms: *antidepressants, augmentation, cognition, cognitive deficits, cognitive dysfunction, functional outcomes, mechanism of action*, and *treatment*. Articles informed by observational studies, clinical trials, and review articles relevant to the discussion of cognition and cognitive impairment in MDD were included for review. Additional terms and citations previously not identified in the initial search were obtained from a manual review of article reference lists.

Results: Cognitive deficits in MDD are replicable, non-specific, and clinically significant. Abnormalities in the domains of learning/memory, executive function, attention, concentration, and processing speed are consistently reported. Only two antidepressants (*i.e.*, duloxetine and vortioxetine) have established procognitive effects utilizing rigorous methodology in MDD. Most antidepressants improve cognitive function(s), but the extent to which they directly exert pro-cognitive effects is not yet understood.

Conclusion: Cognitive dysfunction in MDD is a principal determinant of patient-reported outcomes (*e.g.*, psychosocial function). Healthcare providers are encouraged to screen for cognitive dysfunction in MDD and familiarize themselves with the efficacy profiles of antidepressants on disparate cognitive domains.

ARTICLE HISTORY

Received: January 03, 2017
Revised: July 11, 2017
Accepted: July 11, 2017

DOI:
10.2174/1871527316666170919115100

Keywords: Cognition, domain-based approach, inflammation, Major Depressive Disorder (MDD), pharmacological strategies, unmet needs.

1. INTRODUCTION

The *Diagnostic and Statistical Manual of Mental Disorders, 5th Edition* (DSM-5) characterizes Major Depressive Disorder (MDD) as a syndrome comprised of low mood, apathy, anhedonia, decreased energy, psychomotor disturbances, negative thought patterns, changes in appetite, suicidal ideations, and impaired cognition [1]. Major Depressive

Disorder affects approximately 350 million individuals globally with projections from the World Health Organization (WHO) identifying MDD as the leading cause of disease burden by the year 2030 [2]. Currently, the estimated lifetime prevalence of MDD is 10-15% in North America with annual economic costs of approximately $36.6 billion in the United States and $6.3 billion in Canada [3-5]. The foregoing statistics underscore the debilitating effect of MDD on functional disability and provide the impetus for identifying determinants of health outcome.

MDD is a multidimensional disorder associated with clinically significant impairments in, but not limited to, so-

*Address correspondence to this author at the Mood Disorders Psychopharmacology Unit, University Health Network, 399 Bathurst Street, Toronto, ON, M5T 2S8, Canada; Tel: 416 603 5279; Fax: 416 603 5368; E-mail: roger.mcintyre@uhn.ca

cial, occupational, and cognitive functions. Notably, accumulating evidence indicates that cognitive dysfunction (*e.g.,* memory, executive function, processing speed, and attention) is a critical factor subserving disability in MDD [6]. For example, in a 3-year follow-up study, approximately 44% of individuals with MDD who reported partial/full remission with treatment continued to experience impairments in cognitive function despite the resolution of their depressed mood [7, 8]. Furthermore, epidemiological data suggest that cognitive dysfunction (*i.e.,* concentration, and attention) mediates the association between depression and workplace functioning [9].

Notwithstanding available antidepressant, psychotherapeutic, neuromodulatory, and adjunctive approaches to MDD treatment, "non-mood" symptoms (*e.g.,* cognitive function, anergia, sleep disturbance) and functional outcomes (*e.g.,* quality of life and workplace productivity) remain insufficiently addressed in clinical psychiatry [10]. Furthermore, cognitive dysfunction has been identified as a critical determinant of patient-reported outcomes in MDD (*e.g.,* quality of life, psychosocial normalization, and mental health) [11]. A significant portion of patients in remission from MDD find that they are not able to return to work as a result of their cognitive impairment. Therefore, one of the chief aims of improving patient-, provider-, and societal-defined therapeutic objectives is to target cognitive dysfunction in MDD.

The Research Domain Criteria (RDoC) authored by the National Institute of Mental Health (NIMH) takes an integrative approach to studying psychiatric disorders by converging multiple levels or "units" of analysis to better understand human behaviour [12] (*i.e.,* behaviour with neurocircuitry and vice versa). In contrast with the categorical nosology of the DSM and other available diagnostic tools, the RDoC matrix aims for a dimension-based classification of psychopathology. An example of RDoC-related convergent substrates posits that proinflammatory cytokines play important roles in neuronal integrity [13, 14], with physiologically relevant effects on neurocircuitry and neurotransmitter systems [15]. Indeed, there has been increasing interest in the study of the effects of cytokines on the development and progression of neuropsychiatric diseases. An additional impetus of the RDoC is the insufficient discovery and development of genuinely novel treatment approaches; specifically, the RDoC aims to provide a framework for the discovery and development of novel treatment approaches for mental disorders. Specifically, the strategy is to develop treatments informed by underlying mechanisms and neural substrates and targeting convergent substrates and psychopathological domains. The RDoC framework differentially emphasizes disturbances in cognition and cognitive emotional processes as core and transdiagnostic domains of psychopathology.

The development of therapeutic approaches in MDD has been traditionally focused on improving mood domain severity, with an under-emphasis on "non-mood" dimension-/domain psychopathology [16]. In contrast, screening, assessing, and treating cognitive dysfunction has not been prioritized in the current therapeutic framework in MDD. Herein, we provide a narrative review of cognitive deficits in MDD, with a focused discussion of pharmacological treatment opportunities and related neurobiological substrates.

2. METHOD

An electronic search of PubMed was conducted from inception to November 25, 2016. *Major Depressive Disorder* (and/or variant) was cross-referenced with the following terms (and/or variant): *antidepressants, augmentation, cognition, cognitive deficits, cognitive dysfunction, functional outcomes, mechanism of action,* and *treatment.* Articles informed by observational studies, clinical trials, and review articles relevant to the topic of cognition in MDD were selected for inclusion in this narrative review. Additional terms and citations previously not identified in the initial search were obtained from a manual review of article reference lists.

3. RESULTS AND DISCUSSION

3.1. Cognitive Deficits in MDD

The diagnosis of a DSM-5 -defined Major Depressive Episode (MDE) uses a polythetical list of diagnostic criteria, whereby no single diagnostic criterion is essential for the diagnosis for MDE [17]. A domain-based approach to understanding cognition in MDD may be necessary to determine the contributing role of highly complex phenomenological features. For example, disturbances in concentration, thinking, and/or decision-making are included in the DSM-5 as inclusive criterion items. Domains that involve disparate neurobiological systems (*i.e.,* impulsivity, reward, disturbances relating to suicidality, hopelessness, anhedonia, psychomotor retardation, fatigue) also contribute to cognitive dysfunction [18]. The aforementioned cognitive dysfunctions have been repeatedly replicated in MDD populations in past studies [6]. Additionally, cognitive symptoms in MDD are non-specific (*i.e.,* encompass multiple domains with no established pattern matching particular cognitive deficits with specific mood symptoms).

Several typologies have been proposed to define and operationalize cognitive constructs. For example, the conventional typology would classify cognitive functions into the sub-domains of executive functions, attention, concentration, learning, memory, and processing speed [19]. Although each of the foregoing sub-domains could be viewed as interconnected, they are dissociable phenomena with unique, but overlapping, neurobiological substrates. For example, executive function represents the most complex and multifaceted sub-domain in cognition, involving regulatory systems of planning, initiation, inhibition of thought processes, as well as emotional and behavioural responses [20].

A related, but important discourse is the conceptualization of "cold" and "hot" cognition [21]. "Cold" cognition refers to cognitive processes that are uncoupled from emotional valence (*e.g.,* some aspects of executive function and working memory). Conversely, "hot" cognition refers to cognitive processes that are emotionally-valenced. Processes such as rumination, a domain of "hot" cognition, are often experienced amongst individuals with MDD [22]. In addition, individuals with MDD exhibit increased attentional/memory bias toward negatively valenced stimuli [22]. As discussed in the RDoC, disturbances in negative valence systems contribute to anxiety and fear, and disturbances in positive valence systems phenomenologically overlap with

Table 1.   Common neurocognitive tests.

Cognitive Domain	Neurocognitive Tests
Attention and Processing Speed	Choice Reaction Time (CRT; CANTAB) Continuous Performance Task (CPT) Digit Span Forwards and Backwards (WAIS-R) Digit Symbol Substitution Test (DSST) Paced Auditory Serial Addition Test (PASSAT) Reaction Time (RTI; CANTAB) Serial Sevens Substitution Task (SSST) Simple Reaction Time (SRT; CANTAB)
Cognitive Battery	California Computerized Assessment Package (CalCAP) Cambridge Neuropsychological Test Automated Battery (CANTAB) CNS Vital Signs Delis-Kaplan Executive Function System (D-KEFS) Massachusetts General Hospital Cognitive and Physical Functioning Questionnaire (CPFQ) Victoria Symptom Validity Test (VSVT) Wechsler Adult Intelligence Scale - Revised (WAIS-R) Wechsler Memory Scale - Revised (WMS-R)
Decision-Making and Response Control	Cambridge Gambling Task (CGT; CANTAB) Go/No-Go Association Task (GNAT; CANTAB) Information Sampling Task (IST)
Executive Function	Block Design (WAIS-R) Categories Test Concept Shifting Task (CST) Controlled Oral Word Association Task (COWST) Delis-Kaplan Executive Function System (D-KEFS) Picture Completion (WAIS-R) Spatial Span (SSP; CANTAB) Stroop-Colour Word Interference Test (SCWT) Verbal Fluency, Letter Fluency, Category Fluency Wisconsin Card Sorting Test (WCST)
Language and Verbal Comprehension	Comprehension (WAIS-R) Controlled Oral Word Association Task (COWAT) Information (WAIS-R) Similarities (WAIS-R) Token Test Verbal Fluency, Letter Fluency, Category Fluency Vocabulary (WAIS-R)
Psychomotor Performance	Finger Tapping Grooved Pegboard Test Purdue Pegs
Verbal Learning and Memory	California Verbal Learning Test (CVLT) Digits Span Forwards and Backwards (WAIS-R) Hopkins Verbal Learning Test - Revised (HVLT-R) Luria Verbal Learning Test (LVLT) Rey Auditory Verbal Learning Test (RAVLT) Rivermead Behavioural Memory Test (RBMT) Serial Sevens Subtraction Test (SSST) Verbal Paired Associates (VPA; WMS-R) Verbal Recognition Memory Test (VRM; CANTAB) Visual Verbal Learning Test (VVLT) Visual Reproduction
Visuospatial Processing	Benton Visual Form Discrimination (VFD) Block Design (WAIS-R) Judgement of Line Orientation (JOLO) Visuospatial Span Forwards and Backwards (WMS-R)
Working Memory	Arithmetic (WAIS-R) Delayed Recognition Span Test (DRST) Digit Span Forwards and Backwards (WAIS-R) Letter-Number Sequencing (LNS; WMS-R) Logical Memory (WMS-R) n-Back Test Spatial Working Memory (SWM; CANTAB)

DSM-defined domains of anhedonia, reward, and motivational processing. The RDoC defines emotional valence constructs as highly interwoven with cognitive phenomenology and overlapping substrates [23]. Hence, these examples illustrate the reciprocal role between cognition (*i.e.*, executive function) and emotional states.

3.2. Neurocognitive and Clinical Tools

A significant factor affecting the interpretation of cognitive results is the heterogeneity of available neurocognitive tests. A list of neurocognitive assessment tests and batteries can be found in Table **1**. Tests are organized by the principal domains of cognition assessed. However, there is no accepted "gold standard" psychometric of cognitive function in MDD. In the clinical setting, subjective complaints of cognitive deficits are common [24-26], underscoring the pertinence of the development of a comprehensive, feasible and reliable clinical assessment tool.

Full symptomatic remission is a guiding principle focused on recovery of mood, cognition, and psychosocial function. Table **2** summarizes recommended tools for the screening, diagnosis, and rating of MDD symptom severity.

3.3. Neurobiological Substrates

Disturbances in neural sub/circuit structures, function, and reciprocity comprise the foundation for disease modelling. Brain functions, and their corresponding structures, are segregated, as well as integrated. Adaptive brain function depends on normal reciprocity (*e.g.*, anti-correlation) between such segregated and integrated structures. Anti-correlation, or the selective activation of certain regions and deactivation of others, is required for proper functioning [22]. Dysregulation of normal reciprocity between nodal structures within the default mode network has been implicated in the pathophysiology of cognitive impairment in mood disorders, including MDD [27].

Furthermore, an increase in neural effort may also contribute to impairment in cognitive processes in individuals with MDD [28]. Harvey *et al.* examined cerebral activity and cognitive performance, *via* the n-Back test, in adults with MDD (n=10) compared to healthy controls (n=10) [28]. The n-Back test is a measure of working memory, wherein the subject is asked to determine whether a previous stimulus has been observed. Performance on the n-Back test did not significantly differ between depressed subjects and healthy controls. However, when brain activation patterns were examined (as a function of the 1,2,3-Back tests), significant differences were noted in the activation and deactivation of nodal structures between the MDD and non-MDD subjects. More specifically, the depressed individuals exhibited greater activation of the working memory network as a function of greater n-Back complexity relative to healthy controls, which implies depressed individuals require greater effort to achieve the same level of cognitive performance as healthy controls. The authors also noted reduced deactivation in the medial prefrontal cortex within MDD subjects compared to controls, suggesting abnormal reciprocity/anti-correlation and reduced cognitive efficiency in adults with MDD.

3.4. Treatment Implications

The treatment of cognitive dysfunction in MDD should begin with modifying contributing/exacerbating factors, such as comorbidity management and identification of iatrogenic artifacts). Modifiable determinants of MDD present opportunities for therapeutic intervention for treating the cognitive dysfunctions associated with MDD. Existing treatment modalities on cognitive function will be discussed below.

Cognitive Remediation (CR) is a standardized, psychosocial approach that has been demonstrated to improve measures of cognition in individuals with diverse brain disorders associated with cognitive impairment [*e.g.*, attention deficit hyperactivity disorder (ADHD), autism spectrum disorder, schizophrenia, traumatic brain injury]. In the case of MDD, CR first involves cognitive activation which uses the implementation of a computerized task to enhance learning and stimulates neuroplasticity. These tasks are dynamic and keep players at an 80% success rate despite changes in performance over time to elicit sustained motivation. The next key step in CR is strategy development, monitoring, and pruning. Through the support of therapists and peers, those affected by MDD improve the number of options and approaches to cognitively challenging tasks leading to the pruning of ineffective strategies. The final objective of this therapy is "far-transfer", namely the manifestation of improvements in cognition and problem solving to everyday environments [29]. To date, only the first step of this therapy, cognitive activation, has been applied to MDD. Preliminary results also suggest that CR could improve health outcomes in adults with MDD when combined with pharmacotherapy [30-32].

Computerized working memory tasks have also shown promise in improving cognitive function in MDD. One such example is the Paced Auditory Serial Addition Test, which requires patients to add sequentially presented digits. A study conducted by Siegle *et al.* reported that use of the Paced Auditory Serial Addition Test increased metacognitive skills, decreased maladaptive thought patterns (*i.e.*, rumination), and improved depressive symptom severity [33, 34]. Computer programs focused on sequencing a mental arithmetic have been shown to improve full scale intelligence quotient (IQ) in those with MDD [33]. This mode of therapy has also been shown to increase psychosocial functioning, as well as hippocampal and frontotemporal activation [35].

Manual-based psychotherapies (*e.g.*, CBT, mindfulness-based therapies) are highly effective in the acute treatment of MDEs and in maintenance of stable mood in MDD [36, 37]. These interventions primarily target "hot" cognition, with their effects on "cold" cognition requiring further investigation. Of these therapies, CBT is effective for ADHD, which exhibits significant disturbances in executive function and attention [38]. Alternatively, rTMS, a newer approach, has demonstrated procognitive effects in preliminary studies [39]. The increased patient acceptability, minimal propensity for cognitive impairment, and proven efficacy of rTMS in MDD, compared to ECT, provide reasons to believe that rTMS could be a viable and procognitive neuromodulatory strategy.

Aerobic/resistance exercise presents an adjunctive therapeutic opportunity that is cost effective, self-sustaining, has

Table 2.   Clinical tools for diagnosing MDD and measuring depressive symptom severity.

Screening Tools	Center for Epidemiological Studies – Depression Scale (CES-D)
	Hospital Anxiety and Depression Scale (HADS)
	Patient Health Questionnaire-2 (PHQ-2)
	Patient Health Questionnaire-9 (PHQ-9)
	Zung Self-Rating Depression Scale (Zung-SDS)
Diagnostic Tools	Mini International Neuropsychiatric Interview (MINI)
	Patient Health Questionnaire-9 (PHQ-9)
	Primary Care Evaluation of Mental Disorders (PRIME-MD)
	Psychiatric Diagnostic Screening Questionnaire (PDSQ)
	Structured Clinical Interview for DSM-5 (SCID-5)
Measuring Symptom Severity	Beck Depression Inventory (BDI)
	Clinically Useful Depression Outcome Scale (CUDOS)
	Hospital Anxiety and Depression Scale (HADS)
	Hamilton Depression Rating Scale 7 (HAMD-7)
	Hamilton Depression Rating Scale 17 (HAMD-17)
	Inventory of Depressive Symptomatology (IDS)
	Montgomery-Asberg Depression Rating Scale (MADRS)
	Patient Health Questionnaire-9 (PHQ-9)
	Quick Inventory of Depressive Symptomatology (QIDS)
Cognitive Function	Cognitive and Physical Functioning Questionnaire (CPFQ)
	Digit Symbol Substitution Test (DSST)
	Stroop Test
	Trail Making Test (TMT)
	Rey Auditory Verbal Learning Test (RAVLT)
	Simple Reaction Time Test
	Perceived Deficits Questionnaire (PDQ-20)
	Patient Health Questionnaire-5 (PHQ-5)
Patient-Reported Outcomes	Sheehan Disability Scale
	WHO Disability Assessment Schedule (WHO-DAS)
	Short Form Health Survey (SF-36)

negligible side effects and has the potential to be scaled as a population-level health intervention [40]. A recent review by Stanton and Reaburn found aerobic exercise regimes should occur 3-4 times a week for 9 weeks at moderate intensity to alleviate depressive symptoms [41]. The SMILE study showed lower depression relapse rates for those partaking in an exercise regimen when compared to those taking sertraline, a selective-serotonin reuptake inhibitor (SSRI). [35] Both acute and regular aerobic exercise confer improvements in memory with acute physical activity having a greater impact on short- and long-term memory in comparison to chronic physical activity. Additionally, individuals with mild cognitive impairment also see greater improvements in memory compared to cognitively normal individuals when engaging in regular exercise [40-42]. Modest aerobic exercise (*i.e.*, 40 minutes at 40–60% capacity) has been shown to improve executive control [43]. Improvements in psychomotor speed, attention, visual memory, and spatial planning, as well as dose-dependent changes in some executive function and visual memory tasks after exercise augmentation were also observed in the TREAD study [44].

The catecholamines, norepinephrine and dopamine, are important neuromodulators of memory, executive function, and attention. The foregoing neuromodulators increase peripherally during exercise, yet are unable to cross the blood–brain barrier. Moreover, catecholamines have reciprocal relationships with glutamatergic, GABAergic and other synaptic neurons to increase arousal in relevant brain areas [45]. Increased unbound tryptophan in the blood can cross the blood-brain barrier and be converted to serotonin in the brain. Increased hippocampal and whole brain serotonin concentrations, from disparate therapeutic mechanisms of action, have been linked to neurogenesis, synaptic growth, and greater connectivity between the hippocampus, prefrontal cortex and anterior cingulate gyrus [33, 46]. Brain Derived Neurotrophic Growth Factor (BDNF), Vascular Endothelial Growth Factor (VEGF) and Insulin-Like Growth Factor-1 (IGF-1) are associated with exercise, neurogenesis and long term potentiation [47]. These brain correlates are discussed in greater detail elsewhere [48].

Available evidence concerning conventional antidepressants indicates that improvements in measures of cognitive function in adults ages 18 to 65 are consistent with improvements in conventional depressive outcomes. It is not known, however, whether most conventional antidepressants exert direct, independent, and clinically significant effects on cognitive functions in adults with MDD (*i.e.*, pseudospecificity). There are no current Food and Drug Administration (FDA) approved agents or interventions specifically targeting cognitive dysfunction associated with MDD. No particular antidepressants have been found to be efficacious in all domains of cognition, with some causing concerns on decreased self-reported cognitive performance [33]. The efficacy of several antidepressant agents in improving cognitive function in individuals with MDD has been examined. For example, bupropion XL and escitalopram have been reported to improve verbal memory and delayed free recall [49]. Similarly, sertraline has been associated with improved psycho-motor performance (reviewed elsewhere) [50, 51].

With regard to SNRIs, duloxetine has been found to significantly improve cognitive function when compared to placebo, with a greater effect observed among patients with greater depression severity. Specifically, duloxetine improved verbal learning and memory, while also decreasing general symptoms of depression. In a study by Raskin *et al.*, composite cognition scores increased 90.0% direct and 9.1% indirect on the geriatric depression scale, as well as an 81.3% direct and 18.7% indirect improvement in the Hamilton Depression Rating Scale item 17 (HAMD-17) score for duloxetine [52-53]. Both duloxetine and the multimodal antidepressant, vortioxetine, have been shown to improve scores on the Rey Auditory Verbal Learning Test (RAVLT), showing improvements in acquisition time and delayed recall. In both RAVLT recall and acquisition, vortioxetine demonstrated a higher direct effect than duloxetine despite similar beneficial actions on depressive symptom severity [54]. Additionally, duloxetine is limited to improving measures of learning and memory, while vortioxetine improves a broader range of cognitive functions (*i.e.*, executive function, learning, memory, processing speed, and concentration). Vortioxetine has also been shown to significantly improve scores on cognitive measures after 8 weeks of treatment using either 10 or 20 mg doses when compared to placebo [33, 55, 56].

Psychostimulants have not demonstrated consistent efficacy in treating depressive symptoms in adults with MDD. Lisdexamfetamine, however, has demonstrated an ability to specifically target executive dysfunctions in MDD, particularly among individuals with mild MDD who present with

deficits in executive function [57]. However, in some cases, such as in those that have full or partial depression remission, lisdexamfetamine has been shown to improve executive function; an advantage of lisdexamfetamine is its ability to specifically target executive dysfunctions in MDD [57].

Ketamine has demonstrated efficacy in the treatment of treatment-resistant MDD [58]. Available evidence indicates that cognitive functions may serve as a predictor of response to ketamine and may also improve with ketamine therapy [59-60]. On a related note, it has been hypothesized that the anti-suicide effects of ketamine may be mediated by improvements in executive function [61]. A review written by Lee *et al.* discusses pro-cognitive effects of ketamine in greater detail [61].

Preliminary data also support the hypothesis that incretins may improve cognitive function. Incretins (*e.g.*, glucagon-like peptide-1 [GLP-1]) are synthesized in the Leydig cells of the intestine, are involved in gastric motility, and act as insulin secretion analogues. Exogenously administered GLP-1 agonists (*e.g.*, liraglutide) are FDA-indicated for adults with type II diabetes mellitus. Glucagon-like peptide-1 is also synthesized in the nucleus tractus solitarius and its receptors are distributed throughout the brain, with topographical distribution represented in cognitive control structures. Preliminary evidence indicates that liraglutide administered at a dose of 1.8 mg was capable of improving depressive and cognitive measures in adults with a current MDE (as part of MDD or bipolar disorders) [62]. The foregoing results instantiate previous findings indicating that liraglutide has neuroprotective, neurotrophic, and anti-inflammatory properties.

Intranasal insulin is another promising new approach to improving cognition in those with MDD. Insulin inhibits pro-apoptotic pathways and is critical for brain neuroplasticity, neurogenesis, anti-inflammation, and neuronal growth/ survival. Insulin receptors are found throughout neural circuits involved in cognitive and emotional processing [33]. Intranasal insulin has been shown to improve cognitive performance in Alzheimer's Disease (AD) and Bipolar Disorder (BD).

Elevated levels of circulating pro-inflammatory cytokines have been consistently reported in depressed individuals and have been linked to cognitive impairment. Elevated levels of Tumor Necrosis Factor-alpha (TNF-α) are amongst the most consistently identified pro-inflammatory cytokine abnormalities in MDD [63-67]. Infliximab is a monoclonal antibody that binds to soluble and transmembrane forms of TNF-α and inhibits binding of TNF-α with its receptors [67, 68]. Treatment with TNF antagonists has been associated with lower rates of BD and in individuals with rheumatoid arthritis [68]. Evidence also demonstrates its efficacy in a subgroup of individuals with treatment resistant depression [69, 70]. Efficacy of adjunctive infliximab on cognitive symptoms of depressive disorders has not been determined. However, infliximab offers an exciting avenue of adjunctive pharmacological intervention.

The reviews contained herein are not meant to be comprehensive, but offer an overview of current research and clinical opinions on unmet needs in depression treatment and management. Narrative reviews have limitations in comprehensiveness and the content selection may be viewed as more subjective than other systematic approaches. We acknowledge that the narrative format may result in bias in the selection of data and the interpretation of research. However, we believe the narrative format offers us a timely and valuable opportunity to engage in discourse regarding the importance of cognitive dysfunctions as unmet needs in the treatment of depression.

CONCLUSION

The prevailing disease models implicate cognition as a core psychopathological disturbance in MDD. The pertinence of cognitive dysfunction is that cognition is a principal mediator of psychosocial and workplace functional outcomes. The current clinical paradigms in the treatment and assessment of depressive symptoms have insufficiently addressed cognition with existing multi-modal depression treatments. Several factors modify cognitive functions in MDD, providing opportunities for clinical intervention. Clinicians are encouraged to screen and assess cognitive functions in adults with MDD, and to track performance on cognitive assessments to be fully informed of remission outcomes. The interest in the development of domain-based approaches to treatment provides a pragmatic impetus for therapeutic discovery. Amongst the treatment options in MDD, no single modality or agent has proven to be the gold standard in targeting cognition. The path towards functional recovery for many persons with MDD includes targeting impairment and cognitive function; hitherto a therapeutic target that has not been prioritized.

LIST OF ABBREVIATIONS

ADHD	=	Attention Deficit Hyperactivity Disorder
CBT	=	Cognitive Behavioural Therapy
CR	=	Cognitive Remediation
DSM-5	=	Diagnostic and Statistical Manual of Mental Disorders, 5th Edition
MDD	=	Major Depressive Disorder
MDE	=	Major Depressive Episode
NIMH	=	National Institute of Mental Health
RDoC	=	Research Domain Criteria
rTMS	=	Repetitive Transcranial Magnetic Stimulation

CONSENT FOR PUBLICATION

Not applicable.

CONFLICT OF INTEREST

Roger S. McIntyre is a consultant to speak on behalf of, and/or has received research support from Allergan, Astra-Zeneca, Bayer, Bristol-Myers, Squibb, Janssen-Ortho, Eli Lilly, Lundbeck, Merck, Otsuka, Pfizer, Sunovion, and Takeda. All other authors have no financial disclosures to declare.

ACKNOWLEDGEMENTS

Declared none.

REFERENCES

[1]   Gaillard R, Gourion D, Llorca PM. Anhedonia in depression. L'Encéphale 2013; 39(4): 296.

[2]   Collins PY, Patel V, Joestl SS, *et al.* Grand challenges in global mental health. Nature 2011; 475(7354): 27-30.

[3]   Marcus M, Yasamy MT, van Ommeren M, Chisholm D, Saxena S. Depression: a global public health concern. WHO Department of Mental Health and Substance Abuse. 2012.

[4]   Lépine J-P, Briley M. The increasing burden of depression. Neuropsychiatr Dis Treat 2011; 7(Suppl 1): 3-7.

[5]   Jacobs P, Ohinmaa A, Escober-Doran C, Patterson S, Slomp M. PMH31 measuring the economic burden of depression using patient records. Value in Health 2009; 12(7): A356.

[6]   Carvalho AF, Miskowiak KK, *et al.* Cognitive dysfunction in depression - pathophysiology and novel targets. CNS Neurol Disord Drug Targets 2014; 13(10): 1819-35.

[7]   Conradi HJ, Ormel J, de Jonge P. Presence of individual (residual) symptoms during depressive episodes and periods of remission: a 3-year prospective study. Psychol Med 2011; 41: 1165-1174.

[8]   Lam RW, Kennedy SH, McIntyre RS, Khullar A. Cognitive dysfunction in major depressive disorder: effects on psychosocial functioning and implications for treatment. Can J Psychiatry 2014; 59(12): 649-54.

[9]   Buist-Bouwman MA, Ormel J, de Graaf R, *et al.* Mediators of the association between depression and role functioning. Acta Psychiatr Scand 2008; 118(6): 451-8.

[10]   Howland RH. Sequenced treatment alternatives to relieve depression (STAR*D). Part 2: Study outcomes 1. J Psychosoc Nurs Ment Health Serv 2008; 46(0279-3695): 21-4.

[11]   McIntyre RS, Cha DS, Soczynska JK, *et al.* Cognitive deficits and functional outcomes in major depressive disorder: determinants, substrates, and treatment interventions. Depress Anxiety 2013; 30(6): 515-27.

[12]   Dillon DG, Rosso IM, Pechtel P, Killgore WDS, Rauch SL, Pizzagalli DA. Peril and pleasure: an RDoC-inspired examination of threat responses and reward processing in anxiety and depression. Depress Anxiety 2014; 31(3): 233-49.

[13]   Haroon E, Raison CL, Miller AH. Psychoneuroimmunology meets neuropsychopharmacology: translational implications of the impact of inflammation on behavior. Neuropsychopharmacology 2012; 37: 137-162.

[14]   Maes M. The cytokine hypothesis of depression: inflammation, oxidative and nitrosative stress (IO and NS) and leaky gut as new targets for adjunctive treatments in depression. Neuroendocrinol Lett 2008; 29(3): 287-91.

[15]   Felger JC, Miller AH. Cytokine effects on the basal ganglia and dopamine function: the subcortical source of inflammation malaise. Front Neuroendocrinol 2012; 33(3): 315-27.

[16]   McIntyre RS. A vision for drug discovery and development: novel targets and multilateral partnerships. Adv Ther 2014; 31(3): 245-6.

[17]   American Psychiatric Association. Diagnostic and Statistical Manual of Mental Disorders (DSM-5®). American Psychiatric Publishing; 2013.

[18]   McIntyre RS, Woldeyohannes HO, Soczynska JK, *et al.* Anhedonia and cognitive function in adults with MDD: results from the International Mood Disorders Collaborative Project. CNS Spectr 2015; 1-5.

[19]   Harrison JE, Lam RW, Baune BT, McIntyre RS. Selection of cognitive tests for trials of therapeutic agents 1. Lancet Psychiatry 2016; 3(2215-0374): 499.

[20]   McIntyre RS, Xiao HX, Syeda K, *et al.* The prevalence, measurement, and treatment of the cognitive dimension/domain in major depressive disorder. CNS Drugs 2015; 29(7): 577-89.

[21]   Roiser JP, Sahakian BJ. Hot and cold cognition in depression. CNS Spectr 2013; 18(3): 139-49.

[22]   Hamilton JP, Furman DJ, Chang C, Thomason ME, Dennis E, Gotlib IH. Default-mode and task-positive network activity in major depressive disorder: implications for adaptive and maladaptive rumination. Biol Psychiatry 2011; 15: 327-33.

[23]   Keedwell PA, Andrew C, Williams SC, Brammer MJ, Phillips ML. The neural correlates of anhedonia in major depressive disorder. Biol Psychiatry 2005; 58: 843-53.

[24]   Martinez-Aran A, Vieta E, Colom F, *et al.* Cognitive dysfunctions in bipolar disorder: evidence of neuropsychological disturbances. Psychosom 2000; 69(1): 2-18.

[25]   Martinez-Aran A, Vieta E, Reinares M, *et al.* Cognitive function across manic or hypomanic, depressed, and euthymic states in bipolar disorder. Am J Psychiatry 2004; 161(2): 262-70.

[26]   Grut M, Jorm AF, Fratiglioni L, Forsell Y, Viitanen M, Winblad B. Memory complaints of elderly people in a population survey: variation according to dementia stage and depression. J Am Geriatr Soc 1993; 41(12): 1295-300.

[27]   Cha DS, De Michele F, Soczynska JK, *et al.* The putative impact of metabolic health on default mode network activity and functional connectivity in neuropsychiatric disorders. CNS Neurol Disord Drug Targets 2014; 13(10): 1750-8.

[28]   Harvey P-O, Fossati P, Pochon J-B, *et al.* Cognitive control and brain resources in major depression: an fMRI study using the n-back task. Neuroimage 2005; 26(3): 860-9.

[29]   Medalia A, Revheim N, Herlands T. Cognitive remediation for psychological disorders: therapist guide. Oxford University Press, USA, 2009.

[30]   Bowie CR, McGurk SR, Mausbach B, Patterson TL, Harvey PD. Combined cognitive remediation and functional skills training for schizophrenia: effects on cognition, functional competence, and real-world behavior. Am J Psychiatry 2012; 169(7): 710-8.

[31]   Bowie CR, Gupta M, Holshausen K, Jokic R, Best M, Milev R. Cognitive remediation for treatment-resistant depression: effects on cognition and functioning and the role of online homework. J Nerv Ment Dis 2013; 201(8): 680-5.

[32]   Porter RJ, Bowie CR, Jordan J, Malhi GS. Cognitive remediation as a treatment for major depression: A rationale, review of evidence and recommendations for future research. Aust N Z J Psychiatry 2013; 47(12): 1165-75.

[33]   Cha DS, McIntyre RS. Cognitive impairment in major depressive disorder: clinical relevance, biological substrates, and treatment opportunities. Cambridge University Press, 2016.

[34]   Siegle GJ, Thompson W, Carter CS, Steinhauer SR, Thase ME. Increased amygdala and decreased dorsolateral prefrontal BOLD responses in unipolar depression: related and independent features. Biol Psychiatry 2007; 61(2): 198-209.

[35]   Deckersbach T, Kaur N, Hansen NS. A neurocognitive perspective. Symptom to Synapse: a neurocognitive perspective on clinical psychology. 2015; 278.

[36]   Lam RW, Parikh SV, Ramasubbu R, Michalak EE, Tam EM, Axler A, *et al.* Effects of combined pharmacotherapy and psychotherapy for improving work functioning in major depressive disorder 1. Br J Psychiatry 2013; 203(1472-1465): 358-65.

[37]   Parikh SV, Quilty LC, Ravitz P, *et al.* Canadian Network for Mood and Anxiety Treatments (CANMAT) 2016 Clinical Guidelines for the Management of Adults with Major Depressive Disorder: section 2. Psychological Treatments. Can J Psychiatry 2016; 61(9): 524-39.

[38]   Young S, Khondoker M, Emilsson B, Sigurdsson JF, Philipp-Wiegmann F, Baldursson G, *et al.* Cognitive-behavioural therapy in medication-treated adults with attention-deficit/hyperactivity disorder and co-morbid psychopathology: a randomized controlled trial using multi-level analysis. Psychol Med 2015; 45(13): 2793-804.

[39]   Serafini G, Pompili M, Belvederi Murri M, *et al.* The effects of repetitive transcranial magnetic stimulation on cognitive performance in treatment-resistant depression. A systematic review. Neuropsychobiology 2015; 71(3): 125-39.

[40]   Smith PJ, Blumenthal JA, Hoffman BM, *et al.* Aerobic exercise and neurocognitive performance: a meta-analytic review of randomized controlled trials. Psychosomatic Med 2010; 72(3): 239.

[41]   Stanton R, Reaburn P. Exercise and the treatment of depression: a review of the exercise program variables. J Sci Med Sport 2014; 17(2): 177-82.

[42]   Heyn P, Abreu BC, Ottenbacher KJ. The effects of exercise training on elderly persons with cognitive impairment and dementia: a meta-analysis. Archives of physical medicine and rehabilitation. 2004; 85(10): 1694-704.

[43]   Kubesch S, Bretschneider V, Freudenmann R, *et al.* Aerobic endurance exercise improves executive functions in depressed patients. J Clin Psychiatry 2003; 64(9): 1005-12.

[44]   Greer TL, Grannemann BD, Chansard M, Karim AI, Trivedi MH. Dose-dependent changes in cognitive function with exercise augmentation for major depression: results from the TREAD study. Eur Neuropsychopharmacol 2015; 25(2): 248-56.

[45]   McMorris T. Exercise and cognitive function: a neuroendocrinological explanation. Ex Cogni Function 2009; 41-68.

[46]   Intlekofer KA, Berchtold NC, Malvaez M, *et al.* Exercise and sodium butyrate transform a subthreshold learning event into long-term memory *via* a brain-derived neurotrophic factor-dependent mechanism. Neuropsychopharmacology 2013; 38(10): 2027-2034.

[47]   Carl WC, Nicole CB, Lori-Ann C. Exercise builds brain health: key roles of growth factor cascades and inflammation. Trends Neurosci 2007; 30(9): 464-72.

[48]   Millan MJ, Agid Y, Brune M, *et al.* Cognitive dysfunction in psychiatric disorders: characteristics, causes and the quest for improved therapy. Nat Rev Drug Discov 2012; 11(2): 141-68.

[49]   Soczynska JK, Ravindran LN, Styra R. The effect of bupropion xl and escitalopram on memory and functional outcomes in adults with major depressive disorder: results from a randomized controlled trial. Psychiatry Res 2014; 220(1): 245-50.

[50]   Schrijvers D, Maas YJ, Pier MPBI, Madani Y, Hulstijn W, Sabbe BGC. Psychomotor changes in major depressive disorder during sertraline treatment. Neuropsychobiology 2009; 59(1): 34-42.

[51]   Constant EL, Adam S, Gillain B, Seron X, Bruyer R, Seghers A. Effects of sertraline on depressive symptoms and attentional and executive functions in major depression. Depress Anxiety 2005; 21(2): 78-89.

[52]   Raskin J, George T, Granger RE, Hussain N, Zhao GW, Marangell LB. Apathy in currently nondepressed patients treated with a SSRI for a major depressive episode following randomized switch to either duloxetine or escitalopram. J Psychiatr Res 2012; 46(5): 667-74.

[53]   Raskin J, Wiltse CG, Siegal A, *et al.* Efficacy of duloxetine on cognition, depression, and pain in elderly patients with major depressive disorder: an 8-week, double-blind, placebo-controlled trial. Am J Psychiatry 2007; 164(6): 900-9

[54]   McIntyre RS, Lophaven S, Olsen CK. A randomized, double-blind, placebo-controlled study of vortioxetine on cognitive function in depressed adults. Int J Neuropsychopharmacol 2014; 17(10): 1557-67.

[55]   Mahableshwarkar AR, Zajecka J, Jacobson W, Chen Y, Keefe RS. A randomized, placebo-controlled, active-reference, double-blind, flexible-dose study of the efficacy of vortioxetine on cognitive function in major depressive disorder. Neuropsychopharmacology 2015; 40(8): 2025-37.

[56]   McIntyre RS, Harrison J, Loft H, Jacobson W, Olsen CK. The effects of vortioxetine on cognitive function in patients with major depressive disorder: a meta-analysis of three randomized controlled trials. Int J Neuropsychopharmacol 2016. doi: 10.1093/ijnp/pyw055.

[57]   Madhoo M, Keefe RSE, Roth RM, *et al.* Lisdexamfetamine dimesylate augmentation in adults with persistent executive dysfunction after partial or full remission of major depressive disorder. Neuropsychopharmacology 2014; 39(6): 1388-98.

[58]   Venero C. Pharmacological treatment of cognitive dysfunction in neuropsychiatric disorders. Cognitive enhancement: pharmacologic. Environm Genet Factors 2014; 11: 233.

[59]   Zanos P, Moaddel R, Morris PJ, *et al.* NMDAR inhibition-independent antidepressant actions of ketamine metabolites. Nature 2016; 533(7604): 481-6.

[60]   Price RB, Iosifescu DV, Murrough JW, *et al.* Effects of ketamine on explicit and implicit suicidal cognition: a randomized controlled trial in treatment-resistant depression. Depress Anxiety 2014; 31(4): 335-43.

[61]   Lee Y, Syeda K, Maruschak NA, *et al.* A new perspective on the anti-suicide effects with ketamine treatment: a procognitive effect. J Clin Psychopharmacol 2016; 36(1): 50-6.

[62]   Mansur RB, Ahmed J, Cha DS, *et al.* Liraglutide promotes improvements in objective measures of cognitive dysfunction in individuals with mood disorders: a pilot, open-label study. J Affect Disord 2017; 207: 114-20.

[63]   Craft S, Baker LD, Montine TJ, *et al.* Intranasal insulin therapy for Alzheimer disease and amnestic mild cognitive impairment: a polit clinical trial. Arch Neurol 2012; 69 (1): 29-38.

[64]   McIntyre Rs, Xiao HX, Syeda K, *et al.* The prevalence, measurement, and treatment of the cognitive dimension/domain in major depressive disorder. CNS Drugs 2015; 29 (7): 577-89.

[65]   Kauer-Sant'anna M, Kapczinski F, Andreazza AC, *et al.* Brain-derived neurotrophic factor and inflammatory markers in patients with early- vs. late-stage bipolar disorder. Int J Neuropsychopharmacol 2008; 12(4): 447-58.

[66]   Vevera J, Uhrova J, Benakova H, *et al.* Depression, traumatic stress and interleukin-6. J Affect Disord 2010; 120(1-3): 231-4.

[67]   Raison CL, Rutherford RE, Woolwine BJ, *et al.* A randomized control trial of the tumor necrosis factor antagonist infliximab for treatment-resistant depression: the role of baseline inflammatory biomarkers. JAMA Psychiatry 2013; 70(1): 31-41.

[68]   Loftus EV, Feagan BG, Colombel JF, *et al.* Effects of adalimumab maintenance therapy on health-related quality of life of patients with Crohn's disease: patient-reported outcomes of the CHARM trial. Am J Gastroenterol 2008; 103(12): 3132-41.

[69]   Persoons P, Vermeire S, Demyttenaere K, *et al.* The impact of major depressive disorder on the short- and long-term outcome of Crohn's disease treatment with infliximab. Aliment Pharmacol Ther 2005; 22(2): 101-10.

[70]   Tookman AJ, Jones CL, Dewitte M, Lodge PJ. Fatigue in patients with advanced cancer: a pilot study of an intervention with infliximab. Support Care Cancer 2008; 16(10): 1131-40.

REVIEW ARTICLE

New Trends in the Treatment of Schizophrenia

Herbert Y. Meltzer[*]

Department of Psychiatry and Behavioral Sciences, Northwestern Feinberg School of Medicine, 303 East Chicago Ave, Ward Building 7-101, Chicago, Il 60611, USA

Abstract: ***Objectives***: This article are to describe current trends in the treatment of schizophrenia and the most interesting new approaches to optimizing outcome and fostering the development of new schizophrenia treatments.

Results: Increasing utilization of diverse types of atypical antipsychotic drugs (AAPDs), *e.g.* clozapine-type serotonin (5-HT)$_{2A}$ and weak dopamine (DA) D$_2$ antagonist, amisulpride, a D$_2$/D$_3$/5-HT$_7$ antagonist, and cariprazine, a D$_3$ partial agonist with additional neurotransmitter targets, is occurring as their advantages in efficacy, especially for cognitive impairment and mood symptoms, and side effects are becoming appreciated. Typical APDs, *e.g.* haloperidol, are diminishing in favor because of their EPS, especially, tardive dyskinesia (T D) and appreciation that reducing D$_2$ receptor stimulation is not the only means to treat psychosis. Some of the mechanisms inherent in various AAPDs, *e.g.* 5-HT$_{2A}$ inverse agonism, and D$_3$ receptor partial agonism, are now recognized as effective treatments for psychosis. A new focus on treating the cognitive impairment associated with schizophrenia (CIAS) has emerged *via* mechanisms such as stimulation of acetyldraline receptor with muscarinic and nicotinic receptor agonists, but demonstrating their efficacy in trials is proving elusive. Pharmacogenetic strategies which may lead to personalized treatment of schizophrenia are emerging but have not yet succeeded in being widely reimbursable. Transcranial stimulation and cognitive enhancement therapy are more common but more evidence for their efficacy is needed.

Conclusion: The heterogeneity of the pathophysiology of the various domains of schizophrenia requires a diversity of treatments that are best met by the expert use of AAPDs at the current time. Pharmacogenetic efforts are consistent with new evidence that multiple genes are involved in the risk for schizophrenia and the effectiveness of AAPDs.

ARTICLE HISTORY

Received: January 03, 2017
Revised: July 11, 2017
Accepted: July 11, 2017

DOI:
10.2174/1871527316666170728165355

Keywords: Atypical antipsychotics, cognition, psychosis, glutamate, GABA, dopamine, acetylcholine, pharmacogenetics.

1. INTRODUCTION

Schizophrenia is a syndrome which, in its fully developed form, affects about 1% of the adult population, usually beginning in late adolescence, peaking at the end of the second decade and the first half of the third decade. Early stages of the illness usually appear in a prodromal period which varies in duration from months to years. Rare cases of schizophrenia manifest themselves in very young children as soon as language and social behaviors permit identification of aberrant neurodevelopment. Schizophrenia is now understood as one of the most complex of complex disorders, having become the amalgam of the Kraepelinean view of cognitive disturbances (cognitive impairment associated with schizophrenia (CIAS), the Bleulerian emphasis on psychotic symptoms, as well as deficits in affiliation, motivation and emotional response (negative symptoms). Even though suicide attempts, completed suicide and depression are frequent in schizophrenia, these mood symptoms are not considered core features of the syndrome.

This article will highlight some of the major trends in treating this complex disorder. It is not meant to provide a complete survey of current treatments for schizophrenia. Pharmacotherapy, the most widely used and effective treatment for schizophrenia, will receive the most attention. Adoption of atypical antipsychotic drugs (AAPDs) and the decreasing use of typical APDs (TAPDs), the importance of tardive dyskinesia (TD) and new treatments for TD, addition of non-dopamine (DA) targeting medications for treatment of psychosis, novel AAPDs such as cariprazine, treatments for CIAS, treatments for treatment resistant schizophrenia (TRS), prodromal schizophrenia, prospects for personalized medicine through pharmacogenetics, treatment during the prodromal period to prevent the onset of CIAS and psycho-

*Address correspondence to this author at the Department of Psychiatry and Behavioral Sciences, Northwestern Feinberg School of Medicine, 303 East Chicago Ave, Ward Building 7-101, Chicago, Il 60611, USA; Tel: 312 503 0309; Fax: 312 503 0348; E-mail: h-meltzer@northwestern.edu

sis, and cognitive behavioral therapy as a primary treatment modality, will also be discussed.

2. ATYPICAL *VS.* TYPICAL ANTIPSYCHOTIC DRUGS- DIVERSE MECHANISM OF ACTION, PSYCHOSIS, AND COGNITIVE IMPAIRMENT

The major trends in the pharmacologic treatment of schizophrenia are best understood in the context of TAPDs and AAPDs, sometimes referred to as first and second generation APDs. The TAPDS, *e.g.* chlorpromazine, other phenothiazines, haloperidol, and thiothixene, are DA D_2 receptor blockers, and produce a variety of mechanism-based side effects, *i.e.* the consequences of D_2 receptor blockade which, range from Parkinsonism and plasma prolactin elevations to neuroleptic malignant syndrome and TD. Clinically, AAPDs are distinguished from the TAPDS in producing much less motor side effects than the latter. It is noteworthy that risperidone, the most widely used of the AAPDs, and its active metabolite, 9-hydroxypaliperidone, which is also an approved treatment, paliperidone, produce even greater prolactin elevations than the TAPDs, through a combination of D_2 receptor blockade and other partially identified mechanisms. The AAPDs, of which clozapine is the prototype, were discovered soon after the discovery of chlorpromazine. Their pharmacology is diverse but most share more potent serotonin (5-HT)$_{2A}$ than DA D_2 receptor blockade [1-3]. The AAPDs have a diversity of additional pharmacologic effects which contribute to their efficacy in ways that are still being elucidated and which differentiate them from one another. All share the ability to produce an antipsychotic effect with minimal D_2 receptor-mediated side effects in most patients, but TD may sometimes occur [2]. Aripiprazole is a widely used AAPD which substitutes DA D_2 receptor partial agonism for direct D_2 receptor blockade; this action is enhanced by 5-HT$_{2A}$ receptor blockade, 5-HT$_{1A}$ partial agonism, and DA D_3 partial agonism [4]. Some AAPDs lack 5-HT$_{2A}$ receptor blockade, *e.g.* amisulpride [5], and the recently approved cariprazine [6]. Amisulpride was found to be a potent 5-HT$_7$ antagonist, which conveys important advantages for treating depression and cognitive impairment [6, 7]

The AAPDs are the most widely used agents for treating schizophrenia and in the many other indications where APDs are primary or secondary treatments, *e.g.* bipolar disorder, treatment resistant depression, obsessive-compulsive disorder, and autism spectrum disorder. The main reason for the clinical preference of these drugs is their greater tolerability. The motor side effects of the pharmacologically unopposed D_2 receptor blockade produced by the TAPDs make these drugs far less tolerable to patients. Some of the AAPDs, especially clozapine and olanzapine can produce marked weight gain in many, but not all patients, while others like quetiapine and risperidone, do much less frequently. Other AAPDs, especially aripiprazole, asenapine, cariprazine, and lurasidone, produce much less weight gain, with few exceptions.

There has been extensive investigation of the differences in efficacy for various components of the schizophrenia syndrome between the TAPDs and AAPDs. Registration studies in acutely psychotic, non-treatment resistant patients show no notable differences in the efficacy for treating positive

symptoms. However, a decade ago, three major studies compared TAPDs and AAPDs which substituted effectiveness trials for registration style clinical trial, were conducted: CATIE [8], CUtLASS1 [9], and EUFEST [10]. The CATIE and CUtLASS1 studies in chronic patients did not find advantages of the AAPDs over the TAPDs for such measures as time to discontinuation, with the exception that olanzapine was more tolerable in the CATIE study. The EUFEST study [10] of first episode schizophrenia patients showed a clear advantage for amisulpride, olanzapine, quetiapine, and ziprasidone, over haloperidol for time to discontinuation, but not treatment of psychopathology. It is beyond the scope of this article to critique these studies in detail which have been discontinued by many clinicians and in various peer renewal publications because of problems in their design, execution, data analysis, and politicization [11, 12].

The diversity in mechanism of action of AAPDs makes them of further interest for the treatment of psychosis in patients who do not respond to TAPDs. The mechanism of action of the AAPDs is more than the net combined effects of 5-HT$_{2A}$ and D_2 receptor blockade alone. Direct and indirect stimulation of DA receptors, the latter secondary to the release of DA in multiple forebrain areas, as well as dorsal striatum, and indirect stimulation of muscarinic and nicotinic acetylcholine (ACh) receptors from the release of ACh, is a key contributor to the efficacy of the AAPDs, most certainly for cognition but probably also contributing to antipsychotic effects as well [2, 13]. Some of the AAPDs, especially cariprazine and blonanserin, are D_3 receptor partial agonists or antagonists [14-16]. D_3 receptor modulation is one of the actions of some AAPDs, along with 5-HT$_6$ and 5-HT$_7$ antagonism [13], which enable them to be effective when other AAPDs that lack this action do not achieve desired benefits [17]. For this reason, the rationale for switching to an AAPD, which differs most in pharmacology after an adequate trial of one or more AAPD has failed, and before considering clozapine, should be considered. It has been suggested that duration of clinical trial as short as two weeks may identify the majority of responders to APDs [18]. However, there is evidence that two week trials are insufficient to identify most responders, even in first episode schizophrenia patients [19]. As will be discussed, pharmacogenetic strategies may in some cases permit a priori choice of medication.

3. TREATMENT OF COGNITIVE IMPAIRMENT, TARDIVE DYSKINESIA, TREATMENTS FOR TARDIVE DYSKINESIA RELATED TO TETRABENAZINE, AND ADDITIONAL TREATMENTS FOR COGNITIVE IMPAIRMENT: N-DESMETHYLCLOZAPINE AND OTHER MUSCARINIC AGONISTS

Cognitive impairment ranges from mild to severe in patients with schizophrenia [20] and is often the first and most impactful functional burden produced by the multiple genetic, epigenetic and environmental pathogenic factors which produce schizophrenia [20]. The complexity of the underlying neurobiology of cognition, the myriad of processes that control the development and function of the brain's ability to learn, store, retrieve and manipulate knowledge, is such that many different types of abnormalities can and do lead to CIAS and to major differences in which domains of cognition are affected [21]. A critical issue in assessing CIAS is whether to treat it holistically, *e.g.* focusing on a composite score of the deficit, or on individual domains, such as attention, working memory, speed of processing, social cognition, *etc.* Understanding brain development and function strongly argues for focusing on individual domains, as we have discussed elsewhere [2] The choice of composite cognitive scores in clinical trials of possible treatments for CIAS is one of the major reasons for the failure to obtain positive results in clinical trials for treatments of CIAS [2]. A more effective strategy would be to identify treatments that produce strong effects on specific domains in phase 2 studies and replicate those results in follow-up phase 3 trials. Unlike the treatment of psychosis, where single drug can produce major benefits in high percentages of patients, albeit leaving many patients minimally or only partially responsive, the diversity of underlying pathophysiology of CIAS and the limited efficacy of treatments which are effective for the variety of its causes have led some to conclude that there are no effective treatments for CIAS (see [22]. for discussion). This is not a valid conclusion and has misled both basic scientists and clinicians into thinking that the extensive preclinical literature showing cellular, molecular, and electrophysiological advantages of AAPDs should be discontinued [22]. The evidence that AAPDs improve cognition in animal models of CIAS *via* direct and indirect effects on 5-HT, DA, ACh, GABA and glutamate receptors, on neurotrophins such as BDNF and neuregulin, is robust [2, 23-26]. We have discussed reasons for challenging this negative conclusion about AAPDs for CIAS elsewhere [22]. The most recent meta-analyses of the cognitive data from controlled clinical trials of AAPDs , including the controversial data from the cognition arm of the US CATIE study, demonstrate significant advantages of AAPDs over TAPDs, to improve selected domains of cognition. Additional evidence comes from studies on the effect of clozapine on working memory. N-desmethylclozapine, the major metabolite of clozapine, has been shown to be the basis for clozapine to improve working memory in a subgroup of patients with schizophrenia who produce sufficient levels of NDMC to overcome the M_1 antagonist properties of the parent compound, clozapine [27]. These clinical results are consistent with evidence from preclinical studies with a variety of M_1 agonists and the efforts to develop stand-alone specific M_1 agonists for the treatment of CIAS [27, 28].

The role of the basal ganglia, in particular, the dorsal striatum (dSTR), referred to as the associative striatum, to distinguish it from the limbic striatum (nucleus accumbens, stria terminalis) in the pathophysiology of schizophrenia, has received increasing interest in recent years. Classically, this has been associated with motor disturbances, *e.g.* extrapyramidal side effects. However, in recent years, the role of the dSTR in psychosis and CIAS has received renewed attention [29, 30]. Understanding cortical-striatal and striatal-cortical function and connectivity in CIAS is still relatively limited [31]. Individuals who develop TD when treated with TAPDs or AAPDs, have worse cognitive impairment than those who do not develop TD; TD can diminish the ability of AAPDs to improve cognition in patients with schizophrenia [32, 33] suggesting that the site of action of AAPDs is, in part, the dorsal striatum. This is a major reason for avoiding the use of TAPDs for the treatment of schizophrenia or as augmenta-

tion for AADPs. We have found that additional D_2 receptor blockade from haloperidol can block the ability of AAPDs to improve various memory functions in rodents treated with the NMDAR antagonist, phencyclidine (Rajagopal *et al.*, in preparation). TD is often irreversible but can be suppressed by treatment with drugs such as tetrabenazine, and the recently developed isomers of tetrabenazine or a deuterated form of tetrabenazine [34]. Whether suppression of TD with these agents has any effect on cognition in patients remains to be determined. Both TAPDs and AAPDs can suppress TD, but this could worsen striatal dysfunction in vulnerable individuals. It is clearly best to prevent TD by minimizing the use of TAPDs, especially in those who develop significant EPS during the early stages of treatment, and to consider the ability of mechanisms intrinsic to many AAPDs, such as $5\text{-}HT_{1A}$ receptor stimulation, to minimize the EPS produces by D_2 receptor blockade [35].

4. SEROTONIN INVERSE AGONISTS FOR TREATMENT OF SCHIZOPHRENIA

$5\text{-}HT_{2A}$ receptor stimulation with hallucinogens such as LSD, mescaline, or psilocybin is known to cause psychotic symptoms in both normal individuals and schizophrenia patients. However, the symptoms produced by these drugs are most often delusions and visual hallucinations than auditory hallucinations. $5\text{-}HT_{2A}$ antagonists, *e.g.* ritanserin, counteract the psychotic symptoms of the indole hallucinogens [36].

We showed that $5\text{-}HT_{2A}$ receptor blockade was a key component in the action of clozapine and other AAPDs [3]. All the AAPDs are inverse agonists at $5\text{-}HT_{2A}$ receptors, meaning they block the constitutive activity of $5\text{-}HT_{2A}$ receptors [36]. Two selective $5\text{-}HT_{2A}$ inverse agonists, M100907 and SR43469B, have been shown to be virtually as effective as haloperidol as monotherapy for acutely psychotic schizophrenia patients [37]. The selective $5\text{-}HT_{2A}$ inverse agonist, pimavanserin, in combination with a sub-effective dose of risperidone, was shown to be as effective as full doses of risperidone or haloperidol in acutely psychotic schizophrenia patients, but was effective within two weeks compared to six weeks for the other two treatments which produced more side effects, including more weight gain and EPS, and greater serum prolactin elevations [38]. Pimavanserin did not augment haloperidol, 2 mg. in that study, an indication that $5\text{-}HT_{2A}$ inverse agonism may not be additive when combined with full D_2 receptor blockade and that other aspects of the pharmacology of AAPDs may be needed to fully realize the benefits of $5\text{-}HT_{2A}$ inverse agonism. $5\text{-}HT_{2A}$ inverse agonists could make a major contribution to the treatment of acute psychotic phase of schizophrenia by augmenting sub-effective doses of AAPDs. Olanzapine would be an interesting target for augmentation by pimavanserin because of the proclivity of olanzapine to produce massive weight gain.

Pimavanserin has currently been approved only for the treatment of L-DOPA-induced psychosis in Parkinson' disease [39]. $5\text{-}HT_{2A}$ inverse agonists are more effective in the NMDAR animal models of psychosis than they are in amphetamine-based models, *e.g.* locomotor activity in rodents [40]. Further study is needed to determine if pimavanserin or similar drugs will be effective in the treatment of schizophrenia, including the ability to improve cognition. Pimavanserin, the 5-HT$_{1A}$ partial agonist, tandospirone, and low dose haloperidol, in combination, was shown to improve novel object recognition in subchronic PCP- treated rats [41], evidence that 5-HT$_{2A}$ receptor blockade may make a contribution to ameliorating CIAS. However, in normal volunteers, the indole hallucinogen, N,N-dimethyltryptamine, produced less impairment in cognitive function than did ketamine, an NMDA receptor antagonist [42] which is psychotomimetic for some individuals.

5. CLOZAPINE AND OTHER TREATMENTS FOR TREATMENT RESISTANT SCHIZOPHRENIA (TRS)

TRS refers to the approximately 30% of schizophrenia patients who remain persistently psychotic despite adequate trials with standard doses of TAPDs or AAPDs. Clozapine is the only approved treatment for TRS but is underutilized because of the risk of agranulocytosis, weight gain, and sedation. TAPDs are generally ineffective in schizophrenia patients with persistent psychotic symptoms. Since its introduction, weekly monitoring for agranulocytosis with clozapine has been reduced modestly in various countries, but is still required indefinitely in most countries. Efforts to find genetic biomarkers for clozapine induced-agranulocytosis have been successful to a point, but they are not yet sensitive enough for clinical use [43, 44]. The relevant risk markers are in the HLA region. The time required for clozapine to be effective in many TRS patients is greater than the usual 2-6 weeks for efficacy of TAPDs or AAPDs in non-TRS patients.

When administered as monotherapy, administration of melperone, aripiprazole, long acting injectable risperidone and olanzapine for up to six months has been found to be nearly as effective as clozapine in many TRS patients but large scale randomized, blinded trials comparing these other AAPDs with clozapine are needed to confirm this point [2]. There are still many TRS patients who do not respond to clozapine. Transcranial magnetic stimulation or ECT may sometimes be helpful to some TRS individuals [45, 46] We have observed an extremely resistant TRS patients with a 30 year history of diverse psychopathology who responded dramatically to long-acting injectable risperidone after six months of treatment, accompanied by improvement in grey matter volume in the posterior cingulate. Over the six months, there was a remarkable improvement in cognitive impairment, followed by abrupt disappearance of severe delusions and hallucinations which have not returned in five years (Meltzer, in preparation). This singular case is an indication of the heterogeneity of schizophrenia and a rationale for persistent efforts to treat even the most refractory of patients.

6. LIMITED SUCCESS IN DEVELOPING NOVEL TREATMENTS FOR SCHIZOPHRENIA: WRONG TARGETS OR MISSING OPPORTUNITIES TO HELP SUBGROUPS

There have been numerous efforts to develop novel treatments for schizophrenia in recent years. These include efforts to treat global psychopathology, as do TAPDs and

AAPDs, or components of the disorder, *e.g.* the CIAS and negative symptoms. Highlights include mGluR$_2$ agonists [47]. BL-1020, an unusual compound which covalently linked GABA to perphenazine, [48], estradiol [49], glycine reuptake inhibitors [50], omega 3-unsaturated fatty acids, anti [51] inflammatory agents [52, 53] antioxidants [54], α$_7$ nicotinic receptor agonists [55], the immunosuppressive drug, tocilizumab [56] and a DA D$_1$ agonist [57]. Some of these treatments have been found to be effective as adjunctive treatments in animal models of CIAS, but have only been tried in schizophrenia as monotherapy. Thus, the combination of a 5-HT$_{2A}$ inverse agonist and an mGluR$_2$ agonist was found to restore novel object recognition in subchronic PCP-treated rats [58]. The failure of any of these drugs to successfully meet the requirements for approval by US or European regulatory authorities has led a number of major drug companies to cease efforts to develop drugs for schizophrenia, for CIAS, or for negative symptoms. Their rationale has been that animal models and other screening methods for novel treatments are incapable of identifying valid targets. However, it is more likely that many of these mechanisms are effective but that the effectiveness is limited to subgroups of patients and who cannot be identified using the standard trial design to compare with placebo or an active comparator. Many of trials that are considered to have failed or produced negative results, were unable to identify the true drug responders. It is possible to minimize this type of experimental error. Another source of error is contamination by previous or concomitant treatment with other psychotropic drugs, *e.g.* TAPDs or benzodiazepines, *etc.* which may diminish the efficacy of some novel treatments. Designs which involve identifying subjects who respond well and then subsequently re-testing those subjects with the same compound may be able to identify patients who do respond to a specific narrowly targeted therapy.

7. TARGETING PRE- AND PRODROMAL SCHIZOPHRENIA FOR TREATMENT

The concept that the pathophysiology of schizophrenia may begin to unfold in the earliest days of embryogenesis and develop further during early adolescence, setting the stage for the emergence of cognitive impairment, deficits in social interaction, and eventually psychotic experiences is well-established based on the understanding when and how abnormalities develop in the structure or function of brain regions involved in schizophrenia, *e.g.* the dPFC, dSTR, hippocampus, and ventral striatum [59, 60]. Knowledge of how and when the expression of risk genes for schizophrenia changes during development supports the efforts to intervene at early stages of the evolution of psychopathology rather than waiting for it to emerge in a severe form that may be much more difficult to treat, and are possibly irreversible [61]. Typically, the antipsychotic and other psychotropic drug treatments in these studies have been used at very low doses and in small numbers of subjects. It may be the case that higher doses, higher even than those used to treat manifest schizophrenia, are needed. We have shown that the doses of lurasidone, an AAPD, and tandospirone, a 5-HT$_{1A}$ partial agonist, needed to prevent the development of cognitive impairment in rats by subchronic treatment with the

NMDA receptor antagonist, PCP, are significantly higher than the doses needed to reverse established cognitive impairment [62]. Claims have been made for benefits of psychosocial interventions and cognitive behavior therapy in preventing high risk individuals from converting to a psychotic state. [63] but controlled trial have so far failed to substantiate benefits of CBT [64].

8. COGNITIVE BEHAVIORAL THERAPY FOR SCHIZOPHRENIA

There is great interest in utilization of cognitive behavioral treatments (CBT) for treating overall psychopathology, cognitive impairment, negative symptoms and function in patients with schizophrenia, as well as those still in the prodromal phase [65]. AAPDs have the potential to act with environmental enrichment to restore synaptic function. CBT techniques which have shown promise are diverse, frequently involving many months of computerized learning. Individual interactions with therapists and even group therapy, sometimes involving family members, have also been reported to produce positive outcomes [65-67]. CBT has been shown to increase inhibitory activity in the brain of man [68]. There is also evidence that CBT can change the structure and function of the brain in patients with schizophrenia [69]. CBT has been compared to environmental enrichment in laboratory animals which has been found to improve memory and learning in NMDA receptor antagonist-treated rodents [70].Clinical trials of novel drug treatments to improve cognition in schizophrenia with and without CBT are a priority.

9. PHARMACOGENETICS AND PERSONALIZED MEDICINE

Biomarkers, to identify the best choice of AAPDs for schizophrenia patients would clearly be of value because of the great individual variation in efficacy and side effects for any treatment. Various biological parameters, including genetic and epigenetic measures, plasma levels of metabolomics from brain and peripheral tissues, and EEG measures are among the many measures that have been studied as potential biomarkers [71-73]. Candidate gene studies have been widely tested to predict improvement in general psychopathology, cognitive measures, negative symptoms and positive symptoms, risk for TD, and weight gain. Genes involved in synaptic function, D_1, D_2, 5-HT_{2A}, nicotinic and GABA receptors are among those that have been most frequently related to clinical response. Unfortunately, replication of results has been difficult. Common problems in such studies include small sample sizes, inclusion of multiple races without adequate control for variation in rates of minor alleles between ethnic groups, control for baseline levels of psychopathology, age effects, *etc*. There are a few studies which have utilized genome wide association (GWAS) testing to search the whole genome for predictors of response [74, 75]. The cost of a GWAS has been greatly reduced and is continuing to become cheaper because of technological advances. Because treatment response and side effect vulnerability may be the result of hundreds of genes, a GWAS is the most efficient way to identify the most significant variants. We have recently found that SNPs from genes that are classified as synaptic adhesion genes (*e.g.* NRXN1), other synaptic plasticity related genes (NRG1/3 and KALRN), scaffolding genes (MAGI1), alternative splicing genes (RBFOX1), and ion channel genes (KCNA10 and CACNA2D3) predicted improvement in general psychopathology, positive and negative symptoms, in acutely psychotic schizophrenia patients treated with lurasidone in two registration trials [76]. Although none of the biomarkers reached genome-wide significance, many of the genes and associated pathways were SCZ risk genes, providing additional support for their relevance to clinical response to AAPDs. The top SCZ risk genes which contributed to prediction of response to lurasidone were related to neurodevelopment, synaptic biology, inflammation, and histones. Polygenomic scoring was the most effective means to integrate the large amount of data generated in this study. If results from studies like this replicate, become available for a group of possible APD treatments, and can be found to apply in general clinical practice, it is feasible that a GWAS study would become a practical means to choose AAPDs.

CONCLUSION

The treatment of schizophrenia is mainly based on the use of AAPDs, for which there are now drugs of many different classes. These drugs are highly effective for treating positive symptoms and generally well tolerated. The differences among these drugs coupled with patient specific genetic and epigenetic differences make it reasonable to switch to drugs that are different in some key pharmacologic features when response is unsatisfactory with one drug. While the AAPDs can improve some domains of cognition in many patients, further advances in this area are the most pressing need for treatment. Progress will be quicker in finding treatments for specific domains of cognition rather than composite scores. The first non-DA related APD has been approved (for L-DOPA psychosis) but has not yet been approved for treating schizophrenia. This is pimavanserin, a 5-HT_{2A} inverse agonist. Pharmacogenetic biomarkers have been identified and should be further tested in clinical practice. CBT is showing promise as an added means of address CIAS.

CONSENT FOR PUBLICATION

Not applicable.

CONFLICT OF INTEREST

The author declares no conflict of interest, financial or otherwise.

ACKNOWLEDGEMENTS

Herbert Y. Meltzer is a shareholder of ACADIA (pimavanserin). HYM has received research support from ACADIA, Allergan, Janssen, Neurocrine, Novartis, Otsuka, Sumitomo Dainippon, Sunovion, and TEVA.

REFERENCES

[1]   Gray JA, Roth BL. The pipeline and future of drug development in schizophrenia. Mol Psychiatry 2007; 12(10): 904-22.

[2]   Meltzer HY. Update on typical and atypical antipsychotic drugs. Annu Rev Med 2013; 64: 393-406.

[3]   Meltzer HY, Matsubara S, Lee JC. Classification of typical and atypical antipsychotic drugs on the basis of dopamine D-1, D-2 and serotonin2 pKi values. J Pharmacol Exp Ther 1989; 251(1): 238-46.

[4]   Davies MA, Sheffler DJ, Roth BL. Aripiprazole: a novel atypical antipsychotic drug with a uniquely robust pharmacology. CNS Drug Rev 2004; 10(4): 317-36.

[5]   Abbas AI, Hedlund PB, Huang XP, Tran TB, Meltzer HY, Roth BL. Amisulpride is a potent 5-HT7 antagonist: relevance for antidepressant actions *in vivo*. Psychopharmacology (Berl) 2009; 205(1): 119-28.

[6]   Durgam S, Cutler AJ, Lu K, *et al*. Cariprazine in acute exacerbation of schizophrenia: a fixed-dose, phase 3, randomized, double-blind, placebo- and active-controlled trial. J Clin Psychiatry 2015; 76(12): e1574-82.

[7]   Zareifopoulos N, Papatheodoropoulos C. Effects of 5-HT-7 receptor ligands on memory and cognition. Neurobiol Learn Mem 2016; 136: 204-9.

[8]   Lieberman JA, Stroup TS, McEvoy JP, *et al*. Effectiveness of antipsychotic drugs in patients with chronic schizophrenia. N Engl J Med 2005; 353(12): 1209-23.

[9]   Jones PB, Barnes TR, Davies L, *et al*. Randomized controlled trial of the effect on Quality of Life of second- vs first-generation antipsychotic drugs in schizophrenia: cost Utility of the Latest Antipsychotic Drugs in Schizophrenia Study (CUtLASS 1). Arch Gen Psychiatry 2006; 63(10): 1079-87.

[10]   Kahn RS, Fleischhacker WW, Boter H, *et al*. Effectiveness of antipsychotic drugs in first-episode schizophrenia and schizophreniform disorder: an open randomised clinical trial. Lancet 2008; 371(9618): 1085-97.

[11]   Attard A, Taylor DM. Comparative effectiveness of atypical antipsychotics in schizophrenia: what have real-world trials taught us? CNS drugs 2012; 26(6): 491-508.

[12]   Kraemer HC, Glick ID, Klein DF. Clinical trials design lessons from the CATIE study. Am J Psychiatry 2009; 166(11): 1222-8.

[13]   Meltzer HY, Huang M. *In vivo* actions of atypical antipsychotic drug on serotonergic and dopaminergic systems. Prog Brain Res 2008; 172: 177-97.

[14]   Baba S, Enomoto T, Horisawa T, Hashimoto T, Ono M. Blonanserin extensively occupies rat dopamine D3 receptors at antipsychotic dose range. J Pharmacol Sci 2015; 127(3): 326-31.

[15]   Huang M, Kwon S, Oyamada Y, Rajagopal L, Miyauchi M, Meltzer HY. Dopamine D3 receptor antagonism contributes to blonanserin-induced cortical dopamine and acetylcholine efflux and cognitive improvement. Pharmacol Biochem Behav 2015; 138: 49-57.

[16]   Kiss B, Horvath A, Nemethy Z, *et al*. Cariprazine (RGH-188), a dopamine D(3) receptor-preferring, D(3)/D(2) dopamine receptor antagonist-partial agonist antipsychotic candidate: *in vitro* and neurochemical profile. J Pharmacol Exp Ther 2010; 333(1): 328-40.

[17]   Gross G, Wicke K, Drescher KU. Dopamine D(3) receptor antagonism--still a therapeutic option for the treatment of schizophrenia. Naunyn Schmiedebergs Arch Pharmacol 2013; 386(2): 155-66.

[18]   Kinon BJ, Chen L, Ascher-Svanum H, *et al*. Predicting response to atypical antipsychotics based on early response in the treatment of schizophrenia. Schizophr Res 2008; 102(1-3): 230-40.

[19]   Gallego JA, Robinson DG, Sevy SM, *et al*. Time to treatment response in first-episode schizophrenia: should acute treatment trials last several months? J Clin Psychiatry 2011; 72(12): 1691-6.

[20]   Saykin AJ, Shtasel DL, Gur RE, *et al*. Neuropsychological deficits in neuroleptic naive patients with first-episode schizophrenia. Arch Gen Psychiatry 1994; 51(2): 124-31.

[21]   Horvath S, Mirnics K. Schizophrenia as a disorder of molecular pathways. Biol Psychiatry 2015; 77(1): 22-8.

[22]   Meltzer HY. Pharmacotherapy of cognition in schizophrenia. Curr Opin Behav Sci 2015; 4: 115-21.

[23]   Elsworth JD, Morrow BA, Hajszan T, Leranth C, Roth RH. Phencyclidine-induced loss of asymmetric spine synapses in rodent prefrontal cortex is reversed by acute and chronic treatment with olanzapine. Neuropsychopharmacology 2011; 36(10): 2054-61.

[24]   Meltzer HY, Horiguchi M, Massey BW. The role of serotonin in the NMDA receptor antagonist models of psychosis and cognitive impairment. Psychopharmacology (Berl) 2011; 213(2-3): 289-305.

[25]   Nagai T, Kitahara Y, Ibi D, Nabeshima T, Sawa A, Yamada K. Effects of antipsychotics on the behavioral deficits in human dominant-negative DISC1 transgenic mice with neonatal polyI: C treatment. Behav Brain Res 2011; 225(1): 305-10.

[26]   Neill JC, Barnes S, Cook S, *et al*. Animal models of cognitive dysfunction and negative symptoms of schizophrenia: focus on NMDA receptor antagonism. Pharmacol Ther 2010; 128(3): 419-32.

[27]   Meltzer HY. Attention Must Be Paid: the association of plasma clozapine/ndmc ratio with working memory. Am J Psychiatry 2015; 172(6): 502-4.

[28]   Bradley SR, Lameh J, Ohrmund L, *et al*. AC-260584, an orally bioavailable M(1) muscarinic receptor allosteric agonist, improves cognitive performance in an animal model. Neuropharmacology 2010; 58(2): 365-73.

[29]   Kegeles LS, Abi-Dargham A, Frankle WG, *et al*. Increased synaptic dopamine function in associative regions of the striatum in schizophrenia. Arch Gen Psychiatry 2010; 67(3): 231-9.

[30]   Simpson EH, Kellendonk C. Insights about striatal circuit function and schizophrenia from a mouse model of dopamine d2 receptor upregulation. Biol Psychiatry 2017; 81(1): 21-30.

[31]   Simpson EH, Kellendonk C, Kandel E. A possible role for the striatum in the pathogenesis of the cognitive symptoms of schizophrenia. Neuron 2010; 65(5): 585-96.

[32]   Waddington JL. Psychopathological and cognitive correlates of tardive dyskinesia in schizophrenia and other disorders treated with neuroleptic drugs. Adv Neurol 1995; 65: 211-29.

[33]   Caroff SN, Davis VG, Miller DD, *et al*. Treatment outcomes of patients with tardive dyskinesia and chronic schizophrenia. J Clin Psychiatry 2011; 72(3): 295-303.

[34]   Meyer JM. Forgotten but not gone: new developments in the understanding and treatment of tardive dyskinesia. CNS Spectr 2016; 21(S1): 13-24.

[35]   Newman-Tancredi A. The importance of 5-HT1A receptor agonism in antipsychotic drug action: rationale and perspectives. Curr Opin Investig Drugs 2010; 11(7): 802-12.

[36]   Meltzer HY, Roth BL. Lorcaserin and pimavanserin: emerging selectivity of serotonin receptor subtype-targeted drugs. J Clin Invest 2013; 123(12): 4986-91.

[37]   Meltzer HY, Arvanitis L, Bauer D, Rein W, Meta-Trial Study G. Placebo-controlled evaluation of four novel compounds for the treatment of schizophrenia and schizoaffective disorder. Am J Psychiatry 2004; 161(6): 975-84.

[38]   Meltzer HY, Elkis H, Vanover K, *et al*. Pimavanserin, a selective serotonin (5-HT2A-inverse agonist, enhances the efficacy and safety of risperidone, 2mg/day, but does not enhance efficacy of haloperidol, 2mg/day: comparison with reference dose risperidone, 6mg/day. Schizophr Res 2012; 141(2-3): 144-52.

[39]   Meltzer HY, Mills R, Revell S, *et al*. Pimavanserin, a serotonin(2A) receptor inverse agonist, for the treatment of parkinson's disease psychosis. Neuropsychopharmacology 2010; 35(4): 881-92.

[40]   Millan MJ, Brocco M, Gobert A, *et al*. Contrasting mechanisms of action and sensitivity to antipsychotics of phencyclidine versus amphetamine: importance of nucleus accumbens 5-HT2A sites for PCP-induced locomotion in the rat. Eur J Neurosci 1999; 11(12): 4419-32.

[41]   Oyamada Y, Horiguchi M, Rajagopal L, Miyauchi M, Meltzer HY. Combined serotonin (5-HT)1A agonism, 5-HT(2A) and dopamine D(2) receptor antagonism reproduces atypical antipsychotic drug effects on phencyclidine-impaired novel object recognition in rats. Behav Brain Res 2015; 285: 165-75.

[42]   Heekeren K, Daumann J, Neukirch A, *et al*. Mismatch negativity generation in the human 5HT2A agonist and NMDA antagonist model of psychosis. Psychopharmacology (Berl) 2008; 199(1): 77-88.

[43]   Goldstein JI, Jarskog LF, Hilliard C, *et al*. Clozapine-induced agranulocytosis is associated with rare HLA-DQB1 and HLA-B alleles. Nat Commun 2014; 5: 4757.

[44]   Tiwari AK, Need AC, Lohoff FW, *et al*. Exome sequence analysis of Finnish patients with clozapine-induced agranulocytosis. Mol Psychiatry 2014; 19(4): 403-5.

[45]   Dougall N, Maayan N, Soares-Weiser K, McDermott LM, McIntosh A. Transcranial Magnetic Stimulation for Schizophrenia. Schizophr Bull 2015; 41(6): 1220-2.

[46]   Lally J, Tully J, Robertson D, Stubbs B, Gaughran F, MacCabe JH. Augmentation of clozapine with electroconvulsive therapy in treatment resistant schizophrenia: a systematic review and meta-analysis. Schizophr Res 2016; 171(1-3): 215-24.

[47]   Kinon BJ, Zhang L, Millen BA, et al. A multicenter, inpatient, phase 2, double-blind, placebo-controlled dose-ranging study of LY2140023 monohydrate in patients with DSM-IV schizophrenia. J Clin Psychopharmacol 2011; 31(3): 349-55.

[48]   Geffen Y, Keefe R, Rabinowitz J, Anand R, Davidson M. Bl-1020, a new gamma-aminobutyric acid-enhanced antipsychotic: results of 6-week, randomized, double-blind, controlled, efficacy and safety study. J Clin Psychiatry 2012; 73(9): e1168-74.

[49]   Kulkarni J, Gavrilidis E, Wang W, et al. Estradiol for treatment-resistant schizophrenia: a large-scale randomized-controlled trial in women of child-bearing age. Mol Psychiatry 2015; 20(6): 695-702.

[50]   Umbricht D, Alberati D, Martin-Facklam M, et al. Effect of bitopertin, a glycine reuptake inhibitor, on negative symptoms of schizophrenia: a randomized, double-blind, proof-of-concept study. JAMA Psychiatry 2014; 71(6): 637-46.

[51]   Emsley R, Chiliza B, Asmal L, et al. A randomized, controlled trial of omega-3 fatty acids plus an antioxidant for relapse prevention after antipsychotic discontinuation in first-episode schizophrenia. Schizophr Res 2014; 158(1-3): 230-5.

[52]   Chaudhry IB, Hallak J, Husain N, et al. Minocycline benefits negative symptoms in early schizophrenia: a randomised double-blind placebo-controlled clinical trial in patients on standard treatment. J Psychopharmacol 2012; 26(9): 1185-93.

[53]   Vincenzi B, Stock S, Borba CP, et al. A randomized placebo-controlled pilot study of pravastatin as an adjunctive therapy in schizophrenia patients: effect on inflammation, psychopathology, cognition and lipid metabolism. Schizophr Res 2014; 159(2-3): 395-403.

[54]   Trebaticka J, Durackova Z. Psychiatric disorders and polyphenols: can they be helpful in therapy? Oxid Med Cell Longev 2015; 2015: 248529.

[55]   Walling D, Marder SR, Kane J, et al. Phase 2 Trial of an Alpha-7 Nicotinic Receptor Agonist (TC-5619) in negative and cognitive symptoms of schizophrenia. Schizophr Bull 2016; 42(2): 335-43.

[56]   Miller BJ, Dias JK, Lemos HP, Buckley PF. An open-label, pilot trial of adjunctive tocilizumab in schizophrenia. J Clin Psychiatry 2016; 77(2): 275-6.

[57]   Rosell DR, Zaluda LC, McClure MM, et al. Effects of the D1 dopamine receptor agonist dihydrexidine (DAR-0100A) on working memory in schizotypal personality disorder. Neuropsychopharmacology 2015; 40(2): 446-53.

[58]   Horiguchi M, Huang M, Meltzer HY. Interaction of mGlu2/3 agonism with clozapine and lurasidone to restore novel object recognition in subchronic phencyclidine-treated rats. Psychopharmacology (Berl) 2011; 217(1): 13-24.

[59]   Lewis DA, Levitt P. Schizophrenia as a disorder of neurodevelopment. Annu Rev Neurosci 2002; 25: 409-32.

[60]   Millan MJ, Andrieux A, Bartzokis G, et al. Altering the course of schizophrenia: progress and perspectives. Nat Rev Drug Discov 2016; 15(7): 485-515.

[61]   McGorry PD. Early intervention in psychosis: obvious, effective, overdue. J Nerv Ment Dis 2015; 203(5): 310-8.

[62]   Horiguchi M, Hannaway KE, Adelekun AE, Jayathilake K, Meltzer HY. Prevention of the phencyclidine-induced impairment in novel object recognition in female rats by co-administration of lurasidone or tandospirone, a 5-HT(1A) partial agonist. Neuropsychopharmacology 2012; 37(10): 2175-83.

[63]   Fusar-Poli P, Frascarelli M, Valmaggia L, et al. Antidepressant, antipsychotic and psychological interventions in subjects at high clinical risk for psychosis: OASIS 6-year naturalistic study. Psychol Med 2015; 45(6): 1327-39.

[64]   Stain HJ, Bucci S, Baker AL, et al. A randomised controlled trial of cognitive behaviour therapy vs. non-directive reflective listening for young people at ultra high risk of developing psychosis: the detection and evaluation of psychological therapy (DEPTh) trial. Schizophr Res 2016; 176(2-3): 212-9.

[65]   Sarin F, Wallin L, Widerlov B. Cognitive behavior therapy for schizophrenia: a meta-analytical review of randomized controlled trials. Nord J Psychiatry 2011; 65(3): 162-74.

[66]   Cella M, Preti A, Edwards C, Dow T, Wykes T. Cognitive remediation for negative symptoms of schizophrenia: a network meta-analysis. Clin Psychol Rev 2016; 52: 43-51.

[67]   Fisher M, Loewy R, Carter C, et al. Neuroplasticity-based auditory training via laptop computer improves cognition in young individuals with recent onset schizophrenia. Schizophr Bull 2015; 41(1): 250-8.

[68]   Radhu N, Daskalakis ZJ, Guglietti CL, et al. Cognitive behavioral therapy-related increases in cortical inhibition in problematic perfectionists. Brain Stimul 2012; 5(1): 44-54.

[69]   Penades R, Pujol N, Catalan R, et al. Brain effects of cognitive remediation therapy in schizophrenia: a structural and functional neuroimaging study. Biol Psychiatry 2013; 73(10): 1015-23.

[70]   Nozari M, Shabani M, Hadadi M, Atapour N. Enriched environment prevents cognitive and motor deficits associated with postnatal MK-801 treatment. Psychopharmacology (Berl) 2014; 231(22): 4361-70.

[71]   Hayashi-Takagi A, Vawter MP, Iwamoto K. Peripheral biomarkers revisited: integrative profiling of peripheral samples for psychiatric research. Biol Psychiatry 2014; 75(12): 920-8.

[72]   Light GA, Swerdlow NR. Future clinical uses of neurophysiological biomarkers to predict and monitor treatment response for schizophrenia. Ann N Y Acad Sci 2015; 1344: 105-19.

[73]   Sethi S, Brietzke E. Omics-Based Biomarkers: application of metabolomics in neuropsychiatric disorders. Int J Neuropsychopharmacol 2015; 19(3): 096.

[74]   Lavedan C, Licamele L, Volpi S, et al. Association of the NPAS3 gene and five other loci with response to the antipsychotic iloperidone identified in a whole genome association study. Mol Psychiatry 2009; 14(8): 804-19.

[75]   Need AC, Keefe RS, Ge D, et al. Pharmacogenetics of antipsychotic response in the CATIE trial: a candidate gene analysis. Eur J Hum Genet 2009; 17(7): 946-57.

[76]   Li J, Yoshikawa A, Brennan MD, Ramsey TL, Meltzer HY. Genetic predictors of antipsychotic response to lurasidone identified in a whole genome wide association study and from schizophrenia risk genes. Schiz Res 2017; S0920-9964(17): 30196-2.

Send Orders for Reprints to reprints@benthamscience.ae

RESEARCH ARTICLE

Neural Correlates in Patients with Major Affective Disorders: An fMRI Study

Gianluca Serafini[1], Maurizio Pompili[2,*], Andrea Romano[3], Denise Erbuto[2], Dorian A. Lamis[4], Marta Moraschi[5], Maria Camilla Rossi Espagnet[3], Mario Amore[1], Paolo Girardi[2] and Alessandro Bozzao[3]

[1]Department of Neuroscience, Rehabilitation, Ophthalmology, Genetics, Maternal and Child Health, Section of Psychiatry, University of Genoa, Genoa, Italy; [2]Department of Neurosciences, Suicide Prevention Center, Sant'Andrea Hospital, University of Rome, Rome, Italy; [3]Department of Neuroradiology, S. Andrea Hospital, University Sapienza, Rome, Italy; [4]Department of Psychiatry and Behavioral Sciences, Emory University School of Medicine, Atlanta, GA, USA; [5]Centro Fermi, Museo Storico della Fisica e Centro Studi e Ricerche Enrico Fermi - Rome Italy

Abstract: ***Background & Objective***: Brain areas of functional activation during emotional stimuli and their correlations with affective temperaments evaluated using Temperament Evaluation of Memphis, Pisa, Paris and San Diego (TEMPS-A) and hopelessness levels assessed with the Beck Hopelessness Scale (BHS) have been investigated.

Method: Brain activity in response to emotional stimuli was examined by Nuclear Magnetic Resonance Blood Oxygen Level Dependent (NMR BOLD) signal. Seventeen subjects (mean age ± SD = 57 ± 12), diagnosed with major affective disorders and eighteen healthy controls (HC) (mean age ± SD = 50±11) participated in this study. Higher functional activation of the left amygdala and cingulated gyrus was found in subjects with affective disorders; whereas, the right amygdala was mostly activated in the HC group. Higher BHS scores were associated with reduced BOLD activation throughout the primary somatosensorial cortex and left post-central gyrus.

Conclusion: Conversely, increased BOLD activation throughout the parietal superior lobule and right anterior intraperietal sulcus, occipital cortex, and left optical radiation, right insular cortex, right frontal superior gyrus was correlated with higher BHS total scores. Future studies should investigate the nature of the associations among brain activation, suicide risk, and affective temperaments in larger samples.

ARTICLE HISTORY

Received: January 03, 2017
Revised: July 11, 2017
Accepted: July 11, 2017

DOI:
10.2174/1871527316666170803143006

Keywords: Affective temperaments, fMRI, hopelessness, major affective disorders, neural correlates, suicide risk.

1. INTRODUCTION

Major affective disorders are common and disabling conditions associated with significant psychosocial impairment [1, 2], long-term negative outcomes, incomplete recovery between mood episodes, and persistent functional impairment [3]. To date, the pathophysiology underlying major affective disorders is poorly understood and new therapeutic strategies could be developed if neurobiological mechanisms underlying these disabling conditions were identified [4-6].

Over the last two decades, neuroimaging techniques have been used to investigate structural as well as *in vivo* functional brain abnormalities. Promising research has demonstrated the successful application of these techniques to examine the neural mechanisms underlying major affective disorders [7]. In particular, functional Magnetic Resonance Imaging (fMRI), using Blood-Oxygen-Level-Dependent (BOLD) contrast has provided interesting insights into the pathogenesis of these conditions [8, 9].

According to the current literature, structural neuroimaging techniques have clearly suggested the existence of a link between white matter abnormalities (*e.g.*, periventricular lesions), unipolar, and bipolar disorders, as well as suicide risk [10-13]. Similarly, fMRI studies have found specific brain alterations, especially in the orbitofrontal and dorsolateral prefrontal cortices, anterior cingulate gyrus, subcortical (basal ganglia), and temporal (hyppocampus, amygdala) regions, in patients with both unipolar and bipolar disorders [14, 15]. These brain regions play a fundamental role in

*Address correspondence to this author at the Department of Neurosciences Mental Health and Sensory Organs – Suicide Prevention Center – Sant'Andrea Hospital, Sapienza University of Rome 1035-1039, *Via* di Grottarossa, 00189, Rome, Italy; Tel: 00390633775675 (office), Fax: 00390633775669; E-mail: maurizio.pompili@uniroma1.it

emotion regulation as well as short- and long-term memory consolidation [16].

Multiple studies using various emotional paradigms, such as the Ekman faces [17], have suggested active roles of both the prefrontal cortex and fronto-limbic structures in the pathogenesis of major affective disorders [18]; however, there is conflicting research with regard to this finding. Some researchers [19, 20] have suggested that abnormalities in the fronto-striatal circuitries are actively involved in the pathophysiology of unipolar/bipolar affective disorders. To date, although unipolar and bipolar disorders are clinically well described in diagnostic manuals, these conditions have not been adequately characterized using neuroimaging techniques. Thus, in the present fMRI study, we investigated the prevalence patterns of brain activation in response to emotional stimuli among patients with major affective disorders and specific affective temperaments. We also examined the potential associations among these patterns of brain activation and hopelessness levels.

2. METHOD

2.1. Subjects

Subjects were recruited at the Suicide Prevention Center of Sant'Andrea Hospital (Rome). Inclusion criteria for subjects with major affective disorders were: 1) a DSM IV-TR diagnosis of major affective disorders (*i.e.*, unipolar major depressive disorder (MDD), bipolar disorder type I (BD-I), bipolar disorder type II (BD-II); [21]; 2) the ability to sign an informed consent. Exclusion criteria for all subjects were: 1) presence of severe neurological disorders (*e.g.*, epilepsy, multiple sclerosis, Alzheimer's Disease, dementia); 2) diagnosis of other Axis I and II major psychiatric disorders evaluated using DSM-IV criteria; 3) family history of dementia; 4) presence of structural MRI findings compatible with stroke or other gross brain lesions or malformations; 5) history of electroconvulsive therapy in the past 6 months.

Subjects with major affective disorders were divided into three groups according to the diagnosis of mood disorders. Psychiatric diagnoses were determined by the referring psychiatrists (M.P.) and confirmed using the Mini International Neuropsychiatric Interview (MINI) [22], a clinically administered tool that is currently in use on the psychiatric unit. Clinical and socio-demographic information was collected from medical records by two researchers independently (D.E., G.S.). In cases of disagreement, a third clinician was consulted (P.G.).

Subjects were aware of the purpose of the study and provided a regular written informed consent. The study protocol was approval by the local research ethics review board.

2.2. Clinical Assessment

Patients were assessed using the following empirically validated instruments: 1) Hamilton Depression Rating Scale (HDRS) [23]; 2) Young Mania Rating Scale (YMRS) [24]; 3) Beck Hopelessness Scale (BHS) [25]; 4) Temperament Evaluation of Memphis, Pisa, Paris and San Diego (TEMPS-

A) [26]. Evaluators who administered the HDRS and YMRS were blind to the neuroimaging assessment

2.2.1. HDRS and YMRS

The HDRS [23], a 17-item clinician-rated scale, was used to assess depressive symptom severity. The YMRS [24] is an 11-item rating scale for mania that explores manic symptoms and is considered the gold standard for evaluating the concurrent validity of bipolar mania with newer scales.

2.2.2. BHS

The BHS is a 20-item self-report scale assessing hopelessness/negative attitudes concerning the future [25]. Specifically, the BHS evaluates feelings, loss of motivation, and expectations regarding the future. Subjects are requested to endorse a pessimistic sentence or deny an optimistic sentence. Research has documented the existence of associations among the BHS total score, depressive symptoms, and suicidal intent/ideation. Furthermore, Beck *et al.* [27] conducted a follow-up study on a large sample of outpatients and reported that those with higher BHS total scores (≥ 9) were 11 times more likely to die by suicide than those with lower BHS total scores. Thus, the BHS is a useful predictor of suicidal behavior. The Italian version of the BHS has been validated by Pompili and colleagues [28]. The present study used the cut-off score of ≥ 9 to distinguish those patients who were considered at higher suicide risk.

2.2.3. TEMPS-A

The TEMPS-A is a self-report measure of the affective temperaments, by means of 110 items that define the bipolar spectrum, with depressive (D), cyclothymic (C), hyperthymic (H), irritable (I), and anxious (A) subscales [26]. The scale is different from most other temperament instruments since it taps sub-affective trait expressions as they were conceptualized in Greek psychological medicine and, in recent times, German psychiatry. Additionally, the TEMPS-A is not affected by current mood state (*e.g.*, depressive *vs.* manic) and is able to identify temperament profiles reliably in psychiatric inpatients with severe Axis-I psychopathology, presumably combined with life crises leading to hospitalization [26].

2.3. Data Acquisition

All images were acquired using a 1.5 T Siemens Magnetom Sonata scanner (Erlangen, Germany) equipped with a standard bird-cage volume coil. For all subjects included in the study, conventional MRI (dual-echo multislice turbo SE) sequence, generating proton density and weighted images, and FLAIR (Fluid Attenuated Inversion Recovery) sequence were acquired, and used to test exclusion criteria. T1 weighted images, for anatomical reference, were acquired using a IR-GRE (TR/TE = 2000/4.38 ms, in plane resolution = 1x1 mm^2, slice thickness = 1 mm, FA = 15°, matrix = 250x250, number of slices = 144). Functional images were acquired by means of EPI-SE sequence (TR/TE = 3000/49 ms, in plane resolution = 3.8x3.8 mm^2 slice thickness= 2.5 mm FA = 90°, matrix = 240x240 slices = 36).

2.4. Experimental Paradigm and Procedure

All individuals participated in an event-related experiment lasting 12 minutes. The visual stimulation was presented using a MRI compatible device (CinemaVision, Resonance Technology, Inc, Northridge, CA). The experiment consisted of viewing 40 facial expressions from standardized series [17]. Individuals viewed 20 prototypically fearful, mild and strong, and 20 prototypically neutral facial expressions that were casually alternated to represent the range of intensity of fearful emotion. We used fearful facial expressions as examples of emotional stimuli as demonstrated by previous functional neuroimaging studies [29, 30].

Each facial expression, overlapped on a grey background, was presented for 2 seconds, with an Inter-Stimulus Interval (ISI) of variable duration, according to a Poisson distribution (mean ISI = 4.9s). The ISI consisted of a grey isoluminant screen with a white cross at the center in order of maintain fixation. Moreover, to ensure that attention was maintained and directed to the face, participants were asked to press a button, associated with an auditory signal that may be picked up only by the staff experimenters, each time they saw a male face.

2.5. Statistical Analyses

Data preprocessing and subsequent statistical analyses were conducted using the SPM5 software package (http://www.fil.ion.ucl.ac.uk/spm). Before performing statistical analyses, functional volumes of all participants were realigned to the mean functional volume of the corresponding session and slice timing corrected. For each subject, T1-weighted volume was coregistered to the mean functional volume and matrix of normalization to the MNI atlas (Montreal Neurological Institute) template was generated. Matrix has been applied to both T1-weighted and corresponding functional volumes. Finally, normalized functional volumes, ($2x2x2$ mm^3 resolution in the normalized space) have been convoluted with an isotropic Gaussian Kernel (FWHM=10x 10x10 mm^3).

For each subject, functional analyses have been carried out in the time domain on a voxel-by-voxel basis by modeling the functional signal as the convolution of the standard haemodynamic response function with task paradigm. Realignment parameters have been included as confounding variables, to avoid false positive images due to the eventual subjects' movement occurring simultaneously with the stimulation. Realignment data are generally satisfactory, and only one subject was excluded by the subsequent statistical analysis. For each subject, the pattern of activation associated with visual stimulation has been determined by means of a one-tailed one-sample t-test. Activations are deemed statistically significant at $p < 0.01$ with a minimum clustering of 20 voxels.

2.5.1. Comparison within the Two Main Groups

Common activated regions among subjects in each of the study groups (subjects with affective disorders and HC, respectively) were performed by means of a one-tailed one sample t-test.

2.5.2. Comparison between the three Subgroups of Subjects with Affective Disorders

Statistical comparison tests were conducted between between the subgroups (MDD, BD-I, BD-II) and HC. Voxels that were deemed statistically significant at $p < 0.01$ were included in a cluster of at least 20 contiguous voxels. In addition, an Analysis of Variance (ANOVA) test was carried out between the three affective disorder subgroups.

2.5.3. Correlational Analysis

Multiple Regression analysis between functional response to stimuli, BHS, and TEMPS total scores were conducted within the three affective disorder groups.

3. RESULTS

3.1. Study Sample

Seventeen subjects (6 females, 11 males; mean age ± SD = 57 ± 12) diagnosed with major affective disorders and 18 healthy controls (HC; 8 females, 10 males; mean age ± SD = 50 ± 11) participated in this study. These groups did not differ with regards to age ($t = 1.268$, $p = 0.213$). Among participants, eight (47%) subjects were diagnosed with MDD, three (17.6%) with BD-I, and six (35.4%) with BD-II, respectively. Of the eight subjects with MDD, two (11.8%) reported a single depressive episode, whereas six (35.3%) suffered from a recurrent depressive episode. Moreover, three MDD subjects (37.5%) were affected by a moderate depressive episode and five (62.5%) by a severe depressive episode, respectively. Among those with BD-I, 1 (5.9%) subject was affected by a more recent depressive episode, and two (11.8%) by a more recent manic episode. Finally, among those with BD-II three (17.6%) suffered from a most recent depressive episode, whereas three (17.6%) by a most recent hypomanic episode, respectively.

3.2. Comparison within the two Main Groups

Statistically significant regions of activation within the HC group ($p < 0.01$, cluster 20 voxel) were found in the bilateral amygdala (Fig. **1a**), whereas, significant regions of activation within the group of subjects with affective disorders ($p < 0.01$, cluster 20 voxel) were reported in the left amygdala (Fig. **1b**).

3.3. Comparison between the Three Subgroups of Subjects with Affective Disorders

BD-I and BD-II subjects showed a significantly increased BOLD signal compared to HC subjects signal in the dorsolateral prefrontal cortex (BA9) as reported in Fig. (**2a**) Subjects with MDD showed a significantly decreased BOLD signal compared to HC subjects signal in the right amygdala (Fig. **2b**). ANOVA showed that BOLD activation was significantly different ($p < 0.01$, threshold cluster 20 voxel) among groups in the left subcortical region of amygdala (Fig. **2c**).

Table 1.   Socio-demographic and clinical characteristics of participants (N=17) and healthy controls (N=18).

Categorical Variables	Participants		Healthy Controls			
Gender	N	%	N	%	Statistic (χ^2)	*Significance*
Males	11	64.7	8	44.4	1.446	0.315*
Females	6	35.3	10	65.6		
Psychiatric diagnoses						
MDD, single episode	2	11.8				
MDD, recurrent episode	6	35.3				
MDD (moderate severity)	3	37.5				
MDD (moderate severity)	5	62.5				
BD-I, more recent depressive episode	1	5.9				
BD-I, more recent manic episode	2	11.8				
BD-II, more recent depressive episode	3	17.6				
BD-II, more recent hypomanic episode	3	17.6				
Quantitative variables	Mean	SD			Statistic (Student's t-test)	*Significance*
Age (years)	57	12	50	11	1.268	0.213

Note: MDD=Major Depressive Disorder; BD-I=Bipolar Disorder type I; BD-II=Bipolar Disorder type I; *=Fisher's exact test.

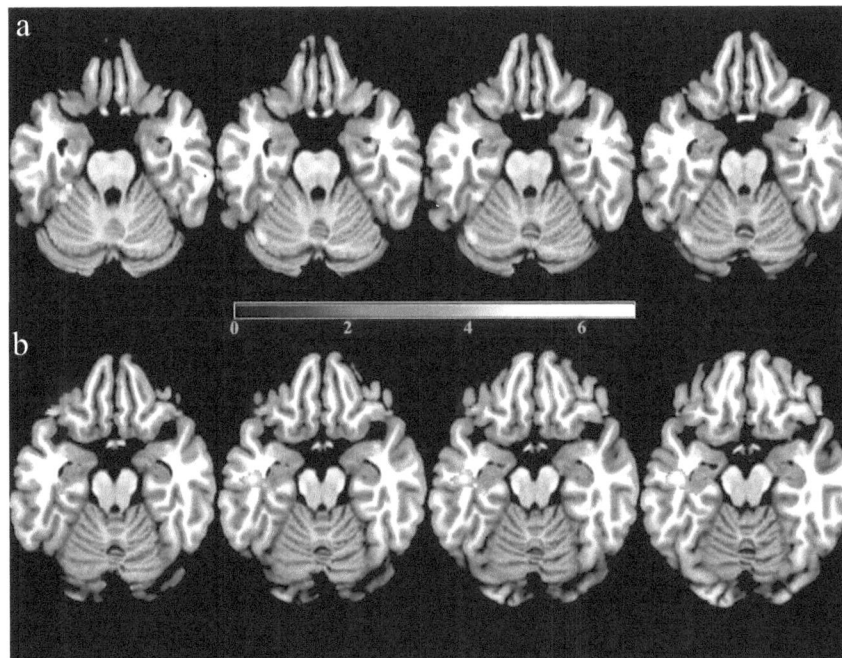

Fig. (1). Common regions of activation (p<0.01, threshold cluster 20 voxel) in HC (bilateral amygdala, **a**) and in subjects with affective disorders (left amygdala, **b**).

3.4. Correlations between BOLD Activation, BHS Total Score, and Affective Temperaments

Reduced BOLD signal throughout the primary somatosensorial cortex and left post-central gyrus was associated with higher BHS total score, ($p < 0.001$) (Fig. **3**), whereas increased BOLD signal within the parietal superior lobule, insular cortex, and right frontal superior gyrus was associated with higher BHS total score ($p < 0.001$) (Fig. **4 a,b,c**). No significant correlations were found between BOLD activation and specific affective temperaments.

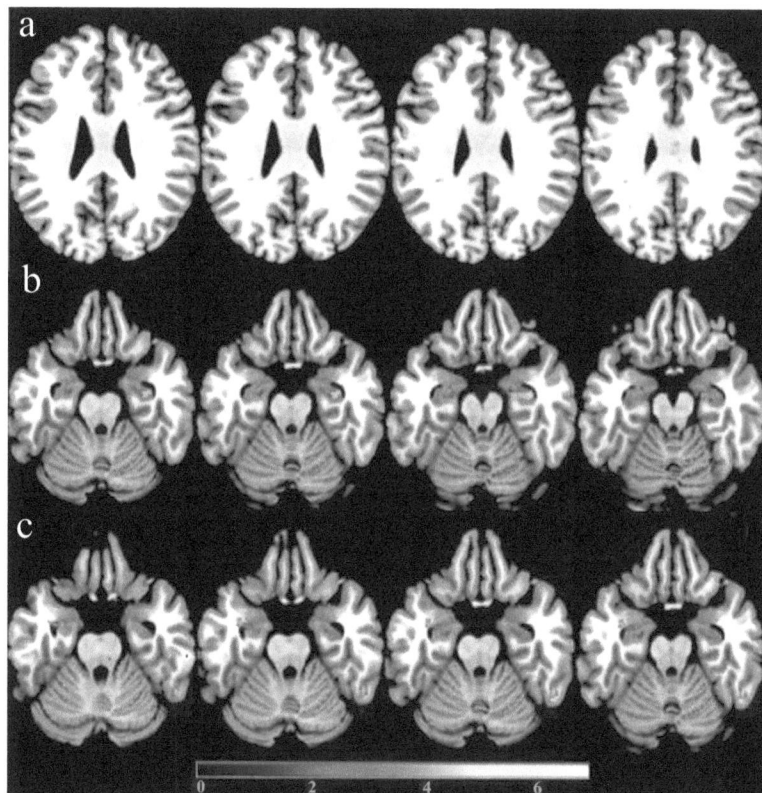

Fig. (2). In a, Brain regions with a significantly greater BOLD activation in BD-I and BD-II subjects (p<0.01, threshold cluster 20 voxel) when compared with the BOLD activation of HC: dorsolateral prefrontal cortex (a). In b, brain regions with a significantly smaller BOLD activation in MDD subjects (p<0.01, threshold cluster 20 voxel) when compared with HC: right amygdala. In c brain regions in which BOLD activation significantly differ (p<0.01, threshold cluster 20 voxel] amnong the three subgroups of subjects with affective disorders (MDD, BD-I, and BD-II): left amygdala.

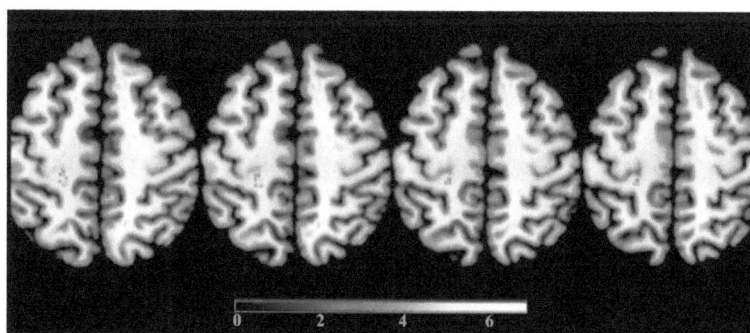

Fig. (3). Correlation between BOLD activation and BHS total score. Bold activation is reduced throughout the primary somatosensorial cortex and left post-central gyrus according to a BHS total score increase (p<0.001).

4. DISCUSSION

This is, to our knowledge, the first fMRI study to investigate the prevalence patterns of brain activation in response to emotional stimuli among patients with major affective disorders and specific affective temperaments together with their association with hopelessness levels.

First, we found that the left amygdala and cingulate gyrus were predominantly activated in subjects with major affective disorders; whereas, the right amygdala was predominantly activated in the HC group. The amygdala [31-33] as well as the cingulate cortex [34-36] have been found to play a relevant role in the pathogenesis of major affective disorders. Recent evidence has demonstrated that the subgenual anterior cingulate cortex plays a pivotal role in major depression where aberrant patterns of resting-state functional connectivity may be revealed. For example, in a sample of 23 MDD adolescents and 36 well-matched control subjects who underwent fMRI, Connolly *et al.* [34] found increased connectivity between the subgenual anterior cingulate cortex and insula as well as between the subgenual anterior cingulate cortex and amygdala in the MDD group compared to controls. The

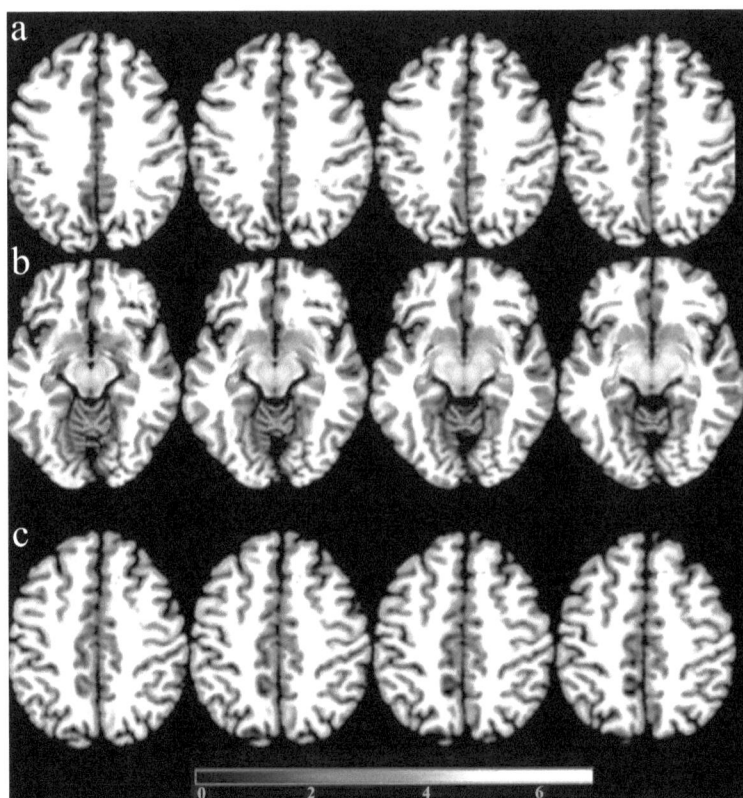

Fig. (4). Correlation between BOLD activation and BHS total score. Bold activation is increased throughout the parietal superior lobule right (**a**) the right insular cortex (**b**) and the right frontal superior gyrus (**c**) according to a BHS total score increase (p<0.001).

authors also reported that higher levels of depression were significantly associated with decreased connectivity between the subgenual anterior cingulate cortex and left precuneus in the MDD group. Additionally, increased rumination has been shown to be significantly associated with decreased connectivity between the subgenual anterior cingulate cortex as well as the middle and inferior frontal gyrus among MDD subjects. More generally, evidence supports a regional dysfunction within a corticolimbic neural system that subserves emotional processing and regulation in subjects with major affective disorders [36].

In the present study, we found that MDD patients had greater BOLD activation in the right amygdala than HC and BD-I and BD-II patients had greater BOLD activation in the dorsolateral prefrontal cortex [BA9] when compared to HC. Previous studies in adults with BD have suggested the existence of abnormalities in specific regions of interest such as amygdala, ventral striatum, temporal lobe, and orbitofrontal cortex that are crucial for the processing of emotional stimuli and behavioural response. Alterations in brain structures such as dorsolateral prefrontal cortex that are supposed to critically regulate initial emotional responses have also been reported [37-39]. Brain regions such as the dorsolateral prefrontal cortex are closely connected with limbic regions and play a fundamental role in processing emotional information [40-43].

Importantly, our results indicated that BOLD activation significantly differed in the left subcortical region of

amygdala among the three subgroups in our sample. As mentioned above, the amygdala is a critical brain region that is mainly involved in the accurate interpretation of emotion, emotional memory, and fear conditioning [44]. Many unipolar and bipolar patients who suffer from anxiety, fear, and worries apprehension, have structural alterations in their amygdala.

In addition, we found that reduced BOLD activation throughout the primary somatosensorial cortex and left postcentral gyrus was associated with higher BHS total scores; whereas, increased BOLD activation throughout the parietal superior lobule and right anterior intraperietal sulcus, occipital cortex and left optical radiation, right insular cortex, right frontal superior gyrus was associated with higher BHS total scores. These findings add to previous research regarding the neural correlates underlying key psychological constructs such as hopelessness. Hopelessness, a negative perspective regarding the future, has been shown to play a key role in the suicidal process, and is an established risk factor for suicidal behavior [25, 27, 45-47]. Hopelessness is also part of the negative cognitive triad to characterize the depressive cognitive style. To the best of our knowledge, no studies have directly focused on the association between specific patterns of BOLD activation and hopelessness levels. Recently, a study using Diffusion Tensor Imaging (DTI) and tractography investigated a sample of 45 patients (of which 13 euthymic suicide attempters, 15 euthymic non-attempters, and 17 HC) and found that lower connectivity strength between the right calcarine fissure and left middle occipital gyrus was associated with higher hopelessness levels (assessed using BHS) and self-reported depressive symptoms [48]. The authors also suggested that reduced connectivity strength in the minor and major forceps, which has been associated with maladaptive clinical characteristics (*e.g.*, hopelessness), may contribute to suicidal behavior. In another fMRI study, abnormally increased greater hippocampal activation during loss events was found to be associated with both self-reported depression and hopelessness [49]. Finally, Zhong *et al.* [33] investigated 29 medication-free MDD subjects, 26 never-depressed subjects with cognitive vulnerability, and 31 never-depressed HC using fMRI, and reported that cognitive vulnerability to depression may be characterized by a failure to engage the prefrontal cortex combined with hyperactivation of the amygdala in response to emotional stimuli.

The present study should be interpreted in the light of several limitations. First, the small sample size did not allow for the generalization of the present findings. These data are preliminary and need to be replicated in future larger samples before the results can be confirmed. Furthermore, patients who have been included in the present study all reported euthymic mood but may significantly differ based on the clinical characteristics of their illness (*e.g.*, number of episodes, polarity of first episode). This is relevant as patients with BD may exhibit different levels of cognitive and emotional processing deficits and functional limitations even during periods of mood stability [50].

Another limitation of our study is that the majority of patients were taking psychoactive medications when they underwent fMRI, which may represent a significant confounding factor potentially precluding the generalization of the main findings. Despite this shortcoming, most of the neuroimaging studies that have investigated brain volumes in patients with major affective disorders included medicated subjects [51]. Importantly, further additional studies analyzing the long-term effects of psychoactive medications on brain activation patterns are necessary in order to understand whether functional alterations may be related to the outcome and neuroprogression of affective conditions, or should be alternatively related to the effect of medications.

CONCLUSION

In conclusion, different regions of activation have been reported within groups of subjects with major affective disorders when compared to HC. Moreover, BD-I, BD-II, and MDD subjects showed a distinct pattern of BOLD activation when compared to that of HC. The comparisons among BD-I, BD-II, and MDD subjects demonstrated significant differences in their BOLD activation. Future fMRI studies should aim to identify and examine the neural correlates underlying major affective disorders in larger samples of patients.

ETHICS APPROVAL AND CONSENT TO PARTICIPATE

The study protocol was regularly approved by the local research ethics review board.

HUMAN AND ANIMAL RIGHTS

No animal were used in this study, Reported experiments on humans were in accordance with the ethical standards of the committee responsible for human experimentation (institutional national), and with the *Helsinki Declaration* of 1975, as revised in 2008 (http://www.wma.net/en/20activities/10ethics/10helsinki/).

CONSENT FOR PUBLICATION

Subjects were aware of the purpose of the study and provided a regular written informed consent.

CONFLICT OF INTEREST

The authors declare no conflict of interest, financial or otherwise.

ACKNOWLEDGEMENTS

Declared none.

CONTRIBUTORS

Dr. Serafini and Prof. Pompili wrote the protocol and the first draft of the manuscript, managed the literature searches, and interpreted the main results of the present paper. Dr. Romano and Dr. Moraschi acquired data, and undertook the statistical analysis. Dr. Erbuto and Dr. Rossi Espagnet recruited the patients. Dr. Lamis reviewed the paper for the quality of language and critically reviewed the manuscript. Prof. Amore, Prof. Girardi and Prof. Bozzao designed the study, supervised the search strategy, and provided the intellectual impetuous to write the manuscript. All authors contributed to and have approved the final manuscript.

REFERENCES

[1]   Pompili M, Innamorati M, Gonda X, *et al.* Affective temperaments and hopelessness as predictors of health and social functioning in mood disorder patients: a prospective follow-up study. J Affect Disord 2013; 150(2): 216-22.

[2]   Judd LL, Schettler PJ, Solomon DA, *et al.* Psychosocial disability and work role function compared across the long-term course of bipolar I, bipolar II and unipolar major depressive disorders. J Affect Disord 2008; 108(1-2): 49-58.

[3]   Tohen M, Hennen J, Zarate CM Jr, *et al.* Two-year syndromal and functional recovery in 219 cases of first episode major affective disorder with psychotic features. Am J Psychiatry 2000; 157(2): 220-8.

[4]   Barbui C, Cipriani A, Brambilla P, Hotopf M. Which bias in antidepressant drug trials? J Clin Psychopharmacol 2004; 24(2): 126-30.

[5]   Brambilla P, Cipriani A, Hotopf M, Barbui C. Side-effect profile of fluoxetine in comparison with other ssris, tricyclic and newer antidepressants: a meta-analysis of clinical trial data. Pharmacopsychiatry 2005; 38(2): 69-77.

[6]   Cipriani A, Brambilla P, Furukawa T, *et al.* Fluoxetine versus other types of pharmacotherapy for depression. Cochrane Database Syst Rev 2005; (4): CD004185.

[7]   Kerestes R, Davey CG, Stephanou K, Whittle S, Harrison BJ. Functional brain imaging studies of youth depression: a systematic review. Neuroimage Clin 2013; 4: 209-31.

[8]   Lener MS, Iosifescu DV. In pursuit of neuroimaging biomarkers to guide treatment selection in major depressive disorder: a review of the literature. Annals N Y Acad Sci 2015; 1344: 50-65.

[9]   Price JL, Drevets WC. Neural circuits underlying the pathophysiology of mood disorders. Trends Cogn Sci 2012; 16(1): 61-71.

[10] Pompili M, Ehrlich S, De Pisa E, *et al.* White matter hyperintensities and their associations with suicidality in patients with major af-

fective disorders. Eur Arch Psychiatry Clin Neurosci 2007; 257(8): 494-9.

[11]   Pompili M, Innamorati M, Mann JJ, *et al.* Periventricular white matter hyperintensities as predictors of suicide attempts in bipolar disorders and unipolar depression. Prog Neuropsychopharmacol Biol Psychiatry 2008; 32(6): 1501-7.

[12]   Serafini G, Pompili M, Innamorati M, *et al.* Affective temperamental profiles are associated with white matter hyperintensity and suicidal risk in patients with mood disorders. J Affect Disord 2011; 129(1-3): 47-55.

[13]   Serafini G, Pompili M, Innamorati M, *et al.* The impact of periventricular white matter lesions in patients with bipolar disorder type I. CNS Spectr 2016; 21(3): 23-34.

[14]   Soloff PH, Lynch KG, Kelly TM. Childhood abuse as a risk factor for suicidal behavior in borderline personality disorder. J Pers Disord 2002; 16(3): 201-21.

[15]   Soloff PH, Lynch KG, Kelly TM, Malone KM, Mann JJ. Characteristics of suicide attempts of patients with major depressive episode and borderline personality disorder: a comparative study. Am J Psychiatry 2000; 157(4): 601-8.

[16]   Soares JC, Mann JJ. The anatomy of mood disorders-review of structural neuroimaging studies. Biol Psychiatry 1997; 41(1): 86-106.

[17]   Ekman P, Friesen WV. Pictures of facial affect. Palo Alto: consulting Psychologist Press, 1976.

[18]   Naismith SL, Lagopoulos J, Ward PB, Davey CG, Little C, Hickie IB. Fronto-striatal correlates of impaired implicit sequence learning in major depression: an frMRI study. J Affect Disord 2010; 125(1-3): 256-61.

[19]   Arnold JF, Zwiers MP, Fitzgerald DA, *et al.* Fronto-limbic microstructure and structural connectivity in remission from major depression. Psychiatry Res 2012; 204(1): 40-8.

[20]   Malykhin NV, Carter R, Hegadoren KM, Seres P, Coupland NJ. Fronto-limbic volumetric changes in major depressive disorder. J Affect Disord 2012; 136(3): 1104-13.

[21]   American Psychiatric Association. Diagnostic and statistical manual of mental disorders, 4th ed. American Psychiatric Association, Washington, DC, 1994.

[22]   Sheehan DV, Lecrubier Y, Sheehan KH, *et al.* The mini-international neuropsychiatric interview (M.I.N.I.): the development and validation of a structured diagnostic psychiatric interview for DSM-IV and ICD-10. J Clin Psychiatry 1998; 59(S20): 22-33 quiz 34-57.

[23]   Hamilton M. A rating scale for depression. J Neurol Neurosurg Psychiatry 1960; 23: 56-62.

[24]   Young RC, Biggs JT, Ziegler VE, Meyer DA. A rating scale for mania: reliability, validity and sensitivity. Br J Psychiatry 1978; 133: 429-35.

[25]   Beck AT, Weissman A, Lester D, Trexler L. The measurement of pessimism: the hopelessness scale. J Consult Clin Psychol 1974; 42(6): 861-5.

[26]   Akiskal HS, Akiskal KK. TEMPS: Temperament Evaluation of Memphis, Pisa, Paris and San Diego. J Affect Disord 2005; 85(1-2): 1-2.

[27]   Beck AT, Brown G, Berchick RJ, Stewart BL, Steer RA. Relationship between hopelessness and ultimate suicide: a replication with psychiatric outpatients. Am J Psychiatry 1990; 147(2): 190-5.

[28]   Pompili M, Tatarelli R, Rogers JR, Lester D. The Hopelessness Scale: a factor analysis. Psychol Rep 2007; 100(2): 375-8.

[29]   Mitchell AE, Dickens GL, Picchioni MM. Facial emotion processing in borderline personality disorder: a systematic review and meta-analysis. Neuropsychol Rev 2014; 24(2): 166-84.

[30]   Sabatinelli D, Fortune EE, Li Q, *et al.* Emotional perception: meta-analyses of face and natural scene processing. Neuroimage 2011; 54(3): 2524-33.

[31]   Tang Y, Kong L, Wu F, *et al.* Decreased functional connectivity between the amygdala and the left ventral prefrontal cortex in treatment-naive patients with major depressive disorder: a resting-state functional magnetic resonance imaging study. Psychol Med 2013; 43(9): 1921-7.

[32]   Perlman SB, Almeida JR, Kronhaus DM, *et al.* Amygdala activity and prefrontal cortex-amygdala effective connectivity to emerging emotional faces distinguish remitted and depressed mood states in bipolar disorder. Bipolar Disord 2012; 14(2): 162-74.

[33]   Zhong M, Wang X, Xiao J, *et al.* Amygdala hyperactivation and prefrontal hypoactivation in subjects with cognitive vulnerability to depression. Biol Psychol 2011; 88(2-3): 233-42.

[34]   Connolly CG, Wu J, Ho TC, *et al.* Resting-state functional connectivity of subgenual anterior cingulate cortex in depressed adolescents. Biol Psychiatry 2013; 74(12): 898-907.

[35]   Davey CG, Harrison BJ, Yücel M, Allen NB. Regionally specific alterations in functional connectivity of the anterior cingulate cortex in majordepressive disorder. Psychol Med 2012; 42(10): 2071-81.

[36]   Wang F, Bobrow L, Liu J, Spencer L, Blumberg HP. Corticolimbic functional connectivity in adolescents with bipolar disorder. PLoS One 2012; 7(11): e50177.

[37]   Davidson RJ. Anxiety and affective style: role of prefrontal cortex and amygdala. Biol Psychiatry 2002; 51(1): 68-80.

[38]   LeDoux J. The emotional brain, fear, and the amygdala. Cell Mol Neurobiol 2003; 23(4-5): 727-38.

[39]   Phillips ML, Drevets WC, Rauch SL, Lane R. Neurobiology of emotion perception, I: the neural basis of normal emotion perception. Biol Psychiatry 2003; 54(5): 504-14.

[40]   Beauregard M, Levesque J, Bourgouin P. Neural correlates of conscious self-regulation of emotion. J Neurosci 2001; 21(18): 1-6.

[41]   Green M, Cahill C, Malhi G. The cognitive and neurophysiological basis of emotion dysregulation in bipolar disorder. J Affect Disord 2007; 103(1-3): 29-42.

[42]   Keightley M, Winocur G, Graham S, Mayberg H, Hevenor S, Grady C. An fMRI study investigating cognitive modulation of brain regions associated with emotional processing of visual stimuli. Neuropsychologia 2003; 41(5): 585-96.

[43]   Ochsner K, Knierim K, Ludlow D, Hanelin J, Ramachandran T, Glover G. Reflecting upon feelings: an fMRI study of neural systems supporting the attribution of emotion to self and other. J Cogn Neurosci 2004; 16(10): 1746-72.

[44]   Dall'Oglio A, Dutra AC, Moreira JE, Rasia-Filho AA. The human medial amygdala: structure, diversity, and complexity of dendritic spines. J Anat 2015; 227(4): 440-59.

[45]   Beck AT, Steer RA, Kovacs M, Garrison B. Hopelessness and eventual suicide: a 10-year prospective study of patients hospitalized with suicidal ideation. Am J Psychiatry 1985; 142(5): 559-63.

[46]   Brown GK, Beck AT, Steer RA, Grisham JR. Risk factors of suicide in psychiatric outpatients. J Consult Clin Psychol 2000; 68(3): 371-7.

[47]   Glanz LM, Haar GL, Sweeney JA. Assessment of Hopelessness in suicidal patients. Clin Psychol Rev 1995; 15: 49-64.

[48]   Bijttebier S, Caeyenberghs K, van den Ameele H, *et al.* The Vulnerability to suicidal behavior is associated with reduced connectivity strength. Front Hum Neurosci 2015; 9: 632.

[49]   Johnston BA, Tolomeo S, Gradin V, Christmas D, Matthews K, Steele JD. Failure of hippocampal deactivation during loss events in treatment-resistant depression. Brain 2015; 138(Pt 9): 2766-76.

[50]   McKenna BS, Eyler LT. Overlapping prefrontal systems involved in cognitive and emotional processing in euthymic bipolar disorder and following sleep deprivation: a review of functional neuroimaging studies. Clin Psychol Rev 2012; 32(7): 650-63.

[51]   Videbech P, Ravnkilde B. Hippocampal volume and depression a meta-analysis of MRI studies. Am J Psychiatry 2004; 161(11): 1957-66.

Send Orders for Reprints to reprints@benthamscience.ae

CNS & Neurological Disorders - Drug Targets, 2017, 16, 915-926 915

REVIEW ARTICLE

Neural Stem Cells and Human Induced Pluripotent Stem Cells to Model Rare CNS Diseases

Lidia De Filippis[1,*], Cristina Zalfa[2] and Daniela Ferrari[2]

[1]Casa Sollievo della Sofferenza, San Giovanni Rotondo (FG), Italy; [2]Department of Biotechnologies and Bioscience, University Milan Bicocca, Milan, Italy

Abstract: *Background & Objective*: Despite the great effort spent over recent decades to unravel the pathological mechanisms underpinning the development of central nervous system disorders, most of them still remain unclear. In particular, the study of rare CNS diseases is hampered by the lack of post-mortem samples and of reliable epidemiological studies, thus the setting of *in vitro* modeling systems appears essential to dissect the puzzle of genetic and environmental alterations affecting neural cells viability and functionality. The isolation and expansion *in vitro* of embryonic (ESC) and fetal neural stem cells (NSC) from human tissue have allowed the modeling of several neurological diseases "in a dish" and have also provided a novel platform to test potential therapeutic strategies in a pre-clinical setting. In recent years, the development of induced pluripotent stem cell (iPS) technology has added enormous value to the aforementioned approach, thanks to their capability for generating disease-relevant cell phenotypes *in vitro* and to their perspective use in autologous transplantation. However, while the potentiality of ESC, NSC and iPS has been widely sponsored, the pitfalls related to the available protocols for differentiation and the heterogeneity of lines deriving from different individuals have been poorly discussed. Here we present *pro* and *contra* of using ESC, NSC or iPS for modeling rare diseases like Lysosomal Storage disorders and Motor Neuron Diseases.

Conclusion: In this view, the advent of gene editing technologies is a unique opportunity to standardize the data analysis in preclinical studies and to tailor clinical protocols for stem cell-mediated therapy.

ARTICLE HISTORY

Received: November 25, 2016
Revised: January 31, 2017
Accepted: March 18, 2017

DOI:
10.2174/1871527316666170615121753

Keywords: Disease modeling, Stem Cells, Embryonic stem cells, Induced pluripotent cells, Neural stem cells, neurological disorders, rare CNS diseases, Motor Neuron Diseases, Lysosomal Storage Diseases, Huntington's Disease, Parkinson's Disease, Alzheimer's Disease, Amyotrophic Lateral Sclerosis, Central Nervous System, Spinal Cord, Sub-granular Zone, Sub-Ventricular zone, Glycosaminoglycans, Mucopolysaccharidosis, Mucopolysaccharidosis Type II or Huner Syndrome, Iduronate 2-Sulfatase, Enzyme Replacement Therapy.

1. INTRODUCTION

1.1. Cell Modeling of Central Nervous System (CNS) Disease From Embryonic Stem Cells (ESC) to Induced Pluripotent Stem Cells (iPSC)

In the last few years, major advances in the identification of genes and proteins and molecules involved in neurological disorders have partially elucidated pathogenic mechanisms and paved the way to novel therapeutic approaches. Despite this, the lack of appropriate models fully representing the complex network of cross-talking pathways involved in disease progression [1, 2], as well as the unfeasible task of extracting live neurons from patients has hampered the investigation of

many disorders [2]. Animal models still play a fundamental role in the study of genetic diseases, thanks to their easy availability, low cost and high reproducibility. However, often the remarkable difference between humans and rodents raises the question of how long rodent model can faithfully reproduce human system and be eligible for a preclinical investigation. For example, genetic mouse models do not represent the pathophysiological neurodegeneration and protein aggregation pattern observed in Parkinson's Disease (PD) patients [3, 4], and are thus limited [5]. This species-to-species mismatch has fostered the exploitation of human cells as a tool to model neurodegenerative disorders *in vitro* (Fig. **1A**).

A major challenge in the translational research is to find a valid cell system that should ideally fulfill the following requirements (Fig. **1B**):

*Address correspondence to this author at the Casa Sollievo della Sofferenza, San Giovanni Rotondo (FG), Italy; Tel: +39 338 2610386;
E-mail: defilippis@operapadrepio.it

1) Safety and reproducibility of culture protocols;

2) Absence of ethical issues;

3) Reduced/null species to species divergence;

4) Proximity of developmental origin to the neural lineage;

5) Expandability, homogeneity and stability of functional properties over *in vitro* expansion;

6) Reduced/null epigenetic or genetic manipulation;

7) Feasible use for cell-mediated therapy.

In this view, the discovery of neural stem cells (NSC) [6] and the generation of iPSC [7, 8] in the last decade have opened a new era (Fig. **1A**). The ability to isolate and culture different sources of stem cells has allowed to mimic *in vitro* the physiological processes that regulate tissue homeostasis

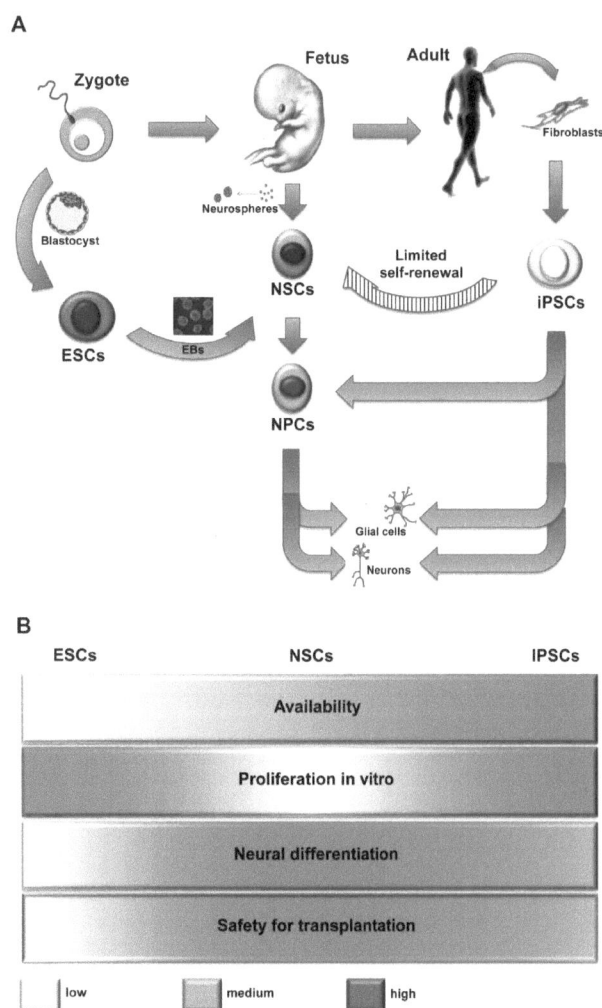

Fig. (1). Cell modeling of rare CNS diseases. **A)** Diagram showing developmental evolution from pluripotent stem cells (ESC from the blastocyst or iPS from adult somatic cells) to fetal neural stem cells to neural progenitors (NPC) to neural phenotypes. **B)** Diagram showing colorimetric index of different stem cell properties required to define a reliable cell modeling system in ESC, NSC and iPSC.

in vivo and to reproduce specific conditions that alter those processes, thus recapitulating the physiopathology of a variety of disorders. Most importantly, SCs have been used for the establishment of drug screening platforms and cell – mediated therapies, leading to new avenues for the cure of previously non-curable diseases.

Three main sources of stem cells are currently being used in biomedical and translational research for the study of neurological disorders: ESC [9], NSC [10] and iPSC [11] (Fig. **1A**).

2. ESC

Neurografts from fetal brain were successfully implanted in Parkinson's Disease (PD) such as HD patients and generated some promising results [12, 13], but objective assessment of benefits in patients revealed no significant long-term efficacy [14]. Since a variety of parameters and principles were very poorly defined such as the optimal source, age, dissection, preparation, implantation, immunoprotection and assessment protocols, the clinical efficacy seemed unreliable [15]. However, these pilot studies suggested that the fetal nervous tissue closely resembles the adult CNS, prompting to explore novel strategies to expand and differentiate neuronal cells from stem cells and, in particular, to use fetal NSC as an alternative strategy to ESC. Different clinical trials were performed by using protocols that were tractable to experimental refinement and multiple recent advances have allowed to tailor more safe and specific therapeutic strategies. Considering the aforementioned criteria (Fig. **1B**) to define the validity of a cell model system, ESC are amenable to easy proliferation *in vitro*, are endowed of great differentiation potential and of stable properties over passaging *in vitro* (Fig. **1A**). However, ethical concerns together with the poor knowledge of the epigenetic changes involved in ESC induction to the neural fate *in vitro*, and of their tumorigenic potential exclude ESC from being an optimal tool for adult disease modeling and a feasible candidate for clinical therapy (Fig. **1B**) [16, 17].

However, ESC still represent a useful tool to model neurodevelopmental disorders by taking advantage of the knowledge gained from studies on ESC, the reprogramming of adult differentiated fibroblast cells to the pluripotent stage (iPS) has opened the potential for an autologous source for transplantation, thus overcoming both the ethical issues related to ESC or the main concern of allograft rejection [18]. Thus, in this review, we will mainly focus our attention on NSC and iPS as feasible sources for the future therapy of neurodegenerative disorders.

3. NSC

The CNS of adult mammals is assembled during developmental neurogenesis and its architectural specificity is maintained through a vast cohort of signaling molecules. The structure of CNS is then sculpted by a synergic interaction of experience with synaptic plasticity through different postnatal developmental stages. In adulthood, neurogenesis reaches a "steady state" where differentiated cellular elements undergo a slow and very balanced turnover. This "dynamic" vision of CNS has been revised, thanks to the identification of NSCs that, in mammals, can be found in the embryonic/fetal neural tissue and in the adult brain tissue. NSCs are unspecialized cells that are able to self-renewal by mitosis, yet are also able to originate the three main neural cell lineages, e.g. neurons, astrocytes and oligodendrocytes [15] and are responsible for tissue homeostasis in the CNS under normal physiological conditions (Fig. **1A**). In particular, adult NSCs reside in specific microenvironments called "niches" and include either NSCs or "bystander" cells that produce supportive signaling for the niche maintenance. The forebrain subventricular zone (SVZ) in the lateral wall of the ventricles, the hippocampal subgranular zone (SGZ) of the dentate gyrus of the hippocampus and olfactory bulbs (OB) have been recognized as the main NSC niches in the adult rodent brain and NSC deriving from these areas have been extensively expanded *in vitro* by the neurosphere assay [19, 20]. Conversely, only SVZ and DG have been recognized as stem cell niche in the adult brain of humans though other "non canonical" niches are currently under investigation [21]. Human NSCs have been efficiently isolated and expanded from the fetal, but not from the post-mortem adult brain [22, 23].

In vivo, NSC are mostly quiescent but allow for tissue homeostasis through the generation of transient amplifying progenitors (NPC) which are endowed with limited self-renewal ability and high proliferation rate and restricted multipotency to the specific neural phenotypes (Fig. **1A**, Fig. **2**). Following a traumatic injury or the onset of a neurodegenerative process, endogenous NSCs are activated to proliferate and to generate increasing amounts of NPCs ready to provide novel neural cells addressed either to replace dead cells or to support degenerating cells [24].

Human NSC/NPCs can be isolated for research from the fetal (*i.e.* abortive tissue [10, 25], or adult brain (resection margins of neurosurgically excised brain lesions involving neurogenic regions) [26] and postmortem brains [27]. However, while NSC isolated from fetal tissue can be extensively expanded and stored in repositories [10, 25], the ability to generate neural cultures from post-mortem human brains or neurosurgical specimen depends greatly on the quality/ quantity of the brain tissue [28], thus in this review, we will mostly focus on the use of fetal NSC.

Human fetal NSC derive from the telencephalic-diencephalic area of the fetal brain (corresponding to 2nd and 3rd ventricles in the adult brain, where highly stem cell-enriched SVZ is located), are endowed with a lower proliferation potential than ESC and are intrinsically committed to the neural lineage, characteristics that have proposed them as an ideal source for cell transplantation in human patients affected by neurological disorders (Fig. **1B**).

Besides having extensive proliferation potential and intrinsic bias to the neural lineage, the great advantage of using human SC deriving from the fetal brain (NSC) rather than from the embryonic stage (ESC) is that they can be derived from spontaneous miscarriages, thus overriding all the ethical issues related to artificial insemination and intentional abortion. Moreover, no tumor development was ever observed after transplantation of NSC in nude mice, indicating a presumably absent tumorigenic potential of NSC [29, 30]. To note, NSCs have been shown to be endowed with a low

immunogenic potential, yet able to provide immunomodulation and neurotrophic support after transplantation [31] and have been recently approved for transplantation in patients affected by neurodegenerative diseases like ALS [32] and HD [33].

However, the paucity of the tissue sources to derive the NSC lines together with the lack of standardization and quality control criteria still represent a hurdle for a wide use of NSC in translational medicine [34]. Also, the onset of sporadic disorders like Huntington Disease (HD) [35], PD [36], Alzheimer's Disease (AD) [37] and Amyotrophic Lateral Sclerosis (ALS) occurs on adulthood and it's still partially unclear whether disease-specific features (together with the environmental conditioning) that usually appear over several years can be reproduced *in vitro* over a period of only a few days to a few months. In this view, fetal NSC may provide only *a priori* model for age-related disorders, suggesting that a parallel clinical investigation and accurate collection of epidemiological data are needed to validate results from *in vitro* modeling cell systems.

4. iPSCs

While human NSC can be currently obtained only from the fetal brain, iPS can be derived from different types of somatic cells (Fig. **1A**). These cells can be reprogrammed to iPS after non-invasive isolation from either healthy or affected adult patients, carrying genetic mutations or genome wide single nucleotide polymorphisms (SNPs). iPSCs represent an ideal tool to dissect the mechanisms underpinning the related pathogenesis and perform therapeutic drug screens on a human genetic background. Being pluripotent, iPSCs offer the unique opportunity to obtain specific cell phenotypes through either genetic or epigenetic protocols [38, 39].

As previously mentioned for fetal NSC, one concern about the exploitation of iPSC in modeling age-related disorders is to correctly reproduce late-onset characteristics and slow progression, since age is a crucial determination factor. As a consequence, iPSCs were initially used to model neurodevelopmental phenotypes and a variety of monogenic early-onset diseases [40-42]. However, later studies using iPSCs from patients affected by age-related disorders have illustrated that, upon differentiation into the neural affected phenotype, iPSCs display the key features of the relative pathophysiology. In this view, it's crucial to use an induction/differentiation method leading to the phenotype of interest through a pipeline of stages as close as possible to the physiological process. The protocols currently used for iPSCs induction to the neural phenotype are basically including genetic [43] or epigenetic [44] manipulation (Fig. **2**). Specific neuronal subtypes can be derived from pluripotent cells [42] through the overexpression of specific lineage-determining transcription factors (TFs) by lentiviral vector/s. Forced expression of a combination of TFs such as Pou3f2, Ascl1, Myt1l and NeuroD1 has been demonstrated to induce both human fibroblasts and iPSCs to functional induced neuronal cells (iNs) as early as 6 days after transgene activation [43].

Alternative to genetic manipulation, several cocktails of small molecules such as neurotrophic factors [45] are available to mimic *in vitro* the signaling produced *in vivo* during

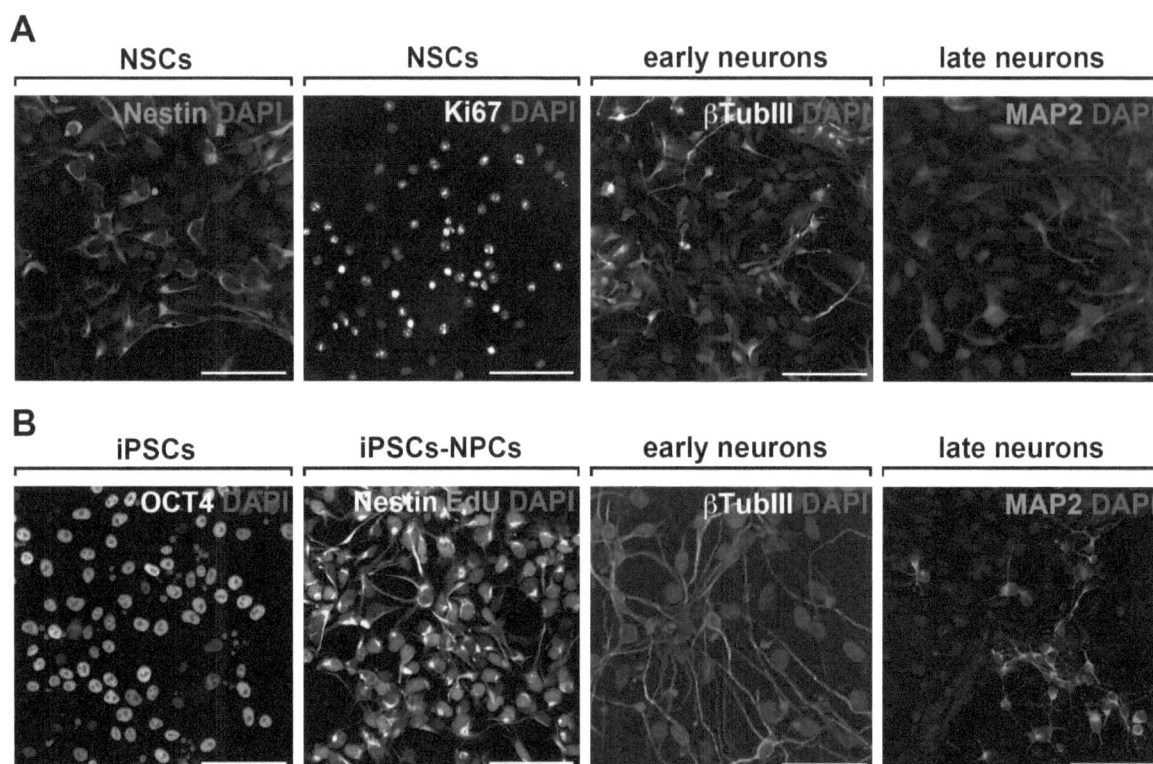

Fig. (2). Differentiation of iPSCs and NSC. Immunofluorescence staining showing markers of **A**) NSC and **B**) iPSCs at different stages of differentiation: Oct4 for iPSCs, nestin for NSC, b-tubIII as early neuronal marker in neural progenitors (NPC) and MAP2 as a dendritic marker of neuronal cells differentiated from NSC or iPSCs. Scale bars: 100μm.

developmental or homeostatic neurogenesis. Dual SMAD inhibitors like Noggin and TGF-β have been shown to induce a rapid and efficient differentiation into neural lineages [46, 47]. Recently a novel strategy using miRNAs in somatic cell reprogramming has been used to obtain pluripotent cells [48] and directly functional neurons [49, 50]. Besides underlying the physiological importance of mi-RNA as regulators of cell proliferation and differentiation, mi-RNA mediated reprogramming represents a groundbreaking frontier for the epigenetic generation of iPSCs as candidates feasible for clinical application.

However, when sporadic and familiar phenotype co-exist, major conclusion deriving from epidemiological studies or meta-analysis are often controversial. This inconsistency is mostly due to the arbitrary patient stratification, meaning subgrouping patients based on the disease severity due to the lack of phenotypic and genetic markers, which is very evident in the variety of neuropsychiatric phenotypes such as Alcohol Use (AUD) [51] and Autism Spectrum (ASD) Disorders [52, 53]. In rare diseases, where diagnostic criteria are still poor and the classification of patients is spread and inconsistent. In general, the patients and the iPS cell lines deriving from them are intrinsically heterogeneous and further data analysis can be found.

The generation of isogenic lines has been proposed as a strategy to overcome the heterogeneity between different iPS lines deriving from different patients. Given the enormous

potential of iPSCs technology, recent studies have been focused on finding effective genomic editing methods besides viral vectors or transposon vectors. Recent genome editing technologies such as zinc finger nucleases, TALEN and CRISPR-Cas 9 system have greatly facilitated the ease of genomic alterations in human iPSCs and, importantly, given that off-targets can be controlled, offers the possibility of correcting pathogenic mutations in iPSCs before autologous transplantation [54]. On the other hand, a variety of induction protocols have allowed the yield of high quantities of functional human neuronal cells *in vitro* that can be used for both diagnostic and translational studies. Accordingly, patient-specific iPSCs are increasingly being considered as alternative cell sources for both disease modeling and cell replacement approaches.

5. REPROGRAMMING AND EPIGENETIC MEMORY

Reprogramming increases cell variability due to the introduction of mutations in the genomic DNA [55] and the insertion of reprogramming genes. Moreover, reprogrammed cells maintain a residual DNA methylation signature characteristic of the somatic tissue of origin [56], which also affects gene expression [57]. This "epigenetic memory" conditions the capacity of a single iPS cell line to originate specific cell phenotypes irrespective of the donor's genotype. However, integrating methods such as lenti- and retro-virus infection for gene transduction, increase reprogramming efficiency but also cell variability since the expression of the reprogramming genes is variably maintained over cell passaging. Since the acquisition of a pluripotent potential is an epigenomic process [58], alternative methods to the integrating vectors have been adopted, such as Sendai virus [59], episomal vectors [60], protein transduction [61], or transfection of modified mRNA transcripts [62]. These are all strategies making feasible the use of iPSCs in future clinical trials.

While an ideal source for disease modeling and personalized medicine would be *bona fide* NSC isolated from patients, yet no efficient protocol does exist for their isolation and expansion from the adult brain, thus the only alternative is represented by iPS-derived NSC. But how are NPCs and neural cells deriving from iPSCs? How have these cells been characterized and which criteria reveal their authenticity? Several studies are urgently needed to answer these questions in order to promote iPSCs to the clinical stage.

Cell modeling becomes particularly relevant when considering rare brain diseases like MNDs and LSDs since epidemiological studies and availability of post-mortem specimen are very poor. To further complicate the study of their pathogenesis is that MNDs and LSDs are multifactorial disorders with genetic or sporadic etiogenesis.

6. RARE MOTOR-NEURONS (MNs) DISEASES

Amyotrophic Lateral Sclerosis (ALS) is a devastating neurodegenerative disease for which currently there are no effective therapies. ALS is the most common and aggressive form of adult MNs degeneration in cortex, brainstem and spinal cord and represent an example of the usefulness of *in vitro* models to elucidate possible mechanisms driving the disease progression in rare diseases.

Clinical features of ALS include muscle weakness, fasciculation, depresses reflexes and extensor plantar responses. The progressive decline of muscular function results in paralysis, speech and swallowing disabilities and failure ultimately, respiratory causing death among most of ALS patients within 2 to 5 years after the onset of symptoms. Pathologically, ALS is characterized by the degeneration of upper motor neurons in the cerebral cortex and of the lower motor neurons in the spinal cord [63]. The few remaining motor neurons are generally atrophic and present abnormal accumulation of neurofilaments, both in their cells bodies and axons. Despite significant advances made in the understanding of molecular and genetic aspects of ALS, causes and mechanisms of the neurodegenerative process typical of this disease are still largely unknown. The heterogeneity of ALS markers and the lack of reliable research models make it difficult to develop successful therapies and currently ALS has no available pharmacological treatments that offer long-term efficacy [64-67]. ALSs are classified in two main categories: the sporadic forms (sALS, 90-95% of ALS cases), with no obvious genetically inherited component and the familiar forms (fALS, 5-10% of ALS cases). Over years, several genes associated with fALS have been identified: C9ORF72 is the cause of about 40% of fALS also associated with FTD cases, 20% of cases are linked to mutations in the superoxide dismutase 1 (SOD1) gene, 5% to mutations in TARDBP and about 5% to mutations in FUS/TLS. The identification of mutated genes associated with ALS has given the opportunity to develop animal [68-71] and cellular models (also Rev in [72]) that have been helpful to dissect some mechanisms in the intricate cascade of events leading to MNs failure, thus providing useful insights also in the pathogenesis of sporadic ALS. However, despite the valuable results achieved with pre-clinical studies, no efficacious treatments have been developed so far.

7. MODELING ALS WITH SC-DERIVED MNs

7.1. MNs from ESC

Several protocols have been established to derive MNs from human pluripotent cells. These differentiation paradigms are intended to faithfully reproduce *in vitro* the sequence of morphogenic signals involved in the development of the spinal cord. Namely, inhibitors of TGF-β and BMP signaling [73] are used to induce early neuroectodermal phenotype while the subsequent addition of retinoic acid (RA) and activation of sonic hedgehog (SHH) pathway promotes caudal and ventral phenotypes respectively [74]. To note, different subtypes of MNs have been identified in different regions of the spinal cord, so that multiple variations of approved differentiation protocols are currently under investigation to target the analysis to specific MN phenotypes. To circumvent these issues mentioned above, the use of NSC and iPSCs in the recent years has gradually replaced that of ESC.

7.2. MNs from NSCs

NSCs can be derived from different region of the developing and adult CNS (SVZ, DG, spinal cord) and expanded with the use of FGF-2 and EGF as neurospheres. Rodent spinal-cord NSCs can generate HB9+/Chat+ MNs even without RA and SHH, although the use of these morphogens seems to improve the final MNs yield in embryonic derived NSCs. Interestingly, MNS carrying the SOD1 mutation have also been derived from NSCs produced from the olfactory bulbs of transgenic SOD1 mice [75]. In a similar fashion, human brain-derived NSCs seem to be able to generate MNs even without the need of SHH and RA [76] and irrespectively of the physiological brain regions of origin [76, 77].

However, given the lower availability and ease of culture of NSC-derived MNs with respect to those derived from iPSCs, the latter represent the presently used high throughput system to model ALS.

7.3. MNs from iPS

The recently developed iPSCs technology, complemented with the growing knowledge of ALS genetic forms, has broadened the spectrum of available *in vitro* ALS models (Rev in [72]). To note, iPSCs-derived MNs can faithfully mirror the unique genetic environment of each patient thus reproducing the inherent variability of ALS progression observed in the clinic. Most important, iPS-derived MNs provide a unique tool to develop more predictive and patient-tailored preclinical drug screening of the disease [78, 79].

The differentiation of iPSCs-derived MNs can be monitored by checking the progressive expression of specific

MNs markers such as Pax-6, NKx6.1, Islet-1, Hb9 and Chat. Within the first phases of the induction process, cells activate the expression of Pax-6 and Nkx6.1 that identify early MNs progenitors. The amount of these transcription factors decreases during differentiation, with a subsequent increase of post-mitotic markers like Islet-1, Hb9, Chat. In addition, the pluripotent stem cells-derived MNs display proper electrophysiological properties [80, 81], thus allowing to model relevant MNs malfunction by patch clamp technique or through a Multielectrode arrays (MEA) recordings.

iPSCs-derived MNs have been generated from fALS patients carrying mutations in SOD1, C9orf72, TDP43 and VAPB genes. Relevant hallmarks indicating the degeneration of neurites have been identified by comparing diseased to wild type MNs, such as NF inclusions [82], reduced soma size, shorter neuronal processes, alterations of mitochondrial morphology and motility, ER stress and altered electrophysiological activity [83]. A correlation between the degree of axonal membrane hyper-excitability and the survival rate of ALS patients has also been shown [84] thus validating iPSC-derived MNs as an appropriate modeling system *in vitro*. In accordance, the therapeutic effects of Riluzole, the only approved treatment for ALS, seems to include the modulation of sodium currents, so far hypothesized as being responsible for membrane hyper-excitability [85-87]. Recently, Wainger *et al.*, 2014 [81] have demonstarted that this altered membrane property is indeed present in iPS-derived MNs obtained from patients bearing three different genetic ALS forms (SOD, C9orf72 and FUS). The specific electrophysiological alterations were evident as early as 4 weeks after induction of iPSCs to MN and the phenotype could be rescued by genetic correction of the mutated gene or by treatment with retigabine, a drug acting on potassium channels, thus suggesting alternative therapeutic targets to modulate MNs excitability [81, 83].

The GGGGCC repeat expansion in C9ORF72 non coding region is one of the most common genetic alterations seen in fALS and sALS [88-90] causing the presence of intranuclear RNA foci both in MNs of the motor cortex and of the spinal cord [91]. Neurons and motor neurons derived from these patients showed an increased susceptibility to common pathogenic ALS mechanisms as glutamate excito-toxicity or choloroquine [88, 89] and altered gene expression profiling [89, 90]. Compelling *in vitro* evidence confirmed the involvement of three pathways in the pathogenic mechanism driven by C9ORF72 mutation: 1. Loss of function of C9ORF72; 2. the intranuclear RNA foci in iPS-derived neurons, that can bind and recruit diverse proteins thus interfering with their functions, such as ADARB2 [89]. 3. The production of non-ATG initiated translation (RAN) peptide, which determines the formation of cytoplasmic RNA foci in iPSCs-derived neurons [88, 89]. The potential toxicity of this phenomenon still needs to be clarified. The additional exceptional advantage of modeling ALS *in vitro* by means of iPSCs is the possibility to easily screen therapeutic strategies in a dish and complement the results obtained with animal models in order to design more efficacious clinical trials for ALS patients and even patient-specific treatments. The results obtained by Egawa *et al.* [79], seem to endorse this possibility. In this study, iPSCs-derived MNs obtained from TDP-43 patients have been used as *in vitro* screening for a

small compound library, finally allowing to the identification of a histone acetyltransferase inhibitor capable of rescuing the abnormal ALS motor neuron phenotype. More recently [78] iPSCs-derived MNs have been validated as a reliable tool to predict the results obtained in clinical studies. In this study, three compounds, kenpaullone, olesoxime and dexpramipexole have been compared for their neuroprotective abilities by a trophic factors deprivation assay. Only kenpaullone was significantly able to prevent MNs degeneration, while the other two had no (dexpramipexole) or limited (olesoxime) survival promoting effect. Interestingly, the results obtained with iPS-derived MNs mirrored those obtained in the phase III ALS clinical trials in which dexpramipexole and olesoxime did not manage to have a favorable impact on the disease.

7.4. Pitfalls of iPSC-MNs as a Cell Modeling System of MNDs: Correct Maturation Stage and Occurrence of Pathogenic Mechanisms

Despite the possibility that MNs from iPSCs represent a valuable tool in dissecting molecular mechanisms of disease progression, there are still limits to this technology, one of them being the level of maturation achieved by the MNs. Indeed, the differentiation protocol developed for ESCs and iPSCs has generated MNs genetically more comparable to their fetal counterpart than to the post-natal tissue [92]. For example they do not express mature markers and do not present the alpha, gamma and functional subclass specification of post-natal differentiated MNs. This *in vitro* to *in vivo* mismatch could be due to different reasons, that may include unknown molecular mechanisms inhibiting the differentiation eventually introduced by the reprogramming protocol (for example de-methylation processes), or the lack of proper environmental factors able to stimulate final maturation (such as feedback signals from target and surrounding cells normally present *in vivo*). The inability to achieve the proper maturation stage, hence the absence of specific proteins potentially involved in the pathogenic process, might limit the validity of this system to model diseases with the onset at the adult stage.

To partially overcome these issues, IPSCs can be induced to a longer maturation process or challenged with multiple disease-related stressing conditions (for example oxidative stress and glutamate overload [93, 94]), that are also useful to reveal selective vulnerability of patients with respect to sane controls.

7.5. Modeling of Non-cell Autonomous Effects in ALS

A general *caveat* of cell disease modeling *in vitro* is the lack of complex networks of environmental factors interacting *in vivo*, from the complexity of tissue architecture to the non-neural phenotypes participating to disease development and progression. For example, neuroinflammation includes an intricate series of events normally involved in most of the neurodegenerative processes [95]. A broad range of studies [64-67], have shown an involvement of non-cell autonomous mechanisms in the pathogenesis of ALS, with inflammatory signals derived from microgliosis and astrogliosis being involved in the degeneration progress of MNs in the spinal cord. To model these putative non-cell autonomous processes, co-culture of stem cell-derived MNs with primary astroglial cells obtained from ALS patients have been developed. These *in vitro* analyses have confirmed the neurotoxicity effect of ALS-astroglial cells on MNs and revealed possible molecular mechanisms driving the noxious activity of mutated astrocytes.

Initial indications came from chimeric animal models that showed how MNs degeneration could be partially counteracted in those SOD1 motor neurons surrounded by non-transgenic supporting cells [96]. In addition, the specific deletion of mutant SOD in astrocytes, significantly slows the progressive phase of the disease [97] thus confirming "bystander" mechanisms as potential therapeutic targets. The altered-toxic functionality of astrocytes bearing the SOD mutation has been efficiently reproduced in the *in vitro* rodent co-culture system, confirming that mutant SOD1 astroglia is harmful *per se* to both wild type and mutated MNs [98, 99].

Human-derived astrocytes and MNs have been used to translate the previous knowledge from a rodent to a human modeling system, thus confirming astrocyte-mediated toxicity also in human ALS [80, 100].

Different from the large-scale protein aggregation detectable in MNs, the effect mediated by the mutated SOD in astrocytes seems to be the induction of an activated phenotype, displaying an increased expression of prostaglandin D2 receptor and of proinflammatory cytokines, production of oxygen radicals, and induction of other factors related to the immune response [80, 100].

These data *in vitro* are corroborated by evidences showing a strong proinflammatory response to ALS in both animal models and patients [101-103]. Mutant astrocytes lead to either human or rodent MN degeneration in co-culture experiments, but the same effect is obtained by treating MNs with astrocyte supernatant, suggesting that astrocyte-produced soluble factors are responsible for the toxic crosstalk between astrocytes and MNs [98].

Antioxidants, growth factors, cell treatment, prostaglandins [80, 100, 104], and also stem cells treatments [105, 106] have then been tested in the same co-culture system to counteract the toxic activity of mutated glia.

In conclusion, MNs derived from iPS cells and glial/MNs co-culture system can model several features of the inherent pathogenic process of ALS, as the hyper-excitability of MNs membranes, vulnerability to excitotoxicity, oxidative stress and non-cell autonomous stimuli, validating these system as useful platforms to test putative therapeutic compounds. Notwithstanding, ALS is a complex multifactorial disease and results obtained *in vitro* still need to be validated *in vivo* by using transgenic mice or human autoptic samples.

8. RARE INHERITED METABOLIC DISORDERS: LYSOSOMAL STORAGE DISEASES

Lysosomal storage diseases (LSDs) are a family of metabolic disorders arising from inherited gene mutations that perturb lysosomal homeostasis [107]. LSDs mainly derive from deficiencies in lysosomal enzymes, but also non-enzymatic lysosomal proteins can be involved leading to abnormal storage of macromolecular substrates [108-110]. The combined incidence of LSDs is estimated to be approximately 1:5,000 live births [109], but the actual figure is likely greater when undiagnosed or misdiagnosed cases are accounted for. The classification of many LSDs can still be made largely on the basis of the kind of substrate accumulation. Common to all LSDs is the initial accumulation of specific macromolecules or monomeric compounds inside organelles of the endosomal–autophagic–lysosomal system. Initial biochemical characterization of stored macromolecules in these disorders led to the implication of defective lysosomal enzymes as a common cause of pathogenesis [108, 111], though a considerable number of these conditions resulting from defects in lysosomal membrane proteins or non-enzymatic soluble lysosomal proteins [112]. Therefore, LSDs offer a window into the normal functions of both enzymatic and non-enzymatic lysosomal proteins.

8.1. The Mucopolysaccharidoses

MPSs are a group of rare genetically inherited lysosomal storage disorders of glycosaminoglycan (GAG) catabolism [113]. Each MPS disorder is caused by a deficiency in the activity of a single, specific lysosomal enzyme required for GAG degradation. These diseases are biochemically characterized by an accumulation of partially degraded GAG within lysosomes and the elevation of GAG fragments in urine, blood [114] and cerebral spinal fluid [115]. The GAG accumulation results in progressive cellular damage, which can affect multiple organ systems and lead to organ failure, cognitive impairment and reduced life expectancy. Of interest to the rheumatologist, skeletal and joint abnormalities are a prominent feature of many of the MPS disorders; patients often present with skeletal dysplasia, decreased joint mobility, short stature and Carpal tunnel syndrome [113]. With the exception of MPS II, the MPS disorders are inherited in an autosomal recessive pattern and affect both males and females equally. Mucopolysaccharidosis type II (MPS II or Hunter Syndrome) is an X-linked recessive disorder that generally affects only males, although rare female patients with MPS II have been described [116]. This can be caused by an X-autosome translocation and non-random X-chromosome inactivation in a carrier female. MPS II is caused by a deficit of the iduronate 2-sulfatase (IDS) enzyme, involved in glycosaminoglycan (GAG) catabolism [113]. The disorder leads to variable progressive organ impairment caused by the lysosomal accumulation of GAGs in all cell types, with incremental neurological deterioration and mental retardation affecting about 50-70% of all patients. Death generally occurs in the first or second decade of life [117].

Over the past two decades, there has been a remarkable expansion in the number of therapeutic strategies for LSDs that target different cellular organelles. The first treatment was Enzyme replacement therapy (ERT), whether by intravenous infusion, gene therapy or hematopoietic or stem cell delivery, has shown potential to treat pathological conditions of the brain [118-122].

However, the clinical limitations of ERT are two-fold. First, product delivery is invasive time-consuming to deliver, and second, lysosomal enzymes do not cross the blood–brain barrier to any significant extent, so cannot effectively treat CNS disease, which is characteristic of most LSDs.

Several alternative therapeutic strategies are currently under investigation in tissue culture models and/or in animal models of LSDs. Small-molecule therapies that readily cross the BBB are also in early trials or in development. Although each therapeutic modality has inherent strengths and weaknesses, perhaps the future of LSD therapy lies in combining different types of treatment [118-120].

Augmentations of enzyme activity by ex vivo gene therapy before cell transplantation [123] simultaneous use of stem cells and small-molecule substrate inhibitors, or HSCT or ERT combined with agents that have the potential to disrupt the BBB are attractive strategies. However, the currently late diagnosis of neuronal dysfunction together with the lack of specimen from early symptomatic patients has limited the elucidation of the neuro-pathogenetic events involved in the development of LSDs. In this view, the identification of affected patients before the onset of symptoms using a tandem mass spectrometry newborn screening approach would be of essence to provide early and more efficacious therapy [124]. Nonetheless, the establishment of reliable *in vitro* model systems would be pivotal to the elucidation of pathogenic mechanisms and to the screening of novel therapeutic strategies.

8.2. Modeling LSDs with NSCs Derived from Animal Models

Considering that the genetic defect in MPS II could compromise the neurogenic properties of NSCs [113], we used NSCs derived from IDS-knock out (IDS-ko) mice to recapitulate MPS II pathogenesis and assess the self-renewal, differentiation and survival properties of these cells [125, 126]. We showed that IDS deficit appears not to affect NSCs proliferation, but glial differentiation and survival leading to later neuronal demise. By a parallel analysis of the correlation between IDS deficit in NSC *in vitro* and abnormal neurogenesis in IDS-ko mouse brain *in vivo,* we showed that MPSII develops through three main stages where the early development of a neuroinflammatory background is followed by glial degeneration and ultimately neuronal death that can be at least partially caused by glial-mediated toxicity. The poor characterization of the CNS in IDS-ko mice and the extremely sporadic availability of samples from human patients has strongly limited the elucidation of MPS II neuropathology in humans. In our study, we also analyzed autoptic specimen from the brain of a Hunter patient. The pattern of a late symptomatic IDS-ko mouse brain was consistent with that of the human Hunter patient, providing an undocumented evidence of the IDS-ko mouse brain as mirroring a human Hunter brain. As a whole, we validated NSCs isolated from IDS-ko mouse brain as an optimal tool to model MPS II brain disease and to potentially investigate novel therapeutic approaches.

8.3. Modeling LSDs with Human iPSC

Murine models of human congenital and acquired diseases are invaluable tools, but do not always faithfully mimic human diseases pathophysiology, especially for human contiguous gene [127, 128]. With regard to this issue, iPSCs

technology offers the opportunity to establish human *in vitro* models of LSDs, derived from patients [7, 8, 97]. Patients-derived iPSCs have permitted the study of early cellular differentiation and phenotypic specification events in a culture system, thus enabling the analysis of the abnormal early developmental impairments likely occurring in these genetic disorders and finally provide an *in vitro* screening tool for therapeutic molecules in disease-relevant cell types [129, 130].

Indeed, patient derived-iPSCs have been differentiated into many cell phenotypes affected by the disease as neurons, hepatocytes, and cardiomyocytes [121, 122, 131] that can be renewed in culture to provide sufficient quantities of differentiated mature cells for phenotypic and karotype screening and evaluation of compound efficacy. Unlike the molecular target-based drug discovery, the possibility to evaluate overall cellular phenotypic impairments within cell culture systems will enable testing of therapeutic agents that are able to counteract those disease features that arise from malfunctioning of multiple interacting pathway often previously unknown, as for example, the formation of storage macromolecules in LSDs [121, 122, 132, 133].

iPSCs have been derived from many LDS: Fabry disease, globoid cell leukodystrophy (GLD or Krabbe disease), Gaucher disease [134], Pompe disease, GM1 gangliosidosis, MPSH1, MPSI [135], MPS IIIB, MPSVII, NPC, Niemann-Pick disease type C (NPC) and Batten disease [121, 122]; MPSII [136], Danon Disease [137] and Metachromatic Leukodistrophy [138].

Of note and in accordance to the early developmental impairments occurring in LDSs, different studies [139] have reported a reduced reprogramming efficiency of somatic cells isolated from affected patients compared to healthy controls. Treatment of the cultures with a specific compound supporting NPCs and the use of higher efficiency reprogramming vectors led to an increased production colonies [121, 122, 128, 133, 140].

Highly predictive cellular and animal models are particularly critical for the clinical development of therapies for LSDs because of the small and mostly juvenile patient populations. Cellular models derived from patient iPSCs and animal models are being used more frequently because they are able to reproduce the pathogenesis of the human disease. The combination of these *in vitro* and *in vivo* models provides a unique translational platform of study to discover new treatments for LSDs including target identification, screening, lead optimization, proof-of-concept studies and preclinical development.

CONCLUDING REMARKS

The elucidation of the mechanisms underpinning the development and progression of rare CNS diseases such as MNDs and LSDs is hindered by the lack of post-mortem specimen and large-scale collection of data from patients. The identification of a reliable cell modeling system is then fundamental to study the pathogenesis of rare CNS diseases and to test novel pharmacological and cell-mediated therapeutic strategies. The advances in the last few years have identified both NSC and iPS as optimal candidates to recapitulate MNDs and LSDs *in vitro* in a human genetic background. However, the collection of clinical data on a large – scale and classification of patients according to uniform criteria still is necessary to validate modeling systems *in vitro.*

LIST OF ABBREVIATIONS

A	=	Alzheimer's Disease,
ALS	=	Amyotrophic Lateral Sclerosis
CNS	=	Central Nervous System
ERT	=	Enzyme Replacement Therapy
ESC	=	Embryonic Stem Cells
GAG	=	Glycosaminoglycans
HD	=	Huntington's Disease
IDS	=	Iduronate 2-sulfatase
iPSC or iPS	=	Induced Pluripotent Stem Cells
LSD	=	Lysosomal Storage Diseases
MN	=	Motor neuron Diseases
MPS II	=	Mucopolysaccharidosis Type II or Hunter Syndrome
MPS	=	Mucopolysaccharidosis
NSC	=	Neural Stem Cells
PD	=	Parkinson's Disease
SC	=	Stem Cells
SGZ	=	Sub-granular Zone
SVZ	=	Sub-ventricular Zone

CONSENT FOR PUBLICATION

Not applicable.

CONFLICT OF INTEREST

The authors declare no conflict of interest, financial or otherwise.

ACKNOWLEDGMENTS

We thank Jason Isaacson for reviewing the quality of written English and precious suggestions.

REFERENCES

[1] Melrose H, Lincoln S, Tyndall G, Dickson D, Farrer M. Anatomical localization of leucine-rich repeat kinase 2 in mouse brain. Neuroscience 2006; 139(3): 791-4.
[2] Dawson TM, Ko HS, Dawson VL. Genetic animal models of Parkinson's disease. Neuron 2010; 66(5): 646-61.
[3] Gispert S, Del Turco D, Garrett L, et al. Transgenic mice expressing mutant A53T human alpha-synuclein show neuronal dysfunction in the absence of aggregate formation. Mol Cell Neurosci 2003; 24(2): 419-29.
[4] Gispert S, Ricciardi F, Kurz A, et al. Parkinson phenotype in aged PINK1-deficient mice is accompanied by progressive mitochondrial dysfunction in absence of neurodegeneration. PLoS One 2009; 4(6): e5777.
[5] Chesselet MF, Richter F. Modelling of Parkinson's disease in mice. Lancet Neurol 2011; 10(12): 1108-18.
[6] Reynolds BA, Weiss S. Generation of neurons and astrocytes from isolated cells of the adult mammalian central nervous system. Science 1992; 255(5052): 1707-10.
[7] Takahashi K, Okita K, Nakagawa M, Yamanaka S. Induction of pluripotent stem cells from fibroblast cultures. Nat Protoc 2007; 2(12): 3081-9.
[8] Takahashi K, Tanabe K, Ohnuki M, et al. Induction of pluripotent stem cells from adult human fibroblasts by defined factors. Cell 2007; 131(5): 861-72.
[9] Hargus G, Ehrlich M, Hallmann AL, Kuhlmann T. Human stem cell models of neurodegeneration: a novel approach to study mechanisms of disease development. Acta Neuropathol 2014; 127(2): 151-73.
[10] Vescovi AL, Snyder EY. Establishment and properties of neural stem cell clones: plasticity in vitro and in vivo. Brain Pathol 1999; 9(3): 569-98.
[11] Yamanaka S. Strategies and new developments in the generation of patient-specific pluripotent stem cells. Cell Stem Cell 2007; 1(1): 39-49.
[12] Rosser AE, Dunnett SB. Neural transplantation in patients with Huntington's disease. CNS Drugs 2003; 17(12): 853-67.
[13] Dunnett SB, Rosser AE. Clinical translation of cell transplantation in the brain. Curr Opin Organ Transplant 2011; 16(6): 632-9.
[14] Barker RA, Mason SL, Harrower TP, et al. The long-term safety and efficacy of bilateral transplantation of human fetal striatal tissue in patients with mild to moderate Huntington's disease. J Neurol Neurosurg Psychiatry 2013; 84(6): 657-65.
[15] Dunnett SB, Rosser AE. Cell transplantation for Huntington's disease should we continue? Brain Res Bull 2007; 72(2-3): 132-47.
[16] Hotta Y. Ethical issues of the research on human embryonic stem cells. J Int Bioethique 2008; 19(3): 77-85, 124-5.
[17] Kamm FM. Ethical issues in using and not using embryonic stem cells. Stem Cell Rev 2005; 1(4): 325-30.
[18] Halevy T, Urbach A. Comparing ESC and iPSC-Based Models for Human Genetic Disorders. J Clin Med 2014; 3(4): 1146-62.
[19] Gil-Perotin S, Duran-Moreno M, Cebrian-Silla A, Ramirez M, Garcia-Belda P, Garcia-Verdugo JM. Adult neural stem cells from the subventricular zone: a review of the neurosphere assay. Anat Rec (Hoboken) 2013; 296(9): 1435-52.
[20] Deleyrolle LP, Reynolds BA. Isolation, expansion, and differentiation of adult Mammalian neural stem and progenitor cells using the neurosphere assay. Methods Mol Biol 2009; 549: 91-101.
[21] Bonfanti L. Adult neurogenesis 50 years later: limits and opportunities in mammals. Front Neurosci 2016; 10: 44.
[22] Lois C, Alvarez-Buylla A. Long-distance neuronal migration in the adult mammalian brain. Science 1994; 264(5162): 1145-8.
[23] Gage FH. Mammalian neural stem cells. Science 2000; 287(5457): 1433-8.
[24] Chaker Z, Codega P, Doetsch F. A mosaic world: puzzles revealed by adult neural stem cell heterogeneity. Wiley Interdiscip Rev Dev Biol 2016; 5(6): 640-58.
[25] Donato R, Miljan EA, Hines SJ, et al. Differential development of neuronal physiological responsiveness in two human neural stem cell lines. BMC Neurosci 2007; 8: 36.
[26] Sanai N, Tramontin AD, Quinones-Hinojosa A, et al. Unique astrocyte ribbon in adult human brain contains neural stem cells but lacks chain migration. Nature 2004; 427(6976): 740-4.
[27] van Strien ME, Sluijs JA, Reynolds BA, Steindler DA, Aronica E, Hol EM. Isolation of neural progenitor cells from the human adult subventricular zone based on expression of the cell surface marker CD271. Stem Cells Transl Med 2014; 3(4): 470-80.
[28] Verwer RW, Hermens WT, Dijkhuizen P, et al. Cells in human postmortem brain tissue slices remain alive for several weeks in culture. Faseb J 2002; 16(1): 54-60.
[29] Li Z, Oganesyan D, Mooney R, et al. L-MYC expression maintains self-renewal and prolongs multipotency of primary human neural stem cells. Stem Cell Reports 2016; 7(3): 483-95.
[30] Ring KL, Tong LM, Balestra ME, et al. Direct reprogramming of mouse and human fibroblasts into multipotent neural stem cells with a single factor. Cell Stem Cell 2012; 11(1): 100-9.
[31] Ulrich H, do Nascimento IC, Bocsi J, Tarnok A. Immunomodulation in stem cell differentiation into neurons and brain repair. Stem Cell Rev 2015; 11(3): 474-86.
[32] Mazzini L, Gelati M, Profico DC, et al. Human neural stem cell transplantation in ALS: initial results from a phase I trial. J Transl Med 2015; 13: 17.
[33] Schwarz SC, Schwarz J. Translation of stem cell therapy for neurological diseases. Transl Res 2010; 156(3): 155-60.

[34] Hsu YC, Chen SL, Wang DY, Chiu IM. Stem cell-based therapy in neural repair. Biomed J 2013; 36(3): 98-105.

[35] Golas MM, Sander B. Use of human stem cells in Huntington disease modeling and translational research. Exp Neurol 2016; 278: 76-90.

[36] Torrent R, De Angelis Rigotti F, Dell'Era P, et al. Using iPS Cells toward the understanding of Parkinson's Disease. J Clin Med 2015; 4(4): 548-66.

[37] Mungenast AE, Siegert S, Tsai LH. Modeling Alzheimer's disease with human induced pluripotent stem (iPS) cells. Mol Cell Neurosci 2016; 73: 13-31.

[38] Liu H, Zeng F, Zhang M, et al. Emerging landscape of cell penetrating peptide in reprogramming and gene editing. J Control Release 2016; 226: 124-37.

[39] Takahashi K, Yamanaka S. A developmental framework for induced pluripotency. Development 2015; 142(19): 3274-85.

[40] Ku S, Soragni E, Campau E, et al. Friedreich's ataxia induced pluripotent stem cells model intergenerational GAATTC triplet repeat instability. Cell Stem Cell 2010; 7(5): 631-7.

[41] Carvajal-Vergara X, Sevilla A, D'Souza SL, et al. Patient-specific induced pluripotent stem-cell-derived models of LEOPARD syndrome. Nature 2010; 465(7299): 808-12.

[42] Rashid ST, Corbineau S, Hannan N, et al. Modeling inherited metabolic disorders of the liver using human induced pluripotent stem cells. J Clin Invest 2010; 120(9): 3127-36.

[43] Zhang Y, Pak C, Han Y, et al. Rapid single-step induction of functional neurons from human pluripotent stem cells. Neuron 2013; 78(5): 785-98.

[44] De Filippis L, Halikere A, McGowan H, et al. Ethanol-mediated activation of the NLRP3 inflammasome in iPS cells and iPS cells-derived neural progenitor cells. Mol Brain 2016; 9(1): 51.

[45] Kriks S, Shim JW, Piao J, et al. Dopamine neurons derived from human ES cells efficiently engraft in animal models of Parkinson's disease. Nature 2011; 480(7378): 547-51.

[46] Wattanapanitch M, Klincumhom N, Potirat P, et al. Dual small-molecule targeting of SMAD signaling stimulates human induced pluripotent stem cells toward neural lineages. PLoS One 2014; 9(9): e106952.

[47] Chambers SM, Fasano CA, Papapetrou EP, Tomishima M, Sadelain M, Studer L. Highly efficient neural conversion of human ES and iPS cells by dual inhibition of SMAD signaling. Nat Biotechnol 2009; 27(3): 275-80.

[48] Adlakha YK, Seth P. The expanding horizon of MicroRNAs in cellular reprogramming. Prog Neurobiol 2017; 148: 21-39.

[49] Richner M, Victor MB, Liu Y, Abernathy D, Yoo AS. MicroRNA-based conversion of human fibroblasts into striatal medium spiny neurons. Nat Protoc 2015; 10(10): 1543-55.

[50] Victor MB, Richner M, Hermanstyne TO, et al. Generation of human striatal neurons by microRNA-dependent direct conversion of fibroblasts. Neuron 2014; 84(2): 311-23.

[51] Jesse S, Brathen G, Ferrara M, et al. Alcohol withdrawal syndrome: mechanisms, manifestations, and management. Acta Neurol Scand 2017; 135(1): 4-16.

[52] Flores-Pajot MC, Ofner M, Do MT, Lavigne E, Villeneuve PJ. Childhood autism spectrum disorders and exposure to nitrogen dioxide, and particulate matter air pollution: a review and meta-analysis. Environ Res 2016; 151: 763-76.

[53] Bottema-Beutel K. Associations between joint attention and language in autism spectrum disorder and typical development: a systematic review and meta-regression analysis. Autism Res 2016; 9(10): 1021-35.

[54] Stone D, Niyonzima N, Jerome KR. Genome editing and the next generation of antiviral therapy. Hum Genet 2016; 135(9): 1071-82.

[55] Gore A, Li Z, Fung HL, et al. Somatic coding mutations in human induced pluripotent stem cells. Nature 2011; 471(7336): 63-7.

[56] Kim K, Doi A, Wen B, et al. Epigenetic memory in induced pluripotent stem cells. Nature 2010; 467(7313): 285-90.

[57] Laurent LC, Ulitsky I, Slavin I, et al. Dynamic changes in the copy number of pluripotency and cell proliferation genes in human ESCs and iPSCs during reprogramming and time in culture. Cell Stem Cell 2011; 8(1): 106-18.

[58] Ma H, Morey R, O'Neil RC, et al. Abnormalities in human pluripotent cells due to reprogramming mechanisms. Nature 2014; 511(7508): 177-83.

[59] Ban H, Nishishita N, Fusaki N, et al. Efficient generation of transgene-free human induced pluripotent stem cells (iPSCs) by tem-perature-sensitive Sendai virus vectors. Proc Natl Acad Sci U S A 2011; 108(34): 14234-9.

[60] Okita K, Matsumura Y, Sato Y, et al. A more efficient method to generate integration-free human iPS cells. Nat Methods 2011; 8(5): 409-12.

[61] Kim D, Kim CH, Moon JI, et al. Generation of human induced pluripotent stem cells by direct delivery of reprogramming proteins. Cell Stem Cell 2009; 4(6): 472-6.

[62] Warren L, Manos PD, Ahfeldt T, et al. Highly efficient reprogramming to pluripotency and directed differentiation of human cells with synthetic modified mRNA. Cell Stem Cell 2010; 7(5): 618-30.

[63] Schuster C, Kasper E, Machts J, et al. Focal thinning of the motor cortex mirrors clinical features of amyotrophic lateral sclerosis and their phenotypes: a neuroimaging study. J Neurol 2013; 260(11): 2856-64.

[64] Valori CF, Brambilla L, Martorana F, Rossi D. The multifaceted role of glial cells in amyotrophic lateral sclerosis. Cell Mol Life Sci 2014; 71(2): 287-97.

[65] Brites D, Vaz AR. Microglia centered pathogenesis in ALS: insights in cell interconnectivity. Front Cell Neurosci 2014; 8: 117.

[66] Rizzo F, Riboldi G, Salani S, et al. Cellular therapy to target neuroinflammation in amyotrophic lateral sclerosis. Cell Mol Life Sci 2014; 71(6): 999-1015.

[67] Papadeas ST, Maragakis NJ. Advances in stem cell research for Amyotrophic Lateral Sclerosis. Curr Opin Biotechnol 2009; 20(5): 545-51.

[68] Dal Canto MC, Gurney ME. Neuropathological changes in two lines of mice carrying a transgene for mutant human Cu,Zn SOD, and in mice overexpressing wild type human SOD: a model of familial amyotrophic lateral sclerosis (FALS). Brain Res 1995; 676(1): 25-40.

[69] Nagai M, Aoki M, Miyoshi I, et al. Rats expressing human cytosolic copper-zinc superoxide dismutase transgenes with amyotrophic lateral sclerosis: associated mutations develop motor neuron disease. J Neurosci 2001; 21(23): 9246-54.

[70] Howland DS, Liu J, She Y, et al. Focal loss of the glutamate transporter EAAT2 in a transgenic rat model of SOD1 mutant-mediated amyotrophic lateral sclerosis (ALS). Proc Natl Acad Sci U S A 2002; 99(3): 1604-9.

[71] Matsumoto A, Okada Y, Nakamichi M, et al. Disease progression of human SOD1 (G93A) transgenic ALS model rats. J Neurosci Res 2006; 83(1): 119-33.

[72] Myszczynska M, Ferraiuolo L. New in vitro models to study amyotrophic lateral sclerosis. Brain Pathol 2016; 26(2): 258-65.

[73] Amoroso MW, Croft GF, Williams DJ, et al. Accelerated high-yield generation of limb-innervating motor neurons from human stem cells. J Neurosci 2013; 33(2): 574-86.

[74] Wichterle H, Lieberam I, Porter JA, Jessell TM. Directed differentiation of embryonic stem cells into motor neurons. Cell 2002; 110(3): 385-97.

[75] Martin LJ, Liu Z, Chen K, et al. Motor neuron degeneration in amyotrophic lateral sclerosis mutant superoxide dismutase-1 transgenic mice: mechanisms of mitochondriopathy and cell death. J Comp Neurol 2007; 500(1): 20-46.

[76] Jordan PM, Ojeda LD, Thonhoff JR, et al. Generation of spinal motor neurons from human fetal brain-derived neural stem cells: role of basic fibroblast growth factor. J Neurosci Res 2009; 87(2): 318-32.

[77] Wu P, Tarasenko YI, Gu Y, Huang LY, Coggeshall RE, Yu Y. Region-specific generation of cholinergic neurons from fetal human neural stem cells grafted in adult rat. Nat Neurosci 2002; 5(12): 1271-8.

[78] Yang N, Ng YH, Pang ZP, Sudhof TC, Wernig M. Induced neuronal cells: how to make and define a neuron. Cell Stem Cell 2011; 9(6): 517-25.

[79] Egawa N, Kitaoka S, Tsukita K, et al. Drug screening for ALS using patient-specific induced pluripotent stem cells. Sci Transl Med 2012; 4(145): 145ra04.

[80] Marchetto MC, Muotri AR, Mu Y, Smith AM, Cezar GG, Gage FH. Non-cell-autonomous effect of human SOD1 G37R astrocytes on motor neurons derived from human embryonic stem cells. Cell Stem Cell 2008; 3(6): 649-57.

[81] Wainger BJ, Kiskinis E, Mellin C, et al. Intrinsic membrane hyperexcitability of amyotrophic lateral sclerosis patient-derived motor neurons. Cell Rep 2014; 7(1): 1-11.

[82]   Chen H, Qian K, Du Z, *et al.* Modeling ALS with iPSCs reveals that mutant SOD1 misregulates neurofilament balance in motor neurons. Cell Stem Cell 2014; 14(6): 796-809.

[83]   Kiskinis E, Sandoe J, Williams LA, *et al.* Pathways disrupted in human ALS motor neurons identified through genetic correction of mutant SOD1. Cell Stem Cell 2014; 14(6): 781-95.

[84]   Geevasinga N, Menon P, Ozdinler PH, Kiernan MC, Vucic S. Pathophysiological and diagnostic implications of cortical dysfunction in ALS. Nat Rev Neurol. 2016; 12(11): 651-61.

[85]   Kuo JJ, Siddique T, Fu R, Heckman CJ. Increased persistent Na(+) current and its effect on excitability in motoneurones cultured from mutant SOD1 mice. J Physiol 2005; 563(Pt 3): 843-54.

[86]   Vucic S, Kiernan MC. Upregulation of persistent sodium conductances in familial ALS. J Neurol Neurosurg Psychiatry 2010; 81(2): 222-7.

[87]   Urbani A, Belluzzi O. Riluzole inhibits the persistent sodium current in mammalian CNS neurons. Eur J Neurosci 2000; 12(10): 3567-74.

[88]   Almeida S, Gascon E, Tran H. Modeling key pathological features of frontotemporal dementia with C9ORF72 repeat expansion in iPSC-derived human neurons. Acta Neuropathol 2013; 126(3): 385-99.

[89]   Donnelly CJ, Zhang PW, Pham JT, *et al.* RNA Toxicity from the ALS/FTD C9ORF72 expansion is mitigated by antisense intervention. Neuron 2013; 80(2): 415-28.

[90]   Sareen D, O'Rourke JG, Meera P, *et al.* Targeting RNA foci in iPSC-derived motor neurons from ALS patients with a C9ORF72 repeat expansion. Sci Transl Med 2013; 5(208): 208ra149.

[91]   DeJesus-Hernandez M, Mackenzie IR, Boeve BF, *et al.* Expanded GGGGCC hexanucleotide repeat in noncoding region of C9ORF72 causes chromosome 9p-linked FTD and ALS. Neuron 2011; 72(2): 245-56.

[92]   Patterson M, Chan DN, Ha I, *et al.* Defining the nature of human pluripotent stem cell progeny. Cell Research 2011; 22(1): 178-93.

[93]   Batista LF, Pech MF, Zhong FL, *et al.* Telomere shortening and loss of self-renewal in dyskeratosis congenita induced pluripotent stem cells. Nature 2011; 474(7351): 399-402.

[94]   Nishitoh H, Kadowaki H, Nagai A, *et al.* ALS-linked mutant SOD1 induces ER stress- and ASK1-dependent motor neuron death by targeting Derlin-1. Genes Dev 2008; 22(11): 1451-64.

[95]   Fakhoury M. Role of immunity and inflammation in the pathophysiology of neurodegenerative diseases. Neurodegener Dis 2015; 15(2): 63-9.

[96]   Clement AM, Nguyen MD, Roberts EA, *et al.* Wild-type nonneuronal cells extend survival of SOD1 mutant motor neurons in ALS mice. Science 2003; 302(5642): 113-7.

[97]   Nakagawa M, Koyanagi M, Tanabe K, *et al.* Generation of induced pluripotent stem cells without Myc from mouse and human fibroblasts. Nat Biotechnol 2008; 26(1): 101-6.

[98]   Di Giorgio FP, Carrasco MA, Siao MC, Maniatis T, Eggan K. Noncell autonomous effect of glia on motor neurons in an embryonic stem cell-based ALS model. Nat Neurosci 2007; 10(5): 608-14.

[99]   Nagai M, Re DB, Nagata T, *et al.* Astrocytes expressing ALS-linked mutated SOD1 release factors selectively toxic to motor neurons. Nat Neurosci 2007; 10(5): 615-22.

[100]   Di Giorgio FP, Boulting GL, Bobrowicz S, Eggan KC. Human embryonic stem cell-derived motor neurons are sensitive to the toxic effect of glial cells carrying an ALS-causing mutation. Cell Stem Cell 2008; 3(6): 637-48.

[101]   Boillee S, Vande Velde C, Cleveland DW. ALS: a disease of motor neurons and their nonneuronal neighbors. Neuron 2006; 52(1): 39-59.

[102]   Almer G, Guegan C, Teismann P, *et al.* Increased expression of the pro-inflammatory enzyme cyclooxygenase-2 in amyotrophic lateral sclerosis. Ann Neurol 2001; 49(2): 176-85.

[103]   Kondo M, Shibata T, Kumagai T, *et al.* 15-Deoxy-Delta(12,14)-prostaglandin J(2): the endogenous electrophile that induces neuronal apoptosis. Proc Natl Acad Sci U S A 2002; 99(11): 7367-72.

[104]   Allodi I, Comley L, Nichterwitz S, *et al.* Differential neuronal vulnerability identifies IGF-2 as a protective factor in ALS. Scientific Reports, Published online: 16 May 2016; | doi: 10.1038/srep25960. 2016.

[105]   Nizzardo M, Simone C, Rizzo F, *et al.* Minimally invasive transplantation of iPSC-derived ALDHhiSSCloVLA4+ neural stem cells effectively improves the phenotype of an amyotrophic lateral sclerosis model. Hum Mol Genet 2014; 23(2): 342-54.

[106]   Nizzardo M, Bucchia M, Ramirez A, *et al.* iPSC-derived LewisX+CXCR4+beta1-integrin+ neural stem cells improve the amyotrophic lateral sclerosis phenotype by preserving motor neurons and muscle innervation in human and rodent models. Hum Mol Genet 2016; 25(15): 3152-3163.

[107]   Burton BK. Inborn errors of metabolism in infancy: a guide to diagnosis. Pediatrics 1998; 102(6): E69.

[108]   Platt FM, Boland B, van der Spoel AC. The cell biology of disease: lysosomal storage disorders: the cellular impact of lysosomal dysfunction. J Cell Biol 2012; 199(5): 723-34.

[109]   Fuller M, Meikle PJ, Hopwood JJ. Epidemiology of lysosomal storage diseases: an overview. 2006.

[110]   Ballabio A, Gieselmann V. Lysosomal disorders: from storage to cellular damage. Biochim Biophys Acta 2009; 1793(4): 684-96.

[111]   Schulze H, Sandhoff K. Lysosomal Lipid Storage Diseases. Cold Spring Harb Perspect Biol 32011.

[112]   Saftig P, Klumperman J. Lysosome biogenesis and lysosomal membrane proteins: trafficking meets function. Nat Rev Mol Cell Biol 2009; 10(9): 623-35.

[113]   Muenzer J. Overview of the mucopolysaccharidoses. Rheumatology (Oxford) 2011; 50 Suppl 5: v4-12.

[114]   Tomatsu S, Sawamoto K, Shimada T, *et al.* Enzyme replacement therapy for treating mucopolysaccharidosis type IVA (Morquio A syndrome): effect and limitations. Expert Opin Orphan Drugs 2015; 3(11): 1279-90.

[115]   Munoz-Rojas MV, Vieira T, Costa R, *et al.* Intrathecal enzyme replacement therapy in a patient with mucopolysaccharidosis type I and symptomatic spinal cord compression. Am J Med Genet A 2008; 146a(19): 2538-44.

[116]   Tuschl K, Gal A, Paschke E, Kircher S, Bodamer OA. Mucopolysaccharidosis type II in females: case report and review of literature. Pediatr Neurol 2005; 32(4): 270-2.

[117]   Scarpa M, Almassy Z, Beck M, *et al.* Mucopolysaccharidosis type II: European recommendations for the diagnosis and multidisciplinary management of a rare disease. Orphanet J Rare Dis 2011; 6: 72.

[118]   Biffi A, Capotondo A, Fasano S, *et al.* Gene therapy of metachromatic leukodystrophy reverses neurological damage and deficits in mice. J Clin Invest 2006; 116(11): 3070-82.

[119]   Biffi A, Cesani M. Human hematopoietic stem cells in gene therapy: pre-clinical and clinical issues. Curr Gene Ther 2008; 8(2): 135-46.

[120]   Biffi A, Montini E, Lorioli L, *et al.* Lentiviral hematopoietic stem cell gene therapy benefits metachromatic leukodystrophy. Science 2013; 341(6148): 1233158.

[121]   Meng XL, Shen JS, Kawagoe S, Ohashi T, Brady RO, Eto Y. Induced pluripotent stem cells derived from mouse models of lysosomal storage disorders. Proc Natl Acad Sci U S A 2010; 107(17): 7886-91.

[122]   Xu M, Motabar O, Ferrer M, Marugan JJ, Zheng W, Ottinger EA. Disease models for the development of therapies for lysosomal storage diseases. Ann N Y Acad Sci 2016; 1371(1): 15-29.

[123]   Visigalli I, Delai S, Politi LS, *et al.* Gene therapy augments the efficacy of hematopoietic cell transplantation and fully corrects mucopolysaccharidosis type I phenotype in the mouse model. Blood 1162010. p. 5130-9.

[124]   Altarescu G, Renbaum P, Eldar-Geva T, *et al.* Preimplantation genetic diagnosis (PGD) for a treatable disorder: gaucher disease type 1 as a model. Blood Cells Mol Dis 2011; 46(1): 15-8.

[125]   Fusar Poli E, Zalfa C, D'Avanzo F, *et al.* Murine neural stem cells model Hunter disease in vitro: glial cell-mediated neurodegeneration as a possible mechanism involved. Cell Death Dis 2013; 1: 12.

[126]   Zalfa C, Verpelli C, D'Avanzo F, *et al.* Oxidative damage with glial degeneration drives neuronal demise in MPSII disease. Cell Death Dis 2016; 7(8): e233.

[127]   Chen M, Tomkins DJ, Auerbach W, *et al.* Inactivation of Fac in mice produces inducible chromosomal instability and reduced fertility reminiscent of Fanconi anaemia. Nat Genet 1996; 12(4): 448-51.

[128]   Nelson DL, Gibbs RA. Genetics. The critical region in trisomy 21. Science 2004; 306(5696): 619-21.

[129]   Huang HP, Chuang CY, Kuo HC. Induced pluripotent stem cell technology for disease modeling and drug screening with emphasis on lysosomal storage diseases. Stem Cell Res Ther 2012; 3(4): 34.

[130]   Yu D, Swaroop M, Wang M, *et al.* Niemann-Pick disease type c: induced pluripotent stem cell-derived neuronal cells for modeling

neural disease and evaluating drug efficacy. J Biomol Screen 2014; 19(8): 1164-73.

[131]   Bellin M, Marchetto MC, Gage FH, Mummery CL. Induced pluripotent stem cells: the new patient? Nat Rev Mol Cell Biol 2012; 13(11): 713-26.

[132]   Zheng W, Thorne N, McKew JC. Phenotypic screens as a renewed approach for drug discovery. Drug Discov Today 2013; 18(21-22): 1067-73.

[133]   Aflaki E, Stubblefield BK, Maniwang E, *et al.* Macrophage models of Gaucher disease for evaluating disease pathogenesis and candidate drugs. Sci Transl Med 2014; 6(240): 240ra73.

[134]   Tiscornia G, Vivas EL, Matalonga L, *et al.* Neuronopathic Gaucher's disease: induced pluripotent stem cells for disease modelling and testing chaperone activity of small compounds. Hum Mol Genet 2013; 22(4): 633-45.

[135]   Tolar J, Park IH, Xia L, *et al.* Hematopoietic differentiation of induced pluripotent stem cells from patients with mucopolysaccharidosis type I (Hurler syndrome). Blood 2011; 117(3): 839-47.

[136]   Varga E, Nemes C, Bock I, *et al.* Generation of Mucopolysaccharidosis type II (MPS II) human induced pluripotent stem cell (iPSC) line from a 3-year-old male with pathogenic IDS mutation. Stem Cell Res 2016; 17(3): 479-81.

[137]   Hashem SI, Perry CN, Bauer M, *et al.* Brief Report: oxidative stress mediates cardiomyocyte apoptosis in a human model of danon disease and heart failure. Stem Cells 2015; 33(7): 2343-50.

[138]   Meneghini V, Frati G, Sala D, *et al.* Generation of human induced pluripotent stem cell-derived bona fide neural stem cells for *ex vivo* gene therapy of metachromatic leukodystrophy. Stem Cells Transl Med 2016; 6(2): 352-368.

[139]   Lemonnier T, Blanchard S, Toli D, *et al.* Modeling neuronal defects associated with a lysosomal disorder using patient-derived induced pluripotent stem cells. Hum Mol Genet 2011; 20(18): 3653-66.

[140]   Lieu PT, Fontes A, Vemuri MC, Macarthur CC. Generation of induced pluripotent stem cells with CytoTune, a non-integrating Sendai virus. Methods Mol Biol 2013; 997: 45-56.

Send Orders for Reprints to reprints@benthamscience.ae

CNS & Neurological Disorders - Drug Targets, 2017, *16,* 927-935

REVIEW ARTICLE

Leber's Hereditary Optic Neuropathy: Novel Views and Persisting Challenges

Jasna Jančić[1], Janko Samardžić[2,*], Stevan Stojanović[1], Amalija Stojanović[3], Ana Marija Milanović[3], Blažo Nikolić[1], Nikola Ivančević[1] and Vladimir Kostić[4]

[1]*Clinic of Neurology and Psychiatry for Children and Youth, Medical Faculty, University of Belgrade, Belgrade, Serbia;* [2]*Institute of Pharmacology, Clinical Pharmacology and Toxicology, Medical Faculty, University of Belgrade, Belgrade, Serbia;* [3]*Medical Faculty, University of Belgrade, Belgrade, Serbia;* [4]*Clinic of Neurology, Medical Faculty, University of Belgrade, Belgrade, Serbia*

ARTICLE HISTORY

Received: May 12, 2017
Revised: July 03, 2017
Accepted: July 18, 2017

DOI:
10.2174/1871527316666170724172455

Abstract: ***Background & Objective***: Leber's hereditary optic neuropathy is an inherited form of optic neuropathy, genetically and pathophysiologically based on mitochondrial insufficiency causing bilateral loss of central vision mostly amongst young adults. Despite being one of the most common mitochondrial diseases, the explanation for its pathophysiological background and effective clinical solutions remain elusive. Widening the scope in the search for pathological findings beyond the optic system has yielded several non-ophthalmologic findings, which might imply that Leber's hereditary optic neuropathy is in fact a multi-systemic disease.

Conclusion: The aim of this review is to provide an overview of literature regarding the epidemiology, etiology, pathogenesis, clinical features, diagnostics and possible treatment options and drug targets, as well as presenting challenges related to the disease and proposing a diagnostic algorithm based on current clinical experience.

Keywords: Leber's hereditary optic neuropathy, epidemiology, etiopathogenesis, clinical features, drug targets, multi-systemic involvement, mitochondrial disease, ophthalmological manifestations.

1. INTRODUCTION

Leber's hereditary optic neuropathy (LHON) is an inherited form of optic neuropathy, genetically and pathophysiologically based on mitochondrial insufficiency causing bilateral loss of central vision mostly amongst young adults. Despite being one of the most common mitochondrial diseases [1, 2], epidemiological estimations of LHON prevalence are scarce and somewhat divergent. In European population over 95% of LHON cases are caused by one of the three most common mutations (m.11778G>A, m.3460G>A and m.14484T>C, affecting ND4, ND1 and ND6 genes, respectively) [3], with additional rare pathogenic variants associated with the disease (*www.mitomap.org*). The prevalence of LHON is 1 in 31 000 in the North UK [4], 1 in 39 000 in the Netherlands [5] and 1 in 50 000 in Finland [6], mostly affecting males (80-90%) [7]. Certain authors [8] have shown a lower prevalence of LHON. The disease occurs at a median of 15-35 years of age, but presentation is possible within a broader age specter of 2 to 80 years [8, 9]. Around 1 in 9000 individuals are carriers of LHON-related mitochondrial mutations and only 20-60% of males and 4-32% of females develop clinical features of the disease [8]. From the perspective of LHON pathogenesis, all pathogenic mutations cause disturbances in mitochondrial complex I (NADH:ubiquinone oxidoreductase) [10], almost exclusively leading to retinal ganglion cell (RGC) loss.

These findings lead to several challenging issues:

- The evident gender bias lacks definitive explanation. The difference in prevalence and male to female ratio amongst the Serbian population [8], when compared to other findings, could be attributed to challenges in the diagnosis of LHON. Alternatively, sequencing efforts in the past used to be riddled with issues leading to the rise of phantom mutations and false positive results [11], potentially hindering the creation of a clear epidemiologic and clinical image of LHON. Next generation mitochondrial genome sequencing has progressed considerably in the past decade, paving the way for other potential explanations.

- The cause of incomplete penetrance is unknown, but might be found in undisclosed genetic, biochemical and environmental factors, possibly revealing a potential target for therapeutic intervention.

*Address correspondence to this author at the Institute of Pharmacology, Clinical Pharmacology and Toxicology, Medical Faculty, University of Belgrade, Belgrade, Serbia; Tel: +381641212849; Fax: +381113643397; E-mails: janko.samardzic@med.bg.ac.rs; jankomedico@yahoo.es

- Despite the general affliction of the cellular energy production amongst all tissues, including highly ATP-demanding cells such as neighboring retinal phosphoreceptor cells, only RGCs seem to be susceptible to cell death, whilst other cells show no histological changes. Expanding beyond the concept of RGC sensitivity, the affliction of other tissues could be clarified by studying LHON-linked syndromes. In a clinical setting LHON is generally considered non-syndromatic, but, albeit rarely, coincides with dystonia [12], multiple-sclerosis-like illness [13] and cerebellar ataxia [14]. Advanced diagnostic tools and imaging techniques might provide insight into extra-optic involvement in LHON.

In this review, we discuss findings revolving around the etiology and pathogenesis of LHON, as well as clinical, diagnostic and treatment issues concerning the disease.

2. ETIOLOGY

Etiology of disease is based on genetic and epigenetic factors.

2.1. Genetic Aspects of LHON

The mitochondria contain their own genome with a procariotic organization - a multi-copied double-stranded circular DNA molecule, containing 37 genes (www.mitomap.org). The origin of this model presumably lies in a primordial symbiotic relationship: a phagocyted prokaryotic organism, the latter mitochondria, enabled efficient ATP synthesis and ROS protection to its eukaryotic host, in exchange for an ideal environment for replication [15]. While mitochondria still provide the same function and replicate independently, they have become heavily reliant on the nuclear genome that encodes most of their components. This means that inherited mitochondrial diseases might develop either from mutations in the mtDNA, which is the case in LHON [16], or the nuclear DNA. The mtDNA in a human organism is entirely of maternal origin after fertilization, the zygote utilizes only ovarial egg mitochondria, disintegrating such organelles from the paternal side via proteolysis [17]. This genetic constellation leads to a maternal inheritance of primary mtDNA mutations causing LHON. However, the phenotype expression depends on mitochondrial (mutation type, heteroplasmy, replicative segregation, the critical threshold) and extra-mitochondrial factors (secondary mutations, environmental factors). The complex inter-reactions between the aforementioned elements are the likely cause of incomplete LHON penetrance.

Heteroplasmy denotes the occurrence of both functionally non-affected (wild-type) and affected mitochondria within the same cell, replicating into two or more strains of organelles. Despite the suboptimal functioning of a certain number of mitochondria, the remaining functional reserve disables disturbances at a cellular level. Segregated randomly during cell division [18, 19], the number of defect mitochondria reaches the critical threshold in some cells, after which phenotype changes arise. When all mitochondria in a cell belong to a single strain, the term homoplasmy is used. Mitochondrial segregation can be mathematically pre-

dicted [19]. In LHON, symptomatic carriers are mostly homoplasmic (80-90%) rare heteroplasmic exceptions [20]. This suggests that a high threshold is the basic requirement for the development of LHON, however different levels of heteroplasmy do not dictate the advent of the disease. This is different when compared to some of the other mitochondrial diseases, where the threshold effect has a significant role.

The role of secondary, non-mitochondrial mutations is controversial. Due to the gender bias favoring males, an involvement of an X-linked factor has been hypothesized. After conducting a pedigree analysis amongst 85 families affected by LHON, Harding *et al.* have concluded that their results show a X-linked susceptibility [20], a finding challenged in other studies [21, 22]. Some association has been found with markers on chromosomes 1, 3, 12, 13 and 18 [23].

2.2. Epigenetic Influences

Given the epidemiological and clinical characteristics of LHON, the disease pathophysiology might not be fully explained by genetically based errors, since several exofactors may play a significant role in the formation of the disease, including smoking [24], light [25], linezolide [26], erythromycin [27], anti-retroviral drugs [28] and ethambutol [29]. Conversely, 17B-estradiol might have a protective effect [30], possibly explaining the gender bias. The Cuban epidemic of a LHON-like disease [31] and the resemblance to tobacco-alcohol amblyopia [32], further fuel claims that LHON is a multifactorial disease.

3. PATHOGENESIS

The oxidative phosphorylation complex I affection and RGC loss are the common denominators when discussing the pathophysiological basis of LHON. Being a part of the respiratory chain, the complex I is a component of an ATP-producing system, functioning in aerobic conditions. Energy depletion is an expected consequence of its malfunction. The exploration of the bioenergetic failure hypothesis has been conducted on several cell lines with inserted mutated ND1, ND4 and ND6 subunit genes in an attempt to mimic the high-demanding energetic metabolism of RGCs. A rapid decrease of ATP concentration has been detected in all three types of mutation-carrying cell cultures [33]. However, only the ND1 subunit mutation is confirmed to actually cause a considerable decrease of NADH:ubiquinone oxidoreductase activity [34, 35], whereas ND4 and ND6 mutations seem not to have the mentioned effect [36, 37].

A concise model of cell death is yet to be established. Due to lack of inflammation of the optic bundle, apoptosis has been the presumed mechanism of RGC loss [38, 39]. In contrast, mtDNA mutation affecting phosphorylation complex V, found in the lethal Leigh disease, leads to brain necrosis mainly without RGC loss [40, 41], although a report of Leigh-like encephalopathy has been identified in LHON, highlighting the significance of the energetic defect model in RGC sensitivity [42]. The explanation behind the selective RGC apoptotic vulnerability to complex I mutations remains elusive. Anyhow, apoptosis is related to mitochondrial activity, being enabled by several pathways intertwined with the organelle. A mechanism connecting ATP depletion and apoptosis was shown to revolve around the release of cytochrome c, apoptosis inducing factor (AIF) and endonuclease G (endo-G) from the mitochondria into the cytosol, following ATP exhaustion [43]. However, these findings might not fully explain the chain of events taking place in RGCs, since most *in vitro* studies were conducted on lymphoblast, fibroblast and cybrid cell lines. Hypothetically, an ideal experimental model would have to fully take into account RGC structural and biochemical distinctiveness.

Another possible cause of cellular deterioration is oxidative stress [44]. Complex 1 is a known source of reactive oxygen species [45] and, when deficient, could further sensitize RGCs to apoptosis. Calcium deregulation [46], increased permeability of the mitochondrial permeability transition pores [47] glutamate excitotoxicity [48] and endoplasmatic reticulum dysfunction [49, 50], are also looked into as possible accomplices in RGC loss.

RGC structural characteristics might also play a role in LHON pathogenesis. Demyelinated initial segments of RGC axons in the papillo-macullar bundle, in the neuronal path preceding the lamina cribrosa, contain significantly larger aggregations of mitochondria then the myelinated segments [51], likely due to the high-energy demand in an absence of saltatory conduction. In an energy deficient circumstance, these regions are first to be under metabolic strain, and first to undergo degeneration in LHON [52]. It should be mentioned that other cells, despite not undergoing morphologic changes, might have functional disruption. This is demonstrated by disturbances in color vision found in some patients, possibly owing to the presence of phosphoreceptor cell dysfunction [52].

However, rapid biogenesis of mitochondria, acting as a compensatory mechanism in bioenergetic depletion, might be a possible cause of incomplete penetrance in LHON, where unaffected carriers seem to have a higher capacity to develop an efficient response [53].

4. CLINICAL FEATURES

In a clinical setting, LHON is a disease usually characterized by an acutely progressing loss of vision and is comprised of three phases: the pre-symptomatic, acute and chronic (atrophic) phase, Table **1**. Additionally, it is possible for LHON to take a subclinical course amongst carriers of LHON mutations, who might possess subtle diagnostic findings [52].

4.1. Symptoms of LHON

The pre-symptomatic phase denotes the beginning of LHON clinical development, being different from the subclinical form due to the lack of clinical and symptomatic progression in the latter [54]. Vision is likely to be perceived as normal by patients, despite the possible presence of small scotomas and/or subtle loss of color vision. Patients are classically considered to be in the acute symptomatic phase when vision blurring arises [8]. However, the earliest sign of the disease can be dyschromatopsia [52], which might not be apparent to patients [55]. As shown by epidemiological data, the disease usually affects young males in a sudden manner, even though individuals can be affected at a wide age spectrum. Vision loss can present within a spectrum from complete loss of light perception on one side, to a positive outcome of 20/20 vision on the other side of the spectrum [8]. Visual field abnormality typically starts centrocecally, unilaterally and without associated pain [56], as seen in 75% of cases [57]. The other eye is subsequently similarly affected, in 97% of cases within one year, mostly with an 8-week delay [58], but a delayed bilateralization of 18 years has been reported [59]. In 25% of cases a simultaneous bilateral vision loss occurs [57], but it is possible that some these are events of diagnoses not made during the monocular phase. Examples of monocular disease forms have also been reported [60]. Vision loss might take 5-8 months to fully prograde [61], which is then marked as a subacute variant of LHON. Rarely, patients might exhibit slow and gradual development lasting longer than 8 months [8, 62]. After the acute phase, LHON patients enter the chronic (atrophic) phase of the disease, usually characterized by a static and permanent loss of central vision causing serious visual impairment.

4.2. LHON-associated Disorders

LHON-MS: Harding *et al.* [63] were first to describe female patients with LHON who have developed an illness indistinguishable from multiple sclerosis (MS). While it is possible that this co-morbidity is coincidental [64], certain traits of the LHON-MS syndrome raise the question if there is a common pathophysiological and clinical ground between these diseases. Firstly, when associated with MS, LHON is far more likely to show atypical clinical features including female predominance [65] and unilateral vision loss [66]. Secondly, LHON and MS share some clinical traits, such as the Uhthoff phenomenon [67, 78] and demyelinating-like lesions on MRI [68]. Due to LHON rarity, it is a challenge to

Table 1.   The clinical features and phases of LHON development.

Presymptomatic	Acute	Chronic
Normal vision	Blurred vision	Visual loss
Normal visual field or small scotomas	Blind spot enlargement	Central scotoma
Dyschromatopsia	Dyschromatopsia	Color blindness
Visual evoked potentials (VEP) - decreased amplitude	VEP - decreased amplitude and latencies prolongation	VEP - absence
Peripapillary telangiectatic microangiopathy	Peripapillary telangiectatic microangiopathy	Optic nerve atrophy
Normal disc or peripapillary telangiectatic microangiopathy	Optic disc pseudoedema	Optic disc paleness

assess if LHON is statistically more common amongst MS patients or, conversely, MS amongst LHON patients. Matthews *et al.* [69] state that MS coexists with LHON about 50 times more frequently than expected by chance.

LHON plus: Other than visual abnormalities, LHON might present with additional neurologic symptoms, then labeled as LHON+. These include tremor [70], dystonia [12] ataxia [14], peripheral neuropathy [57], Parkinsonism [71], epileptic seizures [9], hearing disturbances [72] and thoracic kyphosis [73]. A study has shown that 59% of examined patients presented with neurological signs in addition to the visual symptomatology [74]. It remains unclear if and which of these manifestations are coincidental.

LHON-cardio: LHON and LHON+ can be associated with cardiological manifestations including Wolf-Parkinson-White syndrome [75], hypertrophic [76] or dilatative [14] cardiomyopathy. Therefore, patients with LHON should be cardiologically examined.

4.3. Diagnostic Procedures and Findings

LHON should be considered as a diagnosis in all patients with bilateral optic neuropathy of undetermined origin, whereas a history of acute vision loss within the patient's family is indicative of LHON.

Diagnostic procedures aiding in LHON diagnosis include fundoscopic examination supplemented by fluorescein angiography, optical coherence tomography (OCT) and visual evoked potentials (VEP). Additional methods include neuroimaging, the use of magnetic resonance imaging (MRI), magnetic resonance spectroscopy (MRS), functional magnetic resonance imaging (fMRI), diffusion tensor imaging (DTI) and voxel-based morphometry (VBM). The definitive diagnosis is made through molecular testing (blood mtDNA sequencing) [9].

Fundoscopic examination during the acute phase can reveal different findings: tortuous and telangiectatic retinal blood vessels, circumscriptuous "pseudoedema" surrounding the optic disc without leakage on fluorescein angiography (which helps in the differential diagnosis from real edema, presenting with leakage), optic disc hemorrhage, optic disc hemorrhage, retinal hemorrhage, retinal lining and macular edema [9, 62]. It is possible for LHON patients in the acute phase to lack any fundoscopic findings, possibly delaying diagnosis [56, 77]. Alternatively, the presence of fundus pathology amongst asymptomatic LHON carriers might not prognosticate loss of vision [78, 79]. Coinciding with the progression towards the chronic phase, the fundus findings are resolved and succeeded by optic disc pallor and cupping [80]. It should be noted that the pupillary light reflex is mostly preserved in LHON [81], despite the optic atrophy. This can be explained by melanopsin-RGC preservation [82].

The value of OCT lies in the ability to reveal a temporal thickening of the retinal nerve fiber layer (RNFL) in asymptomatic carriers [83], as well as demonstrating thickening in the acute phase and RNFL thinning in the chronic phase, commencing within the macular region in some cases [84]. A VBM study [85] correlated visual cortex and optic radiation atrophy to average and temporal RNFL thickness reduction.

VEP analysis can be conducted via patterned VEP (PVEP) or flash VEP (FVEP) [86]. VEP seems not to show significant changes in asymptomatic carriers [87]. PVEP findings during the early acute stage of the disease are greatly distorted, with increased P100 latencies and decreased amplitudes [88]. As the disease further progresses and vision fades, only FVEP application is possible, showing further prolongation of latencies and decline of response wave amplitudes. [89]. The use of evoked potentials as a diagnostic and research tool in LHON might also include brain stem auditory evoked potentials (BAEP), since this method has yielded pathological findings in certain patients [72, 89, 90], indicative of extraocular involvement [91].

MRI, MRS, fMRI and DTI analysis might show different extraocular findings. In a 12-year follow up study, Jancic *et al.* [68] utilized MRI and MRS to evaluate LHON patients, detecting infratentorial and supratentorial white mass lesions, along with MRS abnormalities. However, no neurological deterioration was clinically present. Patients with mostly normal appearing white matter on MRI have shown MRS changes [92], implying that MRS could be used as a diagnostic and research tool in detection of occult brain lesions in LHON. Abnormalities in resting state fluctuations have been shown on an fMRI study [93], revealing not only visual, but also auditory pathology. Moreover, in a contrast to a DTI study conducted in 2001 [94], which has found no damage of the calcarine cortex and optic radiations, a newer DTI study [95] has shown the involvement of optic and acoustic regions, which the authors attributed to transsynaptic degeneration.

Therefore, advanced imaging techniques have a high value in the research concerning LHON, and quite possibly might evolve into important diagnostic tools, along with their introduction into clinical practice [96].

4.4. Diagnostic Algorithm

Based on clinical experience with LHON, we introduce diagnostic algorithms for patients suspected to have LHON and for family members at risk of developing LHON.

We suggest the following diagnostic procedures are to be conducted amongst patients suspected to have LHON, as a part of initial disease diagnosis: anamnesis, family tree analysis, neurological examination, neuro-ophthalmologic examination (visual acuity assessment, pupil reaction assessment, fundoscopic examination, visual field examination, color vision examination), fluorescein angiography, electroretinography, VEP, BAEP, audiometry, electromyoneuromyography, lactate and pyruvate blood levels, cerebrospinal fluid oligoclonal band test, brain MRI, optic MRI on STIR frequencies, MRS and fMRI, cardiologic assessment (echocardiography and electrocardiogrpahy), body weight and height measurements and molecular-genetic analysis (detection of mtDNA mutations via PCR and sequencing).

In the case of family members that are at risk of developing LHON, these steps are suggested: neurological examination, neuro-ophthalmologic examination (visual acuity assessment, fundoscopic examination, visual field examination, color vision examination), electroretinography, VEP, BAEP, audiometry, brain MRI, optic MRI on STIR frequencies, (MRS and fMRI, cardiologic assessment (echocardiography and electrocardiogrpahy) and molecular-genetic analysis (detection of mtDNA mutations via PCR and sequencing).

4.5. Differential Diagnosis

Due to their similarity to LHON, several other diseases should be considered in the differential diagnosis [9]: autosomal dominant optic atrophy, tobacco-alcohol amblyopia, nutritive deficiency (B1, B2, folic acid, B12), toxic optic neuropathies in methanol, cyanide poisoning, as well as ethambutol or chloramphenicol-induced neuropathies. It should be noted that a careful deliberation needs to be conducted when differentiating atypical LHON from autosomal dominant optic atrophy, as they both might present with central scotomas and bilateral loss of vision.

4.6. Prognosis

While patients do usually show differing levels of recovery after the acute phase, permanent visual loss is a common consequence, leading to a severe negative impact on the quality of life [97]. However, 82% of LHON patients are successfully employed despite the consequences of the disease [98]. Despite the loss of central visual acuity, patients usually have a relatively good perception of the environment.

Age-wise, LHON with childhood onset at less than 10 years of age might exhibit a more benign clinical form, with a higher level of visual recovery [99]. When comparing the clinical features of the m.11778G>A, m.3460G>A and m.14484T>C mutations in the acute phase, no significant differences are found [9]. However, mutation type does affect prognosis in terms of penetrance and recovery where m.11778G>A, m.3460G>A and m.14484T>C are considered the worst, the intermediate and the mildest variant, respectively [56, 57]. Visual improvement is possible, whereas the m.14484T>C mutation was associated with the highest chance of spontaneous recovery [100, 115].

5. THERAPY OF LHON

The current therapeutic strategies in LHON include the supportive and symptomatic treatment, nutritional supplements, ubiquinone analogues, pharmacological agonists and mitochondrial genesis activators.

5.1. Supportive and Symptomatic Treatment

The significant decline in the quality of life and a current lack of definitive curative options beckon the need for symptomatic therapy designed to ameliorate the LHON patient's condition. Low-vision rehabilitation therapy and counseling might be beneficial [101], possibly encouraging patients to utilize their mostly unaffected peripheral vision to retain functionality. Additionally, patients should be advised to avoid the precipitating factors of the disease such as alcohol, tobacco, heat and certain types of medication. A ketogenic diet has been hypothesized to be helpful [102]. Genetic counseling could also be an important measure for the quality of patients' lives [57, 103].

5.2. Nutritional Supplements

Due to their proposed antioxidant and neuroprotective effects, a number of vitamins (B2, B3, B12, C, E, and folic acid) and supplements (alpha-lipoic acid, carnitine, creatine, L-arginine, and dichloroacetate) have been utilized in the treatment of LHON [104], either individually or combined. However, there is a lack of convincing evidence that these forms of therapy benefit LHON patients [105].

5.3. Ubiquinone Analogues

The utilization of ubiquinone analogues relies on the premise that these agents could enable a circumvention of the blockage in the electron transport chain, caused by the functional disturbance of mitochondrial complex I in LHON. By acting as acceptors of reduction equivalents from the disrupted electron transport, these agents might provide antioxidative [106], pro-energetic [107] and direct anti-apoptotic effects [108]. Coenzyme Q10 (CoQ10), also known as ubiquinone, has a chemical structure of a long chain benzoquinone and often used in the treatment of LHON. The beneficial effect of CoQ10 has been questioned due to the methodological issues noted amongst the studies concerning CoQ10 therapy [105]. It remains unclear if CoQ10 lipofilic chemical properties hinder its therapeutic effects [108, 109].

Idebenone, a short-chained benzoquinone structurally similar to CoQ10, has been shown in an *in vitro* setting to provide better effects than CoQ10 [110]. It is up to debate what kind of benefit can be expected from ibedenone therapy. A trial on a 28 subjects has shown that 180 mg/day idebenone therapy sped up the rate of visual recovery, without increasing the portion of eyes showing visual recovery [111]. A multicentre, double-blind, randomized placebo-controlled study [112] conducted on a larger population of LHON patients with 85 study subjects has shown that a 900 mg/day dosage failed to deliver an increase in visual acuity at the 24th week of treatment, which had been pre-specified as the primary end-point at which best levels of visual recovery were assessed. However, positive effects of therapy were detected post hoc meeting the secondary end-points, with benefits that seem to persist after the cessation of the therapy [113]. Furthermore, a retrospective study has shown idebenone therapy leads to a larger number of patients with visual recovery [114]. Additionally, idebenone has been shown to protect from color vision loss [115], highlighting the importance of early therapy. Yet, idebenone is still not approved for clinical use in LHON therapy in all countries and patients may choose to acquire the substance on their own.

EPI-743, an agent chemically similar to CoQ10, is a drug utilized in a study by Sadun *et al.* [116] for the treatment of LHON amongst 5 patients being acutely affected by vision loss. The improvement of several parameters including visual acuity, vision field and color vision was detected in 4 out of 5 patients, even implicating vision loss reversal. Larger studies yielding higher levels of evidence need to be conducted to further evaluate the effects of EPI-743 in LHON therapy.

5.4. Pharmacological Agonists and Mitochondrial Genesis Activators

Brimonidine, a topical α2 agonist, is used in the therapy of glaucoma for its ability to decrease intraocular pressure. Increased intraocular pressure has been shown to aggravate RGC loss in LHON [117]. In addition the significance of glaucoma-LHON comorbidity, certain direct pathophysiological similarities between LHON and glaucoma related to RGC death [118, 119], as well as anti-apoptotic properties of brimonidine [120], were asserted. These findings have enticed research to evaluate these effects in the therapy of LHON. Brimonidine was used in a 9 patient, open-labeled study to prevent second–eye involvement to no effect, without visual benefit after the emergence of visual loss [121]. A case of Charles Bonnet syndrome triggered by brimonidine in a patient with LHON has been reported [122]. However, this finding might be coincidental.

Stimulating the biogenesis mitochondria by activating certain cellular pathways, and therefore providing a neuroprotective effect, is a conceivable concept. Several pharmacological strategies were experimentally tested, with some promise: bezafibrate [123] to activate the PPAR-PGC-1α axis, the activation of AMPK and SIRT-1 by resveratrol [124] and the use of quercetin as a SIRT-1 agonist [125]. Further researching mitochondrial biogenesis activators might reveal new therapeutic targets [126], but it remains to be seen if these substances will benefit LHON patients in a clinical setting.

RGC-neuroprotective properties of certain agents such as memantine, valproic acid and prostaglandin J2 have been demonstrated on models of optic nerve degeneration [127], opening additional possibilities in the search for pharmacological agonists to be used in LHON therapy.

5.5. Future Technologies and Treatments

Gene therapy is a promising strategy, considering that mitochondrial gene insertion via adenovirus vectors and subsequent allotropic expression has been successfully demonstrated in the treatment of mice with induced LHON [128]. A number of experimental, practical and ethical hurdles need to be traversed before this form of therapy reaches routine clinical practice. Experimental findings concerning stem cell therapy [56] via differentiated RGC transplantation or mesenchymal stem cell neurotrophic support might yield promise in LHON therapy, but also command caution, due to the presence of non-regulated treatments being offered. A study evaluating near-infrared light-emitting diode therapy was commenced, but terminated as LHON subjects are unable to focus on target (https://clinicaltrials.gov/ct2/show/NCT01389817).

Despite the difficulties these technologies face, it is perceivable that they might eventually become a definitive cure for LHON.

5.6. Challenges and Issues Surrounding LHON Treatment

A reliable cure enabling reversal of LHON symptoms is not currently available [129]. LHON is treated with general therapeutic strategies are employed versus mitochondrial diseases as a whole, without taking into account the clinical and pathophysiological specificity of LHON [130], due to the fact that it is still not completely understood.

Clinical trials testing current modalities of treatment are few in number and small in size [103]. Additionally, the results of some of these trials are contradictory. Large, multi-centered trials are needed for sound proof of benefit from certain therapies.

CONCLUSION

Despite a significant amount of knowledge being accumulated, the complete picture of LHON, as a unique mitochondrial disease, is still unclear. The explanation for incomplete penetrance and gender bias is likely to be complex and multi-factorial. As seen in the MRI, MRS and fMRI studies, widening the scope in the search for extra-optic pathology in LHON leads to the hypothesis that the disease might not be confined to the visual system, but actually presents the "tip of the iceberg" of a multi-systemic disease with significant or subtle changes on the nervous system, cardiac muscle and, quite possibly, other organs with a high energetic demand. These changes sometimes might have a clinical manifestation in the form of LHON-MS, LHON+ and LHON-cardio. This view on LHON opens new questions: why do only certain patients have extraocular manifestations, what triggers their emergence, and why are the manifestations heterogeneous? Resolving these enigmatic issues might not only benefit LHON patients, but also provide new incentive in dealing with other mitochondrial diseases.

LIST OF ABBREVIATIONS

ATP	=	Adenosine Triphosphate
BAEP	=	Brain Stem Auditory Evoked Potentials
CoQ10	=	Coenzyme Q10
DTI	=	Diffusion Tensor Imaging
fMRI	=	Functional Magnetic Resonance Imaging
FVEP	=	Flash Visual Evoked Potentials
LHON	=	Leber's Hereditary Optic Neuropathy
MRI	=	Magnetic Resonance Imaging
MRS	=	Magnetic Resonance Spectroscopy
MS	=	Multiple Sclerosis
mtDNA	=	Mitochondrial DNA
OCT	=	Optical Coherence Tomography
PCR	=	Polymerase Chain Reaction
PVEP	=	Patterned Visual Evoked Potentials
RGC	=	Retinal Ganglial Cells
RNFL	=	Retinal nerve Fiber Layer
VBM	=	Voxel-based Morphometry
VEP	=	Visual Evoked Potentials

CONSENT FOR PUBLICATION

Not applicable.

CONFLICT OF INTEREST

No funding or sponsorship was received for this study or publication of this article. Jasna Janičić is supported by the Ministry of Education, Science and Technological Development of the Republic of Serbia (Grant No: 175031). Janko Samardžić is supported by the Ministry of Education, Science and Technological Development of the Republic of Serbia (Grant No: 175076). All authors declare no conflict of interest regarding the content of this manuscript.

ACKNOWLEDGEMENTS

All named authors meet the International Committee of Medical Journal Editors (ICMJE) criteria for authorship for this manuscript, take responsibility for the integrity of the work as a whole, and have given final approval for the version to be published.

This article is based on previously conducted studies and does not involve any new studies of human or animal subjects performed by any of the authors.

REFERENCES

[1]   Chinnery PF, Johnson MA, Wardell TM, *et al.* The epidemiology of pathogenic mitochondrial DNA mutations. Ann Neurol 2000; 48: 188-93.

[2]   Schaefer AM, Mcfarland R, Blakely EL, *et al.* Prevalence of mitochondrial DNA disease in adults. Ann Neurol 2008; 63: 35-9.

[3]   Zhang AM, Yao YG. Research progress of Leber hereditary optic neuropathy. Yi Chuan 2013; 35: 123-35.

[4]   Y-w-man P, Griffiths PG, Brown DT, Howell N, Turnbull DM, Chinnery PF. The epidemiology of Leber hereditary optic neuropathy in the North East of England. Am J Hum Genet 2003; 72: 333-9.

[5]   Spruijt L, Kolbach DN, Decoo RF, *et al.* Influence of mutation type on clinical expression of Leber hereditary optic neuropathy. Am J Ophthalmol 2006; 141: 676-82.

[6]   Puomila A, Hämäläinen P, Kivioja S, *et al.* Epidemiology and penetrance of Leber hereditary optic neuropathy in Finland. Eur J Hum Genet 2007; 15: 1079-89.

[7]   Newman NJ. Hereditary optic neuropathies: from the mitochondria to the optic nerve. Am J Ophthalmol 2005; 140: 517-23.

[8]   Jančić J, Dejanović I, Samardžić J, *et al.* Leber hereditary optic neuropathy in the population of Serbia. Eur J Paediatr Neurol 2014; 18: 354-9.

[9]   Abu-Amero KK. Leber's Hereditary Optic Neuropathy: the Mitochindrial Connection Revisited. Middle East Afr J Ophthalmol 2011; 18: 17-23.

[10]   Kirches E. LHON: mitochondrial mutations and more. Curr Genomics 2011; 12: 44-54.

[11]   Bandelt HJ, Yao YG, Salas A, Kivisild T, Bravi CM. High penetrance of sequencing errors and interpretative shortcomings in mtDNA sequence analysis of LHON patients. Biochem Biophys Res Commun 2007; 352: 283-91.

[12]   Saracchi E, Difrancesco JC, Brighina L, *et al.* A case of Leber hereditary optic neuropathy plus dystonia caused by G14459A mitochondrial mutation. Neurol Sci 2013; 34: 407-8.

[13]   Manjunath V, Bhatti MT. Leber hereditary optic neuropathy and multiple sclerosis: the mitochondrial connection. Can J Ophthalmol 2015; 50: e14-7.

[14]   Watanabe Y, Odaka M, Hirata K. Case of Leber's hereditary optic neuropathy with mitochondrial DNA 11778 mutation exhibiting cerebellar ataxia, dilated cardiomyopathy and peripheral neuropathy. Brain Nerve 2009; 61: 309-12.

[15]   Gray MW, Burger G, Lang BF. The origin and early evolution of mitochondria. Genome Biology 2001; 2: reviews1018.

[16]   Wallace DC, Singh G, Lott MT, *et al.* Mitochondrial DNA mutation associated with Leber's hereditary optic neuropathy. Science 1988; 242: 1427-30.

[17]   Sutovsky P, Moreno RD, Ramalho-santos J, Dominko T, Simerly C, Schatten G. Ubiquitinated sperm mitochondria, selective proteolysis, and the regulation of mitochondrial inheritance in mammalian embryos. Biol Reprod 2000; 63: 582-90.

[18]   Jenuth JP, Peterson AC, Fu K, Shoubridge EA. Random genetic drift in the female germline explains the rapid segregation of mammalian mitochondrial DNA. Nat Genet 1996; 14: 146-51.

[19]   Wonnapinij P, Chinnery PF, Samuels DC. The distribution of mitochondrial DNA heteroplasmy due to random genetic drift. Am J Hum Genet 2008; 83: 582-93.

[20]   Harding AE, Sweeney MG, Govan GG, Riordan-eva P. Pedigree analysis in Leber hereditary optic neuropathy families with a pathogenic mtDNA mutation. Am J Hum Genet 1995; 57: 77-86.

[21]   Pegoraro E, Carelli V, Zeviani M, *et al.* X-inactivation patterns in female Leber's hereditary optic neuropathy patients do not support a strong X-linked determinant. Am J Med Genet 1996; 61: 356-62.

[22]   Chalmers RM, Davis MB, Sweeney MG, Wood NW, Harding AE. Evidence against an X-linked visual loss susceptibility locus in Leber hereditary optic neuropathy. Am J Hum Genet 1996; 59: 103-8.

[23]   Phasukkijwatana N, Kunhapan B, Stankovich J, *et al.* Genome-wide linkage scan and association study of PARL to the expression of LHON families in Thailand. Hum Genet 2010; 128: 39-49.

[24]   Kirkman MA, Yu-wai-man P, Korsten A, *et al.* Gene-environment interactions in Leber hereditary optic neuropathy. Brain 2009; 132: 2317-26.

[25]   Hunter JJ, Morgan JI, Merigan WH, Sliney DH, Sparrow JR, Williams DR. The susceptibility of the retina to photochemical damage from visible light. Prog Retin Eye Res 2012; 31: 28-42.

[26]   Javaheri M, Khurana RN, O'hearn TM, Lai MM, Sadun AA. Linezolid-induced optic neuropathy: a mitochondrial disorder? Br J Ophthalmol 2007; 91: 111-5.

[27]   Luca CC, Lam BL, Moraes CT. Erythromycin as a potential precipitating agent in the onset of Leber's hereditary optic neuropathy. Mitochondrion 2004; 4: 31-6.

[28]   Mackey DA, Fingert JH, Luzhansky JZ, *et al.* Leber's hereditary optic neuropathy triggered by antiretroviral therapy for human immunodeficiency virus. Eye (Lond) 2003; 17: 312-7.

[29]   Ikeda A, Ikeda T, Ikeda N, Kawakami Y, Mimura O. Leber's hereditary optic neuropathy precipitated by ethambutol. Jpn J Ophthalmol 2006; 50: 280-3.

[30]   Giordano C, Montopoli M, Perli E, *et al.* Oestrogens ameliorate mitochondrial dysfunction in Leber's hereditary optic neuropathy. Brain 2011; 134: 220-34.

[31]   Sadun A. Acquired mitochondrial impairment as a cause of optic nerve disease. Trans Am Ophthalmol Soc 1998; 96: 881-923.

[32]   Amaral-Fernandes MS, Marcondes AM, do Amor Divino Miranda PM, Maciel-Guerra AT, Sartorato EL. Mutations for Leber hereditary optic neuropathy in patients with alcohol and tobacco optic neuropathy. Mol Vis 2011; 17: 3175-9.

[33]   Zanna C, Ghelli A, Porcelli AM, Carelli V, Martinuzzi A, Rugolo M. Apoptotic cell death of cybrid cells bearing Leber's hereditary optic neuropathy mutations is caspase independent. Ann N Y Acad Sci 2003; 1010: 213-7.

[34]   Majander A, Huoponen K, Savontaus ML, Nikoskelainen E, Wikström M. Electron transfer properties of NADH:ubiquinone reductase in the ND1/3460 and the ND4/11778 mutations of the Leber hereditary optic neuroretinopathy (LHON). FEBS Lett 1991; 292: 289-92.

[35]   Brown MD, Trounce IA, Jun AS, Allen JC, Wallace DC. Functional analysis of lymphoblast and cybrid mitochondria containing the 3460, 11778, or 14484 Leber's hereditary optic neuropathy mitochondrial DNA mutation. J Biol Chem 2000; 275: 39831-6.

[36]   Carelli V, Ghelli A, Bucchi L, *et al.* Biochemical features of mtDNA 14484 (ND6/M64V) point mutation associated with Leber's hereditary optic neuropathy. Ann Neuro 1999; 45: 320-8.

[37]   Hofhaus G, Johns DR, Hurko O, Attardi G, Chomyn A. Respiration and growth defects in transmitochondrial cell lines carrying the 11778 mutation associated with Leber's hereditary optic neuropathy. J Biol Chem 1996; 271: 13155-61.

[38]   Levin LA. Mechanisms of retinal ganglion specific-cell death in Leber hereditary optic neuropathy. Trans Am Ophthalmol Soc 2007; 105: 379-91.

[39]   Danielson SR, Wong A, Carelli V, Martinuzzi A, Schapira AH, Cortopassi GA. Cells bearing mutations causing Leber's hereditary optic neuropathy are sensitized to Fas-Induced apoptosis. J Biol Chem 2002; 277: 5810-5.

[40] Thorburn DR, Rahman S. Mitochondrial DNA-Associated Leigh Syndrome and NARP. In: Pagon RA, Adam MP, Ardinger HH, *et al.*, Eds.: GeneReviews® [Internet]. Seattle (WA): University of Washington, Seattle; 1993-2017.Available from: https://www.ncbi. nlm.nih.gov/books/NBK1173/

[41] Kirches E. LHON: mitochondrial mutations and more. Curr Genomics 2011; 12: 44-54.

[42] Funalot B, Reynier P, Vighetto A, *et al.* Leigh-like encephalopathy complicating Leber's hereditary optic neuropathy. Annals of Neurology 2002; 52: 374-7.

[43] Zanna C, Ghelli A, Porcelli AM, Martinuzzi A, Carelli V, Rugolo M. Caspase-independent death of Leber's hereditary optic neuropathy cybrids is driven by energetic failure and mediated by AIF and Endonuclease G. Apoptosis 2005; 10: 997-1007.

[44] Hayashi G, Cortopassi G. Oxidative stress in inherited mitochondrial diseases. Free Radic Biol Med 2015; 88: 10-7.

[45] Murphy MP. How mitochondria produce reactive oxygen species. Biochem J 2009; 417: 1-13.

[46] Chinopoulos C, Gerencser AA, Doczi J, Fiskum G, Adam-vizi V. Inhibition of glutamate-induced delayed calcium deregulation by 2-APB and La3+ in cultured cortical neurones. J Neurochem 2004; 91: 471-83.

[47] Vrabec JP, Lieven CJ, Levin LA. Cell-type-specific opening of the retinal ganglion cell mitochondrial permeability transition pore. Invest Ophthalmol Vis Sci 2003; 44: 2774-82.

[48] Sala G, Trombin F, Beretta S, *et al.* Antioxidants partially restore glutamate transport defect in leber hereditary optic neuropathy cybrids. J Neurosci Res 2008; 86: 3331-7.

[48] Pan BX, Ross-Cisneros FN, Carelli V, *et al.* Mathematically modeling the involvement of axons in Leber's hereditary optic neuropathy. Invest Ophthalmol Vis Sci 2012; 53: 7608-17.

[49] Chao de la Barca J, Simard G, Amati-Bonneau P, *et al.* The metabolomic signature of Leber's hereditary optic neuropathy reveals endoplasmic reticulum stress. Brain 2016; 139: 2864-76.

[50] Cortopassi G, Danielson S, Alemi M, *et al.* Mitochondrial disease activates transcripts of the unfolded protein response and cell cycle and inhibits vesicular secretion and oligodendrocyte-specific transcripts. Mitochondrion 2006; 6: 161-75.

[51] Yu-Wai-Man P, Griffiths PG, Chinnery PF. Mitochondrial optic neuropathies - disease mechanisms and therapeutic strategies. Prog Retin Eye Res 2011; 30: 81-114.

[52] Quiros PA, Torres RJ, Salomao S, *et al.* Colour vision defects in asymptomatic carriers of the Leber's hereditary optic neuropathy (LHON) mtDNA 11778 mutation from a large Brazilian LHON pedigree: a case-control study. Br J Ophthalmol 2006; 90: 150-3.

[53] Giordano C, Iommarini L, Giordano L, *et al.* Efficient mitochondrial biogenesis drives incomplete penetrance in Leber's hereditary optic neuropathy. Brain 2014; 137: 335-53.

[54] Kerrison JB. Latent, acute, and chronic Leber's hereditary optic neuropathy. Ophthalmology 2005; 112: 1-2.

[55] Chronister CL, Gurwood AS, Burns CM, Merckle SJ. Leber's hereditary optic neuropathy: a case report. Optometry 2005; 76: 302-8.

[56] Meyerson C, Van Stavern G, Mcclelland C. Leber hereditary optic neuropathy: current perspectives. Clin Ophthalmol 2015; 9: 1165-76.

[57] Yu-Wai-Man P, Chinnery PF. Leber Hereditary Optic Neuropathy. In: Pagon RA, Adam MP, Ardinger HH, *et al.*, Eds.: GeneReviews® [Internet]. Seattle (WA): University of Washington, Seattle; 1993-2017. Available from: https://www.ncbi.nlm.nih.gov/books/ NBK1174.

[58] Yu-Wai-Man P, Turnbull DM, Chinnery PF. Leber hereditary optic neuropathy. J Med Genet 2002; 39: 162-9.

[59] Ohden K, Tang P, Lilley C, *et al.* Atypical leber hereditary optic neuropathy: 18 year interval between eyes. J Neuro-Ophthalmol 2016; 36: 304.

[60] Jacobson DM, Stone EM, Miller NR, *et al.* Relative afferent pupillary defects in patients with Leber hereditary optic neuropathy and unilateral visual loss. Am J Ophthalmol 1998; 126: 291-5.

[61] Mroczek-Tońska K, Kisiel B, Piechota J, Bartnik E. Leber hereditary optic neuropathy-a disease with a known molecular basis but a mysterious mechanism of pathology. J Appl Genet 2003; 44: 529-38.

[62] Nikoskelainen EK, Huoponen K, Juvonen V, Lamminen T, Nummelin K, Savontaus ML. Ophthalmologic findings in Leber hereditary optic neuropathy, with special reference to mtDNA mutations. Ophthalmology 1996; 103: 504-14.

[63] Harding AE, Sweeney MG, Miller DH, *et al.* Occurrence of a multiple sclerosis-like illness in women who have a Leber's hereditary optic neuropathy mitochondrial DNA mutation. Brain 1992; 115: 979-89.

[64] Pénisson-Besnier I, Moreau C, Jacques C, Roger JC, Dubas F, Reynier P. Multiple sclerosis and Leber's hereditary optic neuropathy mitochondrial DNA mutations. Rev Neurol (Paris) 2001; 157: 537-41.

[65] Palace J. Multiple sclerosis associated with Leber's Hereditary Optic Neuropathy. J Neurol Sci 2009; 286: 24-7.

[66] Pfeffer G, Burke A, Yu-Wai-Man P, Compston DA, Chinnery PF. Clinical features of MS associated with Leber hereditary optic neuropathy mtDNA mutations. Neurology 2013; 81: 2073-81.

[67] Hsu TK, Wang AG, Yen MY, Liu JH. Leber's hereditary optic neuropathy masquerading as optic neuritis with spontaneous visual recovery. Clin Exp Optom 2014; 97: 84-6.

[68] Jančić J, Dejanović I, Radovanović S, *et al.* White matter changes in two leber's hereditary optic neuropathy pedigrees: 12-year follow-up. Ophthalmologica 2016; 235: 49-56.

[69] Matthews L, Enzinger C, Fazekas F, *et al.* MRI in Leber's hereditary optic neuropathy: the relationship to multiple sclerosis. J Neurol Neurosurg Psychiatr 2015; 86: 537-42.

[70] Charlmers RM, Harding AE. A case-control study of Leber's hereditary optic neuropathy. Brain 1996; 119: 1481-6.

[71] Vital C, Julien J, Martin-Negrier ML, Lagueny A, Ferrer X, Vital A. Parkinsonism in a patient with Leber hereditary optic neuropathy (LHON). Rev Neurol (Paris) 2015; 171: 679-80.

[72] Rance G, Kearns LS, Tan J, *et al.* Auditory function in individuals within Leber's hereditary optic neuropathy pedigrees. J Neurol 2012; 259: 542-50.

[73] Ceranić B, Luxon LM. Progressive auditory neuropathy in patients with Leber's hereditary optic neuropathy. J Neurol Neurosurg Psychiatr 2004; 75: 626-30.

[74] Nikoskelainen EK, Marttila RJ, Huoponen K, *et al.* Leber's "plus": neurological abnormalities in patients with Leber's hereditary optic neuropathy. J Neurol Neurosurg Psychiatr 1995; 59: 160-4.

[75] Nikoskelainen EK, Savontaus ML, Huoponen K, Antila K, Hartiala J. Pre-excitation syndrome in Leber's hereditary optic neuropathy. Lancet 1994; 344: 857-8.

[76] Sorajja P, Sweeney MG, Chalmers R, *et al.* Cardiac abnormalities in patients with Leber's hereditary optic neuropathy. Heart 2003; 89: 791-2.

[77] Nikoskelainen EK, Huoponen K, Juvonen V, Lamminen T, Nummelin K, Savontaus ML. Ophthalmologic findings in Leber hereditary optic neuropathy, with special reference to mtDNA mutations. Ophthalmology 1996; 103: 504-14.

[78] Riordan-Eva P, Sanders MD, Govan GG, Sweeney MG, Da Costa J, Harding AE. The clinical features of Leber's hereditary optic neuropathy defined by the presence of a pathogenic mitochondrial DNA mutation. Brain 1995; 118: 319-37.

[79] Newman NJ, Lott MT, Wallace DC. The clinical characteristics of pedigrees of Leber's hereditary optic neuropathy with the 11778 mutation. Am J Ophthalmol 1991; 111: 750-62.

[80] Behbehani R. Clinical approach to optic neuropathies. Clin Ophthalmol 2007; 1: 233-46.

[81] Moura AL, Nagy BV, La Morgia C, *et al.* The pupil light reflex in Leber's hereditary optic neuropathy: evidence for preservation of melanopsin-expressing retinal ganglion cells. Invest Ophthalmol Vis Sci 2013; 54: 4471-7.

[82] La Morgia C, Ross-Cisneros FN, Sadun AA, *et al.* Melanopsin retinal ganglion cells are resistant to neurodegeneration in mitochondrial optic neuropathies. Brain 2010; 133: 2426-38.

[83] Savini G, Barboni P, Valentino ML, *et al.* Retinal nerve fiber layer evaluation by optical coherence tomography in unaffected carriers with Leber's hereditary optic neuropathy mutations. Ophthalmology 2005; 112: 127-31.

[84] Mizoguchi A, Hashimoto Y, Shinmei Y, *et al.* Macular thickness changes in a patient with Leber's hereditary optic neuropathy. BMC Ophthalmol 2015; 15: 27.

[85] Barcella V, Rocca MA, Bianchi-Marzoli S, *et al.* Evidence for retrochiasmatic tissue loss in Leber's hereditary optic neuropathy. Hum Brain Mapp 2010; 31: 1900-6.

[86] Whatham AR, Nguyen V, Zhu Y, Hennessy M, Kalloniatis M. The value of clinical electrophysiology in the assessment of the eye and visual system in the era of advanced imaging. Clin Exp Optom 2014; 97: 99-115.

[87] Ziccardi L, Sadun F, De negri AM, *et al.* Retinal function and neural conduction along the visual pathways in affected and unaf-

      fected carriers with Leber's hereditary optic neuropathy. Invest Ophthalmol Vis Sci 2013; 54: 6893-901.

[88]   Jančić J, Ivančević N, Nikolić B, *et al.* Visual evoked potentials-current concepts and future perspectives. Vojnosanit Pregl 2017; [*E-pub Ahead of Print*] doi: 10.2298/VSP160613342J

[89]   Rance G, Kearns LS, Tan J, *et al.* Auditory function in individuals within Leber's hereditary optic neuropathy pedigrees. J Neurol 2012; 259: 542-50.

[90]   Kerrison JB, Newman NJ. Clinical spectrum of Leber's hereditary optic neuropathy. Clin Neurosci 1997; 4: 295-301.

[91]   Mondelli M, Rossi A, Scarpini C, Dotti MT, Federico A. BAEP changes in Leber's hereditary optic atrophy: further confirmation of multisystem involvement. Acta Neurol Scand 1990; 81: 349-53.

[92]   Ostojic J, Jancic J, Kozic D, *et al.* Brain white matter 1 H MRS in Leber optic neuropathy mutation carriers. Acta Neurol Belg 2009; 109: 305-9.

[93]   Rocca MA, Valsasina P, Pagani E, *et al.* Extra-visual functional and structural connection abnormalities in Leber's hereditary optic neuropathy. PLoS ONE 2011; 6: e17081.

[94]   Inglese M, Rovaris M, Bianchi S, Comi G, Filippi M. Magnetization transfer and diffusion tensor MR imaging of the optic radiations and calcarine cortex from patients with Leber's hereditary optic neuropathy. J Neurol Sci 2001; 188: 33-6.

[95]   Manners DN, Rizzo G, La morgia C, *et al.* Diffusion tensor imaging mapping of brain white matter pathology in mitochondrial optic neuropathies. AJNR Am J Neuroradiol 2015; 36: 1259-65.

[96]   Martin AR, Aleksanderek I, Cohen-adad J, *et al.* Translating state-of-the-art spinal cord MRI techniques to clinical use: A systematic review of clinical studies utilizing DTI, MT, MWF, MRS, and fMRI. Neuroimage Clin 2016; 10: 192-238.

[97]   Kirkman MA, Korsten A, Leonhardt M, *et al.* Quality of life in patients with Leber hereditary optic neuropathy. Invest Ophthalmol Vis Sci 2009; 50: 3112-5.

[98]   Newman NJ, Biousse V. Hereditary optic neuropathies. Eye (Lond) 2004; 18: 1144-60.

[99]   Barboni P, Savini G, Valentino ML, *et al.* Leber's hereditary optic neuropathy with childhood onset. Invest Ophthalmol Vis Sci 2006; 47: 5303-9.

[100]   Stone EM, Newman NJ, Miller NR, Johns DR, Lott MT, Wallace DC. Visual recovery in patients with Leber's hereditary optic neuropathy and the 11778 mutation. J Clin Neuroophthalmol 1992; 12: 10-4.

[101]   Markowitz SN. Principles of modern low vision rehabilitation. Can J Ophthalmol 2006; 41: 289-312.

[102]   Zarnowski T, Tulidowicz-Bielak M, Kosior-Jarecka E, Zarnowska I, A turski W, Gasior M. A ketogenic diet may offer neuroprotection in glaucoma and mitochondrial diseases of the optic nerve. Med Hypothesis Discov Innov Ophthalmol 2012; 1: 45-9.

[103]   Huoponen K, Puomila A, Savontaus ML, Mustonen E, Kronqvist E, Nikoskelainen E. Genetic counseling in Leber hereditary optic neuropathy (LHON). Acta Ophthalmol Scand 2002; 80: 38-43.

[104]   Pfeffer G, Majamaa K, Turnbull DM, Thorburn D, Chinnery PF. Treatment for mitochondrial disorders. Cochrane Database Syst Rev 2012; 4: CD004426.

[105]   Pfeffer G, Horvath R, Klopstock T, *et al.* New treatments for mitochondrial disease-no time to drop our standards. Nat Rev Neurol 2013; 9: 474-81.

[106]   Littarru GP, Tiano L. Bioenergetic and antioxidant properties of coenzyme Q10: recent developments. Mol Biotechnol 2007; 37: 31-7.

[107]   Beal MF, Henshaw DR, Jenkins BG, Rosen BR, Schulz JB. Coenzyme Q10 and nicotinamide block striatal lesions produced by the mitochondrial toxin malonate. Ann Neurol 1994; 36: 882-8.

[108]   Papucci L, Schiavone N, Witort E, *et al.* Coenzyme q10 prevents apoptosis by inhibiting mitochondrial depolarization independently of its free radical scavenging property. J Biol Chem 2003; 278: 28220-8.

[109]   Yu-wai-man P, Votruba M, Moore AT, Chinnery PF. Treatment strategies for inherited optic neuropathies: past, present and future. Eye (Lond) 2014; 28: 521-37.

[110]   Fung WY, Liong MT, Yuen KH. Preparation, *in-vitro* and *in-vivo* characterisation of CoQ10 microparticles: electrospraying-enhanced bioavailability. J Pharm Pharmacol 2016; 68: 159-69.

[111]   Mashima Y, Kigasawa K, Wakakura M, Oguchi Y. Do idebenone and vitamin therapy shorten the time to achieve visual recovery in Leber hereditary optic neuropathy? J Neuroophthalmol 2000; 20: 166-70.

[112]   Klopstock T, Yu-wai-man P, Dimitriadis K, *et al.* A randomized placebo-controlled trial of idebenone in Leber's hereditary optic neuropathy. Brain 2011; 134: 2677-86.

[113]   Klopstock T, Metz G, Yu-Wai-Man P, *et al.* Persistence of the treatment effect of idebenone in Leber's hereditary optic neuropathy. Brain 2013; 136: e230.

[114]   Carelli V, La Morgia C, Valentino ML, *et al.* Idebenone treatment in Leber's hereditary optic neuropathy. Brain 2011; 134: e188.

[115]   Rudolph G, Dimitriadis K, Büchner B, *et al.* Effects of idebenone on color vision in patients with leber hereditary optic neuropathy. J Neuroophthalmol 2013; 33: 30-6.

[116]   Sadun AA, Chicani CF, Ross-Cisneros FN, *et al.* Effect of EPI-743 on the clinical course of the mitochondrial disease Leber hereditary optic neuropathy. Arch Neurol 2012; 69: 331-8.

[117]   Thouin A, Griffiths PG, Hudson G, Chinnery PF, Yu-wai-man P. Raised intraocular pressure as a potential risk factor for visual loss in Leber Hereditary Optic Neuropathy. PLoS ONE 2013; 8: e63446.

[118]   Osborne NN. Mitochondria: their role in ganglion cell death and survival in primary open angle glaucoma. Exp Eye Res 2010; 90: 750-7.

[119]   Osborne NN. Pathogenesis of ganglion "cell death" in glaucoma and neuroprotection: focus on ganglion cell axonal mitochondria. Prog Brain Res 2008; 173: 339-52.

[120]   Wheeler L, Woldemussie E, Lai R. Role of alpha-2 agonists in neuroprotection. Surv Ophthalmol 2003; 48: S47-51.

[121]   Newman NJ, Biousse V, David R, *et al.* Prophylaxis for second eye involvement in Leber hereditary optic neuropathy: an open-labeled, nonrandomized multicenter trial of topical brimonidine purite. Am J Ophthalmol 2005; 140: 407-15.

[122]   Santos-Bueso E, Sáenz-Francés F, Porta-Etessam J, García-Sánchez J. Charles Bonnet syndrome triggered by brimonidine in a patient with Leber's hereditary optic neuropathy. Rev Psiquiatr Salud Ment 2014; 7: 152-3.

[123]   Noe N, Dillon L, Lellek V, *et al.* Bezafibrate improves mitochondrial function in the CNS of a mouse model of mitochondrial encephalopathy. Mitochondrion 2013; 13: 417-26.

[124]   Price NL, Gomes AP, Ling AJ, *et al.* SIRT1 is required for AMPK activation and the beneficial effects of resveratrol on mitochondrial function. Cell Metab 2012; 15: 675-90.

[125]   Davis JM, Murphy EA, Carmichael MD, Davis B. Quercetin increases brain and muscle mitochondrial biogenesis and exercise tolerance. Am J Physiol Regul Integr Comp Physiol 2009; 296: R1071-7.

[126]   Valero T. Mitochondrial biogenesis: pharmacological approaches. Curr Pharm Des 2014; 20: 5507-9.

[127]   Yu-wai-man P, Griffiths PG, Chinnery PF. Mitochondrial optic neuropathies - disease mechanisms and therapeutic strategies. Prog Retin Eye Res 2011; 30: 81-114.

[128]   Koilkonda R, Yu H, Talla V, *et al.* LHON gene therapy vector prevents visual loss and optic neuropathy induced by G11778A mutant mitochondrial DNA: biodistribution and toxicology profile. Invest Ophthalmol Vis Sci 2014; 55: 7739-53.

[129]   Peragallo JH, Newman NJ. Is there treatment for Leber hereditary optic neuropathy? Curr Opin Ophthalmol 2015; 26: 450-7.

[130]   Jankauskaitė E, Bartnik E, Kodroń A. Investigating Leber's hereditary optic neuropathy: cell models and future perspectives. Mitochondrion 2017; 32: 19-26.

936 CNS & Neurological Disorders - Drug Targets, 2017, 16, 936-944

REVEIW ARTICLE

Immunomodulatory Strategies for Huntington's Disease Treatment

Gabriela D. Colpo[1,*], Natalia P. Rocha[1], Erin Fur Stimming[2] and Antonio L. Teixeira[1]

[1]Neuropsychiatry Program, Department of Psychiatry and Behavioral Sciences, McGovern Medical School, The University of Texas Health Science Center at Houston, Houston, TX, USA; [2]Department of Neurology, McGovern Medical School, The University of Texas Health Science Center at Houston, Houston, TX, USA

Abstract: ***Background & Objective***: Huntington's disease (HD) is an autosomal-dominant, progressive neurodegenerative disease characterized by selective loss of neurons in the striatum and cortex, which leads to progressive motor dysfunction, cognitive decline and behavioral symptoms. HD is caused by a trinucleotide (CAG) repeat expansion in the gene encoding the protein huntingtin. Despite the fact that the HD gene was identified over 20 years ago, there is no effective disease-modifying therapy for HD and only symptomatic therapies are available to date. Recently, new agents and procedures have been investigated for HD and many of them have focused on immunomodulatory and/or anti- inflammatory strategies.

Conclusion: The objective of the current review is to summarize data on the therapeutic strategies to treat HD that are based on immunomodulatory effects.

ARTICLE HISTORY

Received: April 17, 2017
Revised: May 25, 2017
Accepted: June 05, 2017

DOI:
10.2174/1871527316666170613084801

Keywords: Huntington's disease, inflammation, treatment, symptomatic therapies, disease modifying treatment, stem cells.

1. INTRODUCTION

Huntington's disease (HD) is an autosomal-dominant, progressive neurodegenerative disease, caused by an unstable CAG trinucleotide repeat expansion in exon 1 of the *Huntingtin* gene (*HTT*) encoding a mutant form of the huntingtin protein (HTT) [1]. HD is pathologically characterized by selective loss of neurons in the striatum and cortex, which leads to progressive motor dysfunction, cognitive decline and behavioral symptoms. The most common hyperkinetic movement observed in symptomatic individuals is chorea, although dystonia, tics and myoclonus can also be observed. In addition, patients commonly experience severe psychiatric, cognitive, and metabolic symptoms that might occur even in early stages of the disease [2-5]. Psychiatric symptoms are particularly prevalent, including high rates of depression and anxiety [3, 6, 7]. Cognitive symptoms include deficits in memory, executive function, and impulse control [4, 5]. Patients also show metabolic symptoms such as significant weight loss. [8-10].

The presence of more than 40 CAG repeats is translated into the mutant huntingtin protein (mHTT) which causes the disease within a normal lifespan, while longer repeats can accelerate disease onset [11]. The onset of HD usually occurs in midlife, followed by 15 to 20 years of disease progression. However, non-motor aspects of the disease often occur early in the disease process [2]. The development of these features cannot easily be explained by the pathology in the striatum that constitutes the neurobiological substrate for the motor symptoms of the disease.

The normal HTT is ubiquitously expressed and is crucial for embryonic development. The mechanism of neuronal cell toxicity by mHTT has not been clearly established, possibly involving multiple pathways such as mitochondrial dysfunction, transcriptional dysregulation, protein-protein interaction problems, abnormal protein aggregation, and excitotoxicity [12, 13]. Preclinical studies have used these pathways to identify a plethora of potential targets for disease modifying strategies for HD. However, all the strategies have failed when tested in clinical trials [14].

Despite the fact that the HD gene was identified over 20 years ago, there is no effective disease- modifying therapy for HD and only symptomatic therapies are available to date. There is a great opportunity to identify disease modifying therapies for HD as it is a monogenic disorder, with a well-characterized gene [15]. Recently, new agents and procedures have been investigated for HD and many of them have focused on immunomodulatory and/or anti-inflammatory mechanisms. The objective of the current review is to summarize data on the immune-based therapeutic strategies for HD (Fig. **1**).

*Address correspondence to this author at the Neuropsychiatry Program, Department of Psychiatry and Behavioral Sciences. McGovern Medical School, University of Texas Health Science Center at Houston, 1941 East Road, Houston, TX 77054. BBSB 3270, USA; Tel: +1 713 486 2622; E-mail: gabicolpo@gmail.com

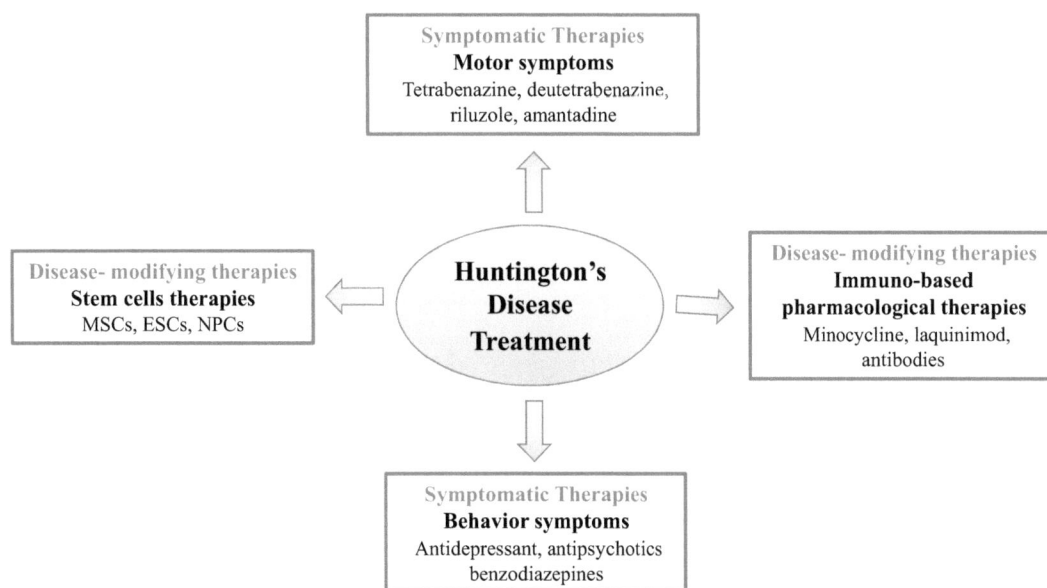

Fig. (1). Therapies for Huntington's disease.

2. NEUROINFLAMMATION IN HUNTINGTON'S DISEASE

A large body of evidence indicates that neuroinflammation plays a key role in the development of neurodegenerative diseases. During the last decade, attention has been drawn to the putative involvement of altered neuroinflammation in HD pathogenesis. Although the primary cause of HD is the mHTT expression in neurons [16, 17], the mutant protein is highly expressed in peripheral immune cells where it can induce immune activation [18, 19]. Once activated, peripheral immune mechanisms may contribute to the physiopathology of HD. Also, in the central nervous system (CNS), HTT is expressed in microglia, and microglial cells are the main mediators of neuroinflammation that, when activated, produce pro-inflammatory cytokines such as TNF-α and IL-1β [20]. Pro-inflammatory cytokines, in turn, promote activation of microglia resulting in an inflammatory flow that further contributes to neuronal toxicity and death [21-23].

In addition, the blood brain barrier (BBB), which regulates the entry and exit of molecules between the CNS and the periphery, in patients with HD present alterations in the cell components [24]. This suggests the probability of crosstalk between the periphery and CNS in HD, potentiating chronic inflammation and contributing to the neurotoxic microenvironment in regions of the brain. Indeed, parabiosis experiments show how systemic inflammatory components act as important factors on aging, neurogenesis, synaptic plasticity, learning and memory in the CNS [25]. However, the precise mechanism by which high systemic levels of pro-inflammatory molecules and dysregulated peripheral cells might affect the HD brain remains unclear.

Activated microglia were found in the brain of HD gene carriers even before the onset of the disease [26]. In addition, positron emission tomography studies (PET) have demonstrated early and significant microglial activation that correlates with the severity of the pathology in HD patients [27] and pre-symptomatic HD gene carriers [28]. Postmortem studies have shown elevated levels of inflammatory markers such as IL-6, IL-8, and IL-10 produced by microglia in the brain of patients with HD [29]. Moreover, increased levels of IL-4, IL-6, IL-8 and TNF-α have been shown in the periphery and cerebrospinal fluid (CSF) of patients with HD [18]. Changes in the levels of inflammatory markers were found not only in the CNS but also in peripheral tissue samples of patients. Peripheral plasma levels of the chemokines eotaxin-3, macrophage inflammatory protein-1B (MIP-1B), eotaxin, monocyte chemotactic protein 1 (MCP-1) and MCP-4 are significantly higher in patients with HD when compared with healthy subjects [30]. It is worth mentioning that animal models of HD also exhibit significant alterations in inflammatory markers and activated microglia [31, 32].

3. SYMPTOMATIC THERAPIES FOR HUNTINGTON'S DISEASE

Most symptomatic therapies for HD target motor symptoms, such as chorea, dystonia, myoclonus and tics through anti-glutamatergic, anti-dopaminergic and GABAergic mechanisms [15]. In 2012, the American Academy of Neurology released its guidelines supporting the use of tetrabenazine (TBZ), amantadine (NMDA antagonist) or riluzole (antiglutamatergic) to treat chorea [33]. However, TBZ and the very recently deutetrabenazine remains the only Food and Drug Administration (FDA) approved medications in the United States for chorea treatment in HD. TBZ reversibly inhibits the vesicular monoamine transporter 2 (VMAT-2) in the CNS. VMAT-2 packages serotonin, dopamine, and norepinephrine from the cytoplasm into presynaptic vesicles, therefore, its inhibition leads to premature degradation of theses monoamines [34]. Similar to TBZ, deutetrabenazine is a VMAT-2 inhibitor, but with prolonged plasma half-life, which may enable less frequent and lower daily doses [35]. Dystonia occurs mainly in juvenile-onset cases and late-stages of the disease. The treatment for dystonia is based on the use of antispastic agents, such as baclofen, as well as benzodiazepines and botulinum toxin [36]. Parkinsonism is another feature of HD, being prominent in juvenile cases and late- stages. Studies suggest that antiparkinsonian medications such as levodopa, dopamine agonists and amantadine might be helpful [37, 38]. Anti-epileptics such as valproic acid, levetiracetam and clonazepam are frequently used for myoclonus [36].

Psychiatric and behavioral symptoms such as aggression, irritability, impulsiveness, anxiety, depression and psychosis are a significant burden for patients with HD. Selective serotonin reuptake inhibitors (SSRIs), serotonin and norepinephrine reuptake inhibitors or tricyclic antidepressants are usually prescribed for depression [39, 40]. Antipsychotics may be used to address aggressiveness and irritability and/or psychosis. Mood stabilizers and benzodiazepines are also commonly used to treat mood lability and anxiety. For cognitive impairment, there are inconsistent data on the potential benefits of cholinesterase inhibition in HD [41, 42].

Nonsteroidal anti-inflammatory drugs (NSAIDs) have been evaluated for behavioral and cognitive symptoms in neurodegenerative diseases and psychiatric disorders with mixed results [43]. One study evaluated acetylsalicylate and rofecoxib in N171-82Q and R6/2 transgenic HD mice with no benefit for the animals [44]. So far, no study investigated NSAIDs in clinical trials in HD.

4. DISEASE MODIFYING TREATMENTS FOR HUNTINGTON'S DISEASE

Several clinical trials have failed to identify a treatment that could alter the progressive motor, cognitive and functional decline characteristic of HD. Recently, new pharmacological agents targeting the inflammatory process present in HD with immunomodulatory and anti- inflammatory compounds have been studied. In addition, treatments with stem cells constitute a promising strategy for HD due to their potential neuroprotective and immunomodulatory activities (Table 1).

4.1. Pharmacological Therapies

Minocycline is a second-generation, semi-synthetic tetracycline antibiotic with proven neuroinflammatory activity [45, 46]. It has been shown to slow disease onset, being neuroprotective in several animal models of CNS disorders, including Parkinson's disease [47], HD [48, 49], amyotrophic lateral sclerosis [50, 51], multiple sclerosis [52], spinal cord injury [53, 54], and traumatic brain injury [55].

Minocycline was described to prevent the up regulation of caspase-1 and caspase-3 expression, and reduce mortality in transgenic R6/2 mice. The transgenic R6/2 mouse has mHTT with CAG repeat expansion (~125 repeats) within the huntingtin gene exon 1. Animals develop HD-like symptoms, being the most commonly used animal model of HD. Increased iNOS expression was detected in R6/2 mouse brains similar to HD patient's brains. Treatment with minocycline reduced iNOS activity by 72% in R6/2 mice [48]. The same group demonstrated that the inhibition of caspase-1 and caspase-3 was necessary for the neuroprotection provided by minocycline in this HD model [48]. Although many of the beneficial effects of minocycline are attributed to its inhibitory actions on anti-inflammatory and apoptotic pathways, the precise mechanism by which minocycline protects from neuronal death has not been identified yet.

A clinical trial in individuals with HD (NCT00277355) showed that minocycline at 100 and 200 mg/day was well tolerated during an eight-week treatment. The study involved 60 patients who were randomly assigned to receive placebo (n = 23), minocycline 100 mg/day (n = 18) or minocycline 200 mg/day (n = 19). Nevertheless, no efficacy was observed based on the UHDRS scores [56]. Conversely, another clinical trial showed a neuroprotective effect of minocycline in HD. Minocycline was administered to 14 patients with HD for 24 months. Different of the natural course of HD, patients showed stabilization in motor performance and neuropsychological tasks at the endpoint, after improvement in the first 6 months. Moreover, a significant amelioration of psychiatric symptoms was reported at the endpoint [57]. Different duration of the trials may explain these discrepant results. A futility study used minocycline 200 mg/d (n=87) or placebo (n=27) for 18 months in HD patients evaluated the Total Functional Capacity (TFC). TFC score declined in the minocycline group but the difference was not significant. Based on in these results, further study of minocycline 200 mg/d in HD was not warranted [58].

More recently laquinomod, a disease modifying therapy for the treatment of relapsing-remitting multiple sclerosis, started being evaluated in HD. Laquinomod is a small molecule that can be given orally with a good safety profile, exerting both immunomodulatory and neuroprotective effects, but the exact mechanism of laquinomod is not clear yet [59]. Laquinomod has been shown to rescue striatal and cortical neurodegeneration and to improve behavior in YAC128 mice (transgenic mice expressing the human HTT containing a 128 CAG repeat expansion and thus an animal model of HD) [60]. Laquinomod decreased NF-kB activation both in the periphery and in the CNS [61], and reduced the levels of secreted pro-inflammatory factors, leading to neuroprotection and improvement in functional outcomes [62]. In addition, laquinomod has been shown to upregulate brain-derived neurotrophic factor (BDNF) [63], a neurotrophic factor with reduced expression and secretion in HD [64]. However, its precise molecular targets remain to be established [62]. A clinical trial (NCT02215616) is currently recruiting participants for testing laquinomod in HD.

As the levels of inflammatory cytokines are increased in HD, Hsiao *et al.* evaluated the role of TNF-α in HD pathogenesis blocking TNF-α signaling using an inhibitor of soluble TNF-α (XPro1595) in two *in vitro* models: i) primary astrocytes-enriched culture isolated from a transgenic mouse model (R6/2) exposed to lipopolysaccharide (LPS); and ii) human astrocyte- enriched culture derived from induced pluripotent stem cells (iPSCs) of patients with HD stimulated with cytokines. XPro1595 effectively inhibited the inflammatory response by blocking TNF-α, protecting the cytokine-induced toxicity in both models. *In vivo*, XPro1595 decreased TNF-α level in the cortex and striatum, enhanced motor function, decreased caspase activation, reduced the total of mHTT aggregates, improving neuronal density and decreasing gliosis in the brain of R6/2 mice [65].

Other compounds with anti-inflammatory / immuno-modulatory proprieties have been studied in HD. Sema-phorin 4D (SEMA4D) is a transmembrane signaling mole-cule that modifies a variety of mechanisms central to neu-roinflammation and neurodegeneration including glial cell activation, neuronal growth cone collapse and apoptosis of neural precursors, as well as inhibition of oligodendrocyte migration, differentiation and process formation [66]. A pre-clinical study evaluated the efficacy of an anti-SEMA4D monoclonal antibody, which prevents the interaction be-tween SEMA4D and its receptors, in the YAC128 HD mouse model. The treatment with anti-SEMA4D improved neuropathological signs, such as striatal, cortical and corpus callosum atrophy and avoided testicular degeneration. In parallel, a subset of behavioral symptoms improved in anti-SEMA4D treated YAC128 mice, including decreased anxi-ety-like behavior and rescue of cognitive deficits. There was, however, no visible effect on motor deficits [66]. At the moment, a clinical trial (NCT02481674) is recruiting partici-pants for testing VX15/2503 (a monoclonal antibody that blocks the activity of Semaphorin 4D) in HD.

There has been increasing interest in the role of trypto-phan (Trp) metabolites and the kynurenine pathway (KP) in neurodegenerative diseases. The KP diverges into two branches that can lead to the production of either neuropro-tective or neurotoxic metabolites. In one branch, kynurenine (Kyn) produced as a result of tryptophan (Trp) catabolism is further metabolized to neurotoxic metabolites such as 3-hydroxykunurenine (3-HK) and quinolinic acid (QA). In the other branch, Kyn is converted to the neuroprotective me-tabolite kynurenic acid (KA) [67]. There are several lines of evidence suggesting that this pathway is imbalanced in HD. For instance, patients with HD exhibited an increased neostriatal QA/KA ratio, caused by a rise in QA levels [68]. Also, a reduction in the levels of neuroprotective KA has been observed in the brain of HD patients [69]. In serum of HD patients, Trp levels are reduced, and the Kyn/Trp is elevated, coinciding with increased production of pro-inflammatory cytokines [70]. Based in these results, Zwill-ing *et al.*, studied in a mouse model of HD the effects of 2-(3,4-dimethoxybenzenesulfonylamino)- 4-(3- nitrophenyl)-5-(piperidin-1-yl) methylthiazole (JM6), an orally bioavailable inhibitor of kynurenine 3-monooxygenase (KMO). KMO is the enzyme required for the synthesis of QA, a neurotoxic metabolite. Treatment with JM6 prevented spatial memory deficits, anxiety-related behavior, and synaptic loss. JM6 also extended life span, prevented synaptic loss, and de-creased microglial activation in the HD experimental model [71]. No clinical trial has been planned with this drug so far.

Cannabinoids have been studied as a potential therapeu-tic approach in HD due to their anti- inflammatory properties among others [72]. A clinical trial was performed to test cannabidiol for 6 weeks in 15 patients with HD. Cannabidiol was considered safe and well tolerated, but no significant improvement in clinical outcomes was observed [73]. How-ever, a case-report described a great improvement in chorea

and behavioral symptoms, mainly irritability, with nabilone, a synthetic cannabinoid used as an antiemetic and as an add-on analgesic for neuropathic pain [74].

Another strategy that is appealing in HD is the idea to lower mutant huntingtin. There are preclinical studies to support the concept of RNA silencing, but, to date, no clini-cal studies have been performed in HD. Two viable treat-ments could decrease huntingtin mRNA and thereby mutant huntingtin protein: antisense oligonucleotide (ASO) and RNA interference (RNAi). ASOs are DNA-based small molecules [75] that do not cross the BBB. They are injected into the lumbar space to reach the CNS [76], determining knockdown of huntingtin mRNA and protein. RNAi uses a series of events in which a small RNA (siRNA) forms a complex with mRNA, bringing an assembly of proteins to the targeted mRNA. siRNA can be introduced into the brain directly, influencing huntingtin expression [77, 78]. It is un-certain the interaction of these approaches with immune-based mechanisms.

4.2. Stem Cells Therapy

Stem cell therapy is potentially a promising treatment for neurodegenerative diseases [79, 80]. During the past years, preclinical studies have proven the efficacy of stem cells in providing functional recovery in various pre-clinical models of HD [81, 82].

Stem cells are undifferentiated cells that can be differen-tiated into different types of cells. The goals of stem cell therapy involve the replenishment of lost cells and the in-crease in cell survival, reversing the disease phenotype or delaying disease progression over time. Theoretically, stem cells can provide therapeutic benefit through two main mechanisms. First, stem cells would differentiate into the lost cell type based on environmental cues, and would be able to reconnect with local circuits. In the second, cell transplantation should be able to work synergistically with the endogenous microenvironment to upregulate intrinsic cell proliferation or neuromodulation through neutrophic factors release and immunomodulation, potentially improv-ing the overall regenerative ability of the transplanted tissue [83, 84]. The second proposed mechanism is the most ac-cepted following stem cell transplantation in HD as these cells are able to provide trophic support, such as BDNF. In addition to the trophic support, immunomodulatory and anti-inflammatory properties of stem cells are very important mechanisms of action of these cells, which can contribute to decreasing the neuroinflammatory process present in HD [85].

Different types of stem cells are being studied in HD. Below we describe the most commonly studied stem cells and a summary of the results obtained in HD studies.

4.2.1. Mesenchymal Stem Cells

Mesenchymal stem cells (MSCs) are multipotent stem cells that are commonly found in umbilical cord, bone mar-row, and adipose tissue [86]. MSCs have the ability to dif-ferentiate into diverse types of cells and are easily culti-vated. MSCs also have paracrine effects as they secrete a variety of bioactive proteins such as neurotrophic factors and anti-inflammatory cytokines, which are thought to have neuroprotective and immunomodulatory activities, respectively. Therefore, it is proposed that the MSCs can promote a regenerative environment and they can act by decreasing inflammation, inhibiting apoptosis and increasing cell survival [87-89].

Several pre-clinical studies were performed using MSCs in animal models of HD. Human MSCs were capable of reducing striatal degeneration, prolonging survival and ameliorating motor deficits through trophic support in HD mouse models (both quinolinic acid (QA)-induced excitotoxicity model and R6/2 mice) [90]. Another study showed that human MSCs implanted into the striatum of N171-82Q mice (transgenic mice expressing an N-terminally truncated human HTT cDNA) increased trophic factors such as FGF-2 (fibroblast growth factor 2), VEGF (vascular endothelial growth factor) and NGF (nerve growth factor), and reduced striatal degeneration and atrophy observed in this animal model [91]. Reduced striatal degeneration and formation of ubiquitin-positive aggregates was also observed following MSCs transplantation in QA-induced striatal degeneration rats as well as in R6/2 mice. MSC transplantation also resulted in behavior improvement in these animals [92]. An additional study showed that R6/2 mice that received MSCs presented significantly less neuropathological changes than the untreated animals, but no motor benefits were observed [93]. Rat derived-MSCs were also tested in animal models of HD, resulting in reduced brain atrophy, increased levels of neurotrophic factors and improvement in behavior [94, 95]. Although MSCs improved behavior and neuropathological signs and increased the levels of neurotrophic factors in animal models of HD, information about the immunodulatory actions of MSCs is lacking. Immunomodulatory and anti-inflammatory are important mechanisms by which MSCs work, and hence further studies in HD are needed in this regard.

4.2.2. Embryonic Stem Cells

Embryonic stem cells (ESCs) are pluripotent stem cells that have the ability to differentiate into cells from all germ layers (ectoderm, mesoderm or endoderm). Human ESCs (hESCs) are derived from the internal cell mass of the blastocyst and have the potential to differentiate into any cell type from human body [96]. The blastocysts are derived from *in vitro* fertilized embryos that were donated to research, but the use of hESCs has important ethical concerns and it is subject to legal restrictions that may be different depending on the country [97, 98].

The transplantation of forebrain GABA neurons and their progenitors derived from hESCs in the striatum of QA-lesioned mice resulted in the generation of GABAergic neurons, corresponding to correction of motor deficits [99]. These neurons were positive for DARPP32 (dopamine- and cyclic-AMP-regulated phosphoprotein of molecular weight 32,000), which is a marker of medium spiny neurons (MSNs) and characterizes most striatal neurons [99]. Another study successfully used hESCs to generate MSNs. When MSNs were transplanted into the striatum of QA-lesioned rats, human derived neurons survived and they were DARPP32+, leading to a restoration of apomorphine-induced rotation behavior [100]. It is worth mentioning that these neurons not only expressed typical neuronal markers, but also carried dopamine and adenosine receptors.

4.2.3. Neural Stem Cells

In mammals, neural stem cells (NSCs) or neural precursor cells (NPCs) are isolated for research from three sources: fetal neural tissue (*i.e.* from aborted fetuses) [101, 102], resection margins of neurosurgically excised brain lesions involving neurogenic regions [103] and postmortem brains [104]. NSCs/NPCs have the potential to differentiate into neurons, astrocytes, and oligodendrocytes [105-107]. Some NSCs/NPSs have been immortalized by viral transduction or immortalized conditionally with transcription factor/mutant estrogen receptor system [101, 108, 109].

Previous studies have shown that NSCs isolated from fetal or adult mammalian brain can propagate *in vitro* [110] and be subsequently implanted in the brain of animals presenting human-like neurological disorders, including HD [111, 112]. In HD animal models, some cells differentiated *in vivo* into DARPP32+ neurons, replacing neurons primarily targeted in this disorder [111].

A study by McBride *et al.* showed that NSCs improved motor function in a rat model of HD [113]. Similarly, Ryu *et al.* showed that NSCs implantation reduce cellular damage and improved motor functions by increasing BDNF secretion [114]. A different group showed that i.v. administered NSCs are capable of migrating to the lesion site, reducing cellular damage and inducing functional recovery in the QA-induced lesion rat model of HD [115]. The same group also showed that NSCs can migrate into the striatum from both ventricle and systemic circulation [116]. Also, NPCs transplantation reduced rotational asymmetry and impairment of spontaneous exploratory forelimb use [117]. In addition, a study using NPCs pretreated with lithium accelerated the sensorimotor function recovery and increased the cellular survival in the QA- lesion rat model of HD [118]. Although, none of these studies evaluated immune and/or inflammatory mechanisms directly, it is highly possible that part of the benefits observed of NSCs in the animals with HD is mediated by their immunomodulatory properties.

4.2.4. Fetal Neural Tissue

Fetal neural tissue has been used in clinical studies with HD patients [119-122]. Neural tissue is isolated from aborted human fetuses that were donated to research. The use of fetal tissue has ethical concerns with respect to the donor and the patient [123]. Therefore, ethical guidelines for the use of fetal tissues have been established [124].

Initial studies on the safety of this procedure reported promising results, including patient tolerance to the transplantation procedure and the immunosuppressant drugs to avoid rejection of the transplant [125]. Patients with HD showed improvement of motor and cognitive symptoms following bilateral neurograft one year after transplantation [119]. During the long-term follow-up of these patients, three patients were in remission for 4-6 years, but thereafter, disease progression resumed [119]. A subsequent collabora-

Table 1.   Clinical trials performed for testing anti-inflammatory- / immunomodulatory-based therapies in Huntington's disease.

Trial	Intervention	Design	Endpoint classification	Outcomes	Status
NCT00029874	Minocycline	Randomized, double blind, placebo controlled, phase 1 / phase 2 trial (n=63)	Safety / Efficacy	No published results	Completed
NCT00277355	Minocycline	Multicenter, randomized, double blind, placebo controlled, phase 2 / phase 3 trial (n=114)	Safety/Efficacy	Minocycline at 100 and 200 mg/day for 8 weeks was well tolerated. Adverse events were not observed with minocycline	Completed
NCT02215616	Laquinimod	Multicenter, randomized, double blind, placebo controlled, phase 2 trial (n=400)	Safety / Efficacy	No published results	Currently recruiting. Estimated primary completion date: August 2017
NCT01834053	Autologous Stem Cell (100 millions per dose)	Open Label, phase 1/phase 2 (n=50)	Safety / Efficacy	No published results	Completed
NCT02481674	VX15/2503	Multicenter, randomized, double blind, placebo controlled, phase 2 trial (n=84)	Safety / Efficacy	No published results	Currently recruiting. Estimated primary completion date: August 2018
NCT01502046	Cannabinoids: delta-9-tetrahydrocannabinol (THC) and cannabidiol (CBD)	Randomized, double blind, cross over, placebo controlled, phase 2 trial (n = 25)	Safety	No published results	Completed

tive effort failed to demonstrate a functional benefit of neurograft during the long-term follow-up of transplanted patients, and this may have been due to the lesser amount of transplanted tissue [126]. Safety concerns also emerged based on adverse effects, [127] such as graft overgrowth, cyst development, and subdural hematoma [122, 128]. With just a few numbers of treated HD patients and substantial differences in the study protocols, it is not possible to draw definite conclusions about the efficacy and long-term safety of fetal neurograft for HD.

CONCLUSION

Despite the discovery of the *huntingtin* gene more than 20 years ago, a disease modifying agent for the disease remains elusive. Therefore, further studies are necessary to discover new therapeutic targets to slow or halt disease progression.

There are promising avenues to HD treatment with anti-inflammatory and immunomodulatory- based strategies. However, it is necessary to better understand the specific immune/inflammatory mechanisms that are involved in HD pathophysiology. Besides immune-based pharmacological interventions, stem cells are also promising due to their immunomodulatory and/or anti- inflammatory properties.

LIST OF ABBREVIATIONS

BDNF   =   Brain-derived Neurotrophic Factor
CNS   =   Central Nervous System
DARPP32 =   Dopamine- and Cyclic-AMP-regulated Phosphoprotein of Molecular Weight 32,000
iPSCs   =   Induced Pluripotent Stem Cells
KA   =   Kynurenic Acid
MSCs   =   Mesenchymal Stem Cell
MSNs   =   Medium Spiny Neurons
NPSs   =   Neural Precursor Cells
NSCs   =   Neural Stem Cells
QA   =   Quinolinic Acid
SEMA4D =   Semaphorin-4D

TNF-α   =   Tumor Necrosis Factor-α

Trp   =   Tryptophan

VMAT-2   =   Vesicular Monoamine Transporter 2

CONSENT FOR PUBLICATION

Not applicable.

CONFLICT OF INTEREST

The authors declare no conflict of interest, financial or otherwise.

ACKNOWLEDGEMENTS

The Neuropsychiatry Program is funded by the Department of Psychiatry and Behavioral Sciences, UT Health Houston. The UT Health Center of Excellence in Huntington's Disease is partly funded by the Huntington's Disease Society of America.

REFERENCES

[1]   MacDonald ME, Barnes G, Srinidhi J, *et al.* Gametic but not somatic instability of CAG repeats length in Huntington's disease. J Med Genet 1993; 30(12): 982-6.

[2]   Hult S, Schultz K, Soylu R, Petersen A. Hypothalamic and neuroendocrine changes in Huntington's disease. Curr Drug Targets 2010; 11(10): 1237-49.

[3]   Anderson KE, Marder KS. An overview of psychiatric symptoms in Huntington's disease. Current Psychiatry Reports 2001; 3(5): 379-88.

[4]   Lawrence AD, Sahakian BJ, Hodges JR, *et al.* Executive and mnemonic functions in early Huntington's disease. Brain 1996; 119 (Pt 5): 1633-45.

[5]   Tabrizi SJ, Langbehn DR, Leavitt BR, *et al.* Biological and clinical manifestations of Huntington's disease in the longitudinal TRACK-HD study: cross- sectional analysis of baseline data. Lancet Neurol 2009; 8(9): 791-801.

[6]   Reedeker W, van der Mast RC, Giltay EJ, *et al.* Psychiatric disorders in Huntington's disease: a 2-year follow-up study. Psychosomatics 2012; 53(3): 220-9.

[7]   Pflanz S, Besson JA, Ebmeier KP, Simpson S. The clinical manifestation of mental disorder in Huntington's disease: a retrospective case record study of disease progression. Acta psychiatrica Scandinavica 1991; 83(1): 53-60.

[8]   Aziz NA, van der Burg JM, Landwehrmeyer GB, *et al.* Weight loss in Huntington disease increases with higher CAG repeat number. Neurology 2008; 71(19): 1506-13.

[9]   Petersen A, Bjorkqvist M. Hypothalamic-endocrine aspects in Huntington's disease. Eur J Neuro Sci 2006; 24(4): 961-7.

[10]   van der Burg JM, Bjorkqvist M, Brundin P. Beyond the brain: widespread pathology in Huntington's disease. Lancet Neurol 2009; 8(8): 765-74.

[11]   Langbehn DR, Hayden MR, Paulsen JS, Group P-HIotHS. CAG-repeat length and the age of onset in Huntington disease (HD): a review and validation study of statistical approaches. Am J Med Genet B Neuropsychiatr Genet 2010; 153B(2): 397-408.

[12]   Heng MY, Detloff PJ, Wang PL, Tsien JZ, Albin RL. *In vivo* evidence for NMDA receptor-mediated excitotoxicity in a murine genetic model of Huntington disease. J Neurosci 2009; 29(10): 3200-5.

[13]   Gil-Mohapel J, Brocardo PS, Christie BR. The role of oxidative stress in Huntington's disease: are antioxidants good therapeutic candidates? Curr Drug Targets 2014; 15(4): 454-68.

[14]   Wild EJ, Tabrizi SJ. Targets for future clinical trials in Huntington's disease: what's in the pipeline? Mov Disord 2014; 29(11): 1434-45.

[15]   Shannon KM, Fraint A. Therapeutic advances in Huntington's Disease. Mov Disord 2015; 30(11): 1539-46.

[16]   Trottier Y, Devys D, Imbert G, *et al.* Cellular localization of the Huntington's disease protein and discrimination of the normal and mutated form. Nature Genet 1995; 10(1): 104-10.

[17]   Ferrante RJ, Gutekunst CA, Persichetti F, *et al.* Heterogeneous topographic and cellular distribution of huntingtin expression in the normal human neostriatum. J Neuro Sci 1997; 17(9): 3052-63.

[18]   Bjorkqvist M, Wild EJ, Thiele J, *et al.* A novel pathogenic pathway of immune activation detectable before clinical onset in Huntington's disease. J Exp Med 2008; 205(8): 1869-77.

[19]   Crotti A, Benner C, Kerman BE, *et al.* Mutant Huntingtin promotes autonomous microglia activation via myeloid lineage-determining factors. Nature Neuro Sci 2014; 17(4): 513-21.

[20]   Kreutzberg GW. Microglia: a sensor for pathological events in the CNS. Trends Neuro Sci 1996; 19(8): 312-8.

[21]   Melton LM, Keith AB, Davis S, *et al.* Chronic glial activation, neurodegeneration, and APP immunoreactive deposreuits following acute administration of double-stranded RNA. Glia 2003; 44(1): 1-12.

[22]   Nakanishi H. Microglial functions and proteases. Mol Neurobiol 2003; 27(2): 163-76.

[23]   Rocha NP, Ribeiro FM, Furr-Stimming E, Teixeira AL. Neuroimmunology of Huntington's Disease: revisiting evidence from human studies. Mediators Inflamm 2016; 2016: 8653132.

[24]   Drouin-Ouellet J, Sawiak SJ, Cisbani G, *et al.* Cerebrovascular and blood-brain barrier impairments in Huntington's disease: potential implications for its pathophysiology. Ann Neurol 2015; 78(2): 160-77.

[25]   Villeda SA, Luo J, Mosher KI, *et al.* The ageing systemic milieu negatively regulates neurogenesis and cognitive function. Nature 2011; 477(7362): 90-4.

[26]   Crotti A, Glass CK. The choreography of neuroinflammation in Huntington's disease. Trends Immunol 2015; 36(6): 364-73.

[27]   Pavese N, Gerhard A, Tai YF, *et al.* Microglial activation correlates with severity in Huntington disease: a clinical and PET study. Neurology 2006; 66(11): 1638-43.

[28]   Tai YF, Pavese N, Gerhard A, *et al.* Microglial activation in presymptomatic Huntington's disease gene carriers. Brain 2007; 130(Pt 7): 1759-66.

[29]   Silvestroni A, Faull RL, Strand AD, Moller T. Distinct neuroinflammatory profile in post-mortem human Huntington's disease. Neuroreport 2009; 20(12): 1098-103.

[30]   Wild E, Magnusson A, Lahiri N, *et al.* Abnormal peripheral chemokine profile in Huntington's disease. PLoS Curr 2011; 3: RRN1231.

[31]   Franciosi S, Ryu JK, Shim Y, *et al.* Age-dependent neurovascular abnormalities and altered microglial morphology in the YAC128 mouse model of Huntington disease. Neurobiol Dis 2012; 45(1): 438-49.

[32]   Ribeiro FM, Camargos ER, de Souza LC, Teixeira AL. Animal models of neurodegenerative diseases. Rev Bras Psiquiatr 2013; 35 Suppl 2: S82-91.

[33]   Armstrong MJ, Miyasaki JM. Evidence-based guideline: pharmacologic treatment of chorea in Huntington disease: report of the guideline development subcommittee of the American Academy of Neurology. Neurology 2012; 79(6): 597-603.

[34]   Hayden MR, Leavitt BR, Yasothan U, Kirkpatrick P. Tetrabenazine. Nat Rev Drug Discov 2009; 8(1): 17-8.

[35]   Huntington G, Frank S, Testa CM, *et al.* Effect of deutetrabenazine on chorea among patients with huntington disease: a randomized clinical trial. JAMA 2016; 316(1): 40-50.

[36]   Adam OR, Jankovic J. Symptomatic treatment of Huntington disease. Neurotherapeutics 2008; 5(2): 181-97.

[37]   Bonelli RM, Niederwieser G, Diez J, Gruber A, Koltringer P. Pramipexole ameliorates neurologic and psychiatric symptoms in a Westphal variant of Huntington's disease. Clin Neuropharmacol 2002; 25(1): 58-60.

[38]   Racette BA, Perlmutter JS. Levodopa responsive parkinsonism in an adult with Huntington's disease. J Neurol 1998; 65(4): 577-9.

[39]   Frank S. Treatment of Huntington's disease. Neurotherapeutics 2014; 11(1): 153-60.

[40]   Pla P, Orvoen S, Saudou F, David DJ, Humbert S. Mood disorders in Huntington's disease: from behavior to cellular and molecular mechanisms. Front Behav Neurosc 2014; 8: 135.

[41]   Vattakatuchery JJ, Kurien R. Acetylcholinesterase inhibitors in cognitive impairment in Huntington's disease: A brief review. World J Psychiatry 2013; 3(3): 62-4.

[42]   Antonio LT. Revisiting the neuropsychiatry of Huntington's disease. Neuropsychologia 2016; 10(4): 261-6.

[43]   Terzi M, Altun G, Sen S, *et al.* The use of non-steroidal anti-inflammatory drugs in neurological diseases. J Chem Neuroanat 2017; S0891-0618(16): 30289-7

[44]   Norflus F, Nanje A, Gutekunst CA, *et al.* Anti- inflammatory treatment with acetylsalicylate or rofecoxib is not neuroprotective in Huntington's disease transgenic mice. Neurobiol Dis 2004; 17(2): 319-25.

[45]   Noble W, Garwood CJ, Hanger DP. Minocycline as a potential therapeutic agent in neurodegenerative disorders characterised by protein misfolding. Prion 2009; 3(2): 78-83.

[46]   Familian A, Boshuizen RS, Eikelenboom P, Veerhuis R. Inhibitory effect of minocycline on amyloid beta fibril formation and human microglial activation. Glia 2006; 53(3): 233-40.

[47]   Du Y, Ma Z, Lin S, *et al.* Minocycline prevents nigrostriatal dopaminergic neurodegeneration in the MPTP model of Parkinson's disease. Proc Natl Acad Sci U S A 2001; 98(25): 14669-74.

[48]   Chen M, Ona VO, Li M, *et al.* Minocycline inhibits caspase-1 and caspase-3 expression and delays mortality in a transgenic mouse model of Huntington disease. Nature Med 2000; 6(7): 797-801.

[49]   Wang X, Zhu S, Drozda M, *et al.* Minocycline inhibits caspase-independent and -dependent mitochondrial cell death pathways in models of Huntington's disease. Proc Natl Acad Sci U S A 2003; 100(18): 10483-7.

[50]   Kriz J, Nguyen MD, Julien JP. Minocycline slows disease progression in a mouse model of amyotrophic lateral sclerosis. Neurobiol Dis 2002; 10(3): 268-78.

[51]   Zhu S, Stavrovskaya IG, Drozda M, *et al.* Minocycline inhibits cytochrome release and delays progression of amyotrophic lateral sclerosis in mice. Nature 2002; 417(6884): 74-8.

[52]   Popovic N, Schubart A, Goetz BD, *et al.* Inhibition of autoimmune encephalomyelitis by a tetracycline. Ann Neurol 2002; 51(2): 215-23.

[53]   Stirling DP, Khodarahmi K, Liu J, *et al.* Minocycline treatment reduces delayed oligodendrocyte death, attenuates axonal dieback, and improves functional outcome after spinal cord injury. J Neurosci 2004; 24(9): 2182-90.

[54]   Teng YD, Choi H, Onario RC, *et al.* Minocycline inhibits contusion-triggered mitochondrial cytochrome c release and mitigates functional deficits after spinal cord injury. J Neurosci 2004; 101(9): 3071-6.

[55]   Sanchez MRO, Ona VO, Li M, Friedlander RM. Minocycline reduces traumatic brain injury-mediated caspase-1 activation, tissue damage, and neurological dysfunction. Neurosurgery 2001; 48(6): 1393-9.

[56]   Huntington G. Minocycline safety and tolerability in Huntington disease. Neurology 2004; 63(3): 547-9.

[57]   Bonelli RM, Hodl AK, Hofmann P, Kapfhammer HP. Neuroprotection in Huntington's disease: a 2-year study on minocycline. Int Clin Psychopharmacol 2004; 19(6): 337-42.

[58]   Huntington DI. A futility study of minocycline in Huntington's disease. Mov Disord 2010; 25(13): 2219-24.

[59]   Kolb-Sobieraj C, Gupta S, Weinstock-Guttman B. Laquinimod therapy in multiple sclerosis: a comprehensive review. Neurol Ther 2014; 3(1): 29-39.

[60]   Garcia-Miralles M, Hong X, Tan LJ, *et al.* Laquinimod rescues striatal, cortical and white matter pathology and results in modest behavioural improvements in the YAC128 model of Huntington disease. Sci Rep 2016; 6: 31652.

[61]   Bruck W, Vollmer T. Multiple sclerosis: oral laquinimod for MS-bringing the brain into focus. Nat Rev Neurol 2013; 9(12): 664-5.

[62]   Varrin-Doyer M, Zamvil SS, Schulze-Topphoff U. Laquinimod, an up-and-coming immunomodulatory agent for treatment of multiple sclerosis. Exp Neurol 2014; 262: 66-71.

[63]   Thone J, Ellrichmann G, Seubert S, *et al.* Modulation of autoimmune demyelination by laquinimod *via* induction of brain-derived neurotrophic factor. Am J Pathol 2012; 180(1): 267-74.

[64]   Zuccato C, Cattaneo E. Role of brain-derived neurotrophic factor in Huntington's disease. Prog Neurobiol. 2007; 81(5-6): 294-330.

[65]   Hsiao HY, Chiu FL, Chen CM, *et al.* Inhibition of soluble tumor necrosis factor is therapeutic in Huntington's disease. Hum Mol Genet 2014; 23(16): 4328-44.

[66]   Southwell AL, Franciosi S, Villanueva EB, *et al.* Anti-semaphorin 4D immunotherapy ameliorates neuropathology and

[67]   some cognitive impairment in the YAC128 mouse model of Huntington disease. Neurobiol Dis 2015; 76: 46-56.

[67]   Mazarei G, Leavitt BR. Indoleamine 2, 3 Dioxygenase as a potential therapeutic target in Huntington's disease. J Huntingtons Dis 2015; 4(2): 109-18.

[68]   Guidetti P, Luthi-Carter RE, Augood SJ, Schwarcz R. Neostriatal and cortical quinolinate levels are increased in early grade Huntington's disease. Neurobiol Dis 2004; 17(3): 455-61.

[69]   Sapko MT, Guidetti P, Yu P, Tagle DA, Pellicciari R, Schwarcz R. Endogenous kynurenate controls the vulnerability of striatal neurons to quinolinate: implications for Huntington's disease. Exp Neurol 2006; 197(1): 31-40.

[70]   Stoy N, Mackay GM, Forrest CM, *et al.* Tryptophan metabolism and oxidative stress in patients with Huntington's disease. J Neurochem 2005; 93(3): 611-23.

[71]   Zwilling D, Huang SY, Sathyasaikumar KV, *et al.* Kynurenine 3-monooxygenase inhibition in blood ameliorates neurodegeneration. Cell 2011; 145(6): 863-74.

[72]   Saito VM, Rezende RM, Teixeira AL. Cannabinoid modulation of neuroinflammatory disorders. Curr Neuropharmacol 2012; 10(2): 159-66.

[73]   Consroe P, Laguna J, Allender J, *et al.* Controlled clinical trial of cannabidiol in Huntington's disease. Pharmacol Biochem Behav 1991; 40(3): 701-8.

[74]   Curtis A, Rickards H. Nabilone could treat chorea and irritability in Huntington's disease. J Neuropsychiatry Clin Neurosci 2006; 18(4): 553-4.

[75]   Aronin N, DiFiglia M. Huntingtin-lowering strategies in Huntington's disease: antisense oligonucleotides, small RNAs, and gene editing. Mov Disord 2014; 29(11): 1455-61.

[76]   Kordasiewicz HB, Stanek LM, Wancewicz EV, *et al.* Sustained therapeutic reversal of Huntington's disease by transient repression of huntingtin synthesis. Neuron 2012; 74(6): 1031-44.

[77]   DiFiglia M, Sena-Esteves M, Chase K, *et al.* Therapeutic silencing of mutant huntingtin with siRNA attenuates striatal and cortical neuropathology and behavioral deficits. Proc Natl Acad Sci USA 2007; 104(43): 17204-9.

[78]   Stiles DK, Zhang Z, Ge P, *et al.* Widespread suppression of huntingtin with convection-enhanced delivery of siRNA. Exp Neurol 2012; 233(1): 463-71.

[79]   Dutta S, Singh G, Sreejith S, *et al.* Cell therapy: the final frontier for treatment of neurological diseases. CNS Neurosci Ther 2013; 19(1): 5-11.

[80]   Colpo GD, Ascoli BM, Wollenhaupt-Aguiar B, *et al.* Mesenchymal stem cells for the treatment of neurodegenerative and psychiatric disorders. An Acad Bras Cienc 2015; 87(2 Suppl): 1435-49.

[81]   Hosseini M, Moghadas M, Edalatmanesh MA, Hashemzadeh MR. Xenotransplantation of human adipose derived mesenchymal stem cells in a rodent model of Huntington's disease: motor and non-motor outcomes. Neurol Res 2015; 37(4): 309-19.

[82]   Kerkis I, Haddad MS, Valverde CW, Glosman S. Neural and mesenchymal stem cells in animal models of Huntington's disease: past experiences and future challenges. Stem Cell Res Ther 2015; 6: 232.

[83]   Sadan O, Shemesh N, Barzilay R, *et al.* Migration of neurotrophic factors-secreting mesenchymal stem cells toward a quinolinic acid lesion as viewed by magnetic resonance imaging. Stem Cells 2008; 26(10): 2542-51.

[84]   Uccelli A, Benvenuto F, Laroni A, Giunti D. Neuroprotective features of mesenchymal stem cells. Best Pract Res Clin Haematol 2011; 24(1): 59-64.

[85]   Politis M, Lahiri N, Niccolini F, *et al.* Increased central microglial activation associated with peripheral cytokine levels in premanifest Huntington's disease gene carriers. Neurobiol Dis 2015; 83: 115-21.

[86]   A.I. C. Mesenchymal stem cells: Handbook of stem cells. . Atala A LR, editor 2004.

[87]   Caplan AI, Dennis JE. Mesenchymal stem cells as trophic mediators. J Cell Biochem 2006; 98(5): 1076-84.

[88]   Bianco P, Cao X, Frenette PS, *et al.* The meaning, the sense and the significance: translating the science of mesenchymal stem cells into medicine. Nat Med 2013; 19(1): 35-42.

[89]   Caplan AI, Correa D. The MSC: an injury drugstore. Cell Stem Cell 2011; 9(1): 11-5.

[90] Lin YT, Chern Y, Shen CK, *et al.* Human mesenchymal stem cells prolong survival and ameliorate motor deficit through trophic support in Huntington's disease mouse models. PloS One 2011; 6(8): e22924.

[91] Snyder BR, Chiu AM, Prockop DJ, Chan AW. Human multipotent stromal cells (MSCs) increase neurogenesis and decrease atrophy of the striatum in a transgenic mouse model for Huntington's disease. PloS One 2010; 5(2): e9347.

[92] Lee ST, Chu K, Jung KH, *et al.* Slowed progression in models of Huntington disease by adipose stem cell transplantation. Ann Neurol 2009; 66(5): 671-81.

[93] Fink KD, Rossignol J, Crane AT, *et al.* Transplantation of umbilical cord-derived mesenchymal stem cells into the striata of R6/2 mice: behavioral and neuropathological analysis. Stem Cell Res Ther 2013; 4(5): 130.

[94] Moraes L, Vasconcelos-dos-Santos A, Santana FC, *et al.* Neuroprotective effects and magnetic resonance imaging of mesenchymal stem cells labeled with SPION in a rat model of Huntington's disease. Stem Cell Res 2012; 9(2): 143-55.

[95] Rossignol J, Boyer C, Leveque X, *et al.* Mesenchymal stem cell transplantation and DMEM administration in a 3NP rat model of Huntington's disease: morphological and behavioral outcomes. Behav Brain Res 2011; 217(2): 369-78.

[96] Thomson JA, Marshall VS, Trojanowski JQ. Neural differentiation of rhesus embryonic stem cells. APMIS 1998; 106(1): 149-56.

[97] Hovatta O, Stojkovic M, Nogueira M, Varela-Nieto I. European scientific, ethical, and legal issues on human stem cell research and regenerative medicine. Stem Cells 2010; 28(6): 1005-7.

[98] Lo B, Zettler P, Cedars MI, *et al.* A new era in the ethics of human embryonic stem cell research. Stem Cells 2005; 23(10): 1454-9.

[99] Ma L, Hu B, Liu Y, *et al.* Human embryonic stem cell- derived GABA neurons correct locomotion deficits in quinolinic acid-lesioned mice. Cell Stem Cell 2012; 10(4): 455-64.

[100] Delli Carri A, Onorati M, Lelos MJ, *et al.* Developmentally coordinated extrinsic signals drive human pluripotent stem cell differentiation toward authentic DARPP-32+ medium-sized spiny neurons. Develop 2013; 140(2): 301-12.

[101] Donato R, Miljan EA, Hines SJ, *et al.* Differential development of neuronal physiological responsiveness in two human neural stem cell lines. BMC Neurosci 2007; 8: 36.

[102] Monni E, Cusulin C, Cavallaro M, Lindvall O, Kokaia Z. Human fetal striatum-derived neural stem (NS) cells differentiate to mature neurons *in vitro* and *in vivo*. Curr Stem Cell Res Ther 2014; 9(4): 338-46.

[103] Sanai N, Tramontin AD, Quinones-Hinojosa A, *et al.* Unique astrocyte ribbon in adult human brain contains neural stem cells but lacks chain migration. Nature 2004; 427(6976): 740-4.

[104] van Strien ME, Sluijs JA, Reynolds BA, *et al.* Isolation of neural progenitor cells from the human adult subventricular zone based on expression of the cell surface marker CD. Stem Cells Transl Med 2014; 3(4): 470-80.

[105] Eriksson PS, Perfilieva E, Bjork-Eriksson T, *et al.* Neurogenesis in the adult human hippocampus. Nat Med 1998; 4(11): 1313-7.

[106] Reynolds BA, Weiss S. Generation of neurons and astrocytes from isolated cells of the adult mammalian central nervous system. Science 1992; 255(5052): 1707-10.

[107] Temple S. Division and differentiation of isolated CNS blast cells in microculture. Nature 1989; 340(6233): 471-3.

[108] El-Akabawy G, Medina LM, Jeffries A, Price J, Modo M. Purmorphamine increases DARPP-32 differentiation in human striatal neural stem cells through the Hedgehog pathway. Stem Cells Dev 2011; 20(11): 1873-87.

[109] Flax JD, Aurora S, Yang C, *et al.* Engraftable human neural stem cells respond to developmental cues, replace neurons, and express foreign genes. Nat Biotechnol 1998; 16(11): 1033-9.

[110] Gage FH. Mammalian neural stem cells. Science 2000; 287(5457): 1433-8.

[111] Armstrong RJ, Watts C, Svendsen CN, Dunnett SB, Rosser AE. Survival, neuronal differentiation, and fiber outgrowth of propagated human neural precursor grafts in an animal model of Huntington's disease. Cell Trans 2000; 9(1): 55-64.

[112] Mothe AJ, Zahir T, Santaguida C, Cook D, Tator CH. Neural stem/progenitor cells from the adult human spinal cord are multipotent and self-renewing and differentiate after transplantation. PloS One 2011; 6(11): e27079.

[113] McBride JL, Behrstock SP, Chen EY, *et al.* Human neural stem cell transplants improve motor function in a rat model of Huntington's disease. J Comp Neurol 2004; 475(2): 211-9.

[114] Ryu JK, Kim J, Cho SJ, *et al.* Proactive transplantation of human neural stem cells prevents degeneration of striatal neurons in a rat model of Huntington disease. Neurobiol Dis 2004; 16(1): 68-77.

[115] Lee ST, Chu K, Park JE, *et al.* Intravenous administration of human neural stem cells induces functional recovery in Huntington's disease rat model. Neurosci Res 2005; 52(3): 243-9.

[116] Lee ST, Park JE, Lee K, *et al.* Noninvasive method of immortalized neural stem-like cell transplantation in an experimental model of Huntington's disease. J Neurosci Methods 2006; 152(1-2): 250-4.

[117] Vazey EM, Chen K, Hughes SM, Connor B. Transplanted adult neural progenitor cells survive, differentiate and reduce motor function impairment in a rodent model of Huntington's disease. Exp Neurol 2006; 199(2): 384-96.

[118] Vazey EM, Dottori M, Jamshidi P, *et al.* Comparison of transplant efficiency between spontaneously derived and noggin-primed human embryonic stem cell neural precursors in the quinolinic acid rat model of Huntington's disease. Cell Transplant 2010; 19(8): 1055-62.

[119] Bachoud-Levi AC, Remy P, Nguyen JP, *et al.* Motor and cognitive improvements in patients with Huntington's disease after neural transplantation. Lancet 2000; 356(9246): 1975-9.

[120] Gallina P, Paganini M, Lombardini L, *et al.* Human striatal neuroblasts develop and build a striatal-like structure into the brain of Huntington's disease patients after transplantation. Exp Neurol 2010; 222(1): 30-41.

[121] Reuter I, Tai YF, Pavese N, *et al.* Long-term clinical and positron emission tomography outcome of fetal striatal transplantation in Huntington's disease. J Neurol Neurosurg Psychiatry 2008; 79(8): 948-51.

[122] Hauser RA, Sandberg PR, Freeman TB, Stoessl AJ. Bilateral human fetal striatal transplantation in Huntington's disease. Neurology 2002; 58(11): 170.

[123] Boer GJ. Ethical issues in neurografting of human embryonic cells. Theor Med Bioeth 1999; 20(5): 461-75.

[124] Boer GJ. Ethical guidelines for the use of human embryonic or fetal tissue for experimental and clinical neurotransplantation and research. Network of European CNS Transplantation and Restoration (NECTAR). J Neurol 1994; 242(1): 1-13.

[125] Kopyov OV, Jacques S, Lieberman A, Duma CM, Eagle KS. Safety of intrastriatal neurotransplantation for Huntington's disease patients. Exp Neurol 1998; 149(1): 97-108.

[126] Barker RA, Mason SL, Harrower TP, *et al.* The long- term safety and efficacy of bilateral transplantation of human fetal striatal tissue in patients with mild to moderate Huntington's disease. J Neurol Neurosurg Psychiatry 2013; 84(6): 657-65.

[127] Freeman TB, Cicchetti F, Bachoud-Levi AC, Dunnett SB. Technical factors that influence neural transplant safety in Huntington's disease. Exp Neurol 2011; 227(1): 1-9.

[128] Keene CD, Chang RC, Leverenz JB, *et al.* A patient with Huntington's disease and long-surviving fetal neural transplants that developed mass lesions. Acta Neuropathol 2009; 117(3): 329-38.

Send Orders for Reprints to reprints@benthamscience.ae

REVIEW ARTICLE

Interrelationships Among Gut Microbiota and Host: Paradigms, Role in Neurodegenerative Diseases and Future Prospects

Javier Caballero-Villarraso[1,2,3], Alberto Galván[1,2], Begoña María Escribano[2,4] and Isaac Túnez[1,2,*]

[1]Departamento de Bioquimica y Biologia Molecular, Facultad de Medicina y Enfermeria, Universidad de Cordoba, Spain; [2]Instituto Maimonides de Investigacion Biomedica de Cordoba (IMIBIC), Spain; Red Tematica de Investigacion Cooperativa en Envejecimiento y Fragilidad (RETICEF), Spain; [3]Unidad de Gestion Clinica de Analisis Clinicos, Hospital Universitario Reina Sofia, Cordoba, Spain; Departamento de Biologia Celular, Fisiologia e Inmunologia, Facultad de Veterinaria, Universidad de Cordoba, Spain

Abstract: ***Background & Objective***: Advances in the knowledge of the microbiota and concepts related to it have triggered a wake-up call in biomedicine. The development in various scientific areas has enabled a better and broader approach to everything concerning the set of families of microorganisms that coexist with an individual and are able to function as one or more organs in its body. Among the aforementioned scientific areas, those worth mentioning are the advances/progress in biotechnological resources and, in particular, molecular biology and related areas. This has given rise to the era of "omics", marking a turning point in the understanding of numerous physiologic and pathophysiologic processes of the organism.

The current theory is that the microbiota and the host maintain an intimate relationship that is of a markedly bilateral nature. This continuous feedback has different connotations between one individual and another, but also within the same individual throughout its life span, which is determined by its own conditioning factors (such as its genetic profile), and environmental ones (mainly diet and lifestyles). Both elements (microbiota and host) coexist harmoniously, maintaining a balance, which can be altered and give rise to different morbid entities. Among these is its relation to chronic processes, and especially those of an autoimmune origin.

Such may be neurological diseases situations and, specifically, those of a neurodegenerative nature. In disorders such as multiple sclerosis, amyotrophic lateral sclerosis, Huntington's chorea and Alzheimer's disease, among others, it has been found that a disharmonic coexistence between microbiota and host may have implications in their etiology and pathogenesis. A better understanding of those implications has led to the development of actions on the gut microbiota as a target to slow down the advancement or establishment of neurodegeneration.

Conclusion: In this scenario, several treatment strategies have emerged, such as probiotic food intake and stool transplantation. Their real potentialities remain to be elucidated, although current scientific evidence infers that the development of those therapeutic approaches could offer a ray of hope in the prospects of tackling neurodegenerative diseases.

ARTICLE HISTORY

Received: April 10, 2017
Revised: June 18, 2017
Accepted: July 01, 2017

DOI:
10.2174/1871527316666170714120118

Keywords: Brain-gut-microbiota axis, microbiota, neurodegenerative diseases, nutritional therapy, stool transplant, targeted therapy.

1. INTRODUCTION

In the last two decades, in the field of biosciences, everything concerning the concept of microbiota and the elements identified in relation to it has become increasingly relevant. This term has replaced the old notion of flora or microflora, in the light of the continuous development of knowledge on the quantitative and qualitative composition of microorganism populations integrated into the economy of other multicellular organisms [1-3].

It can be said that the microbiota is inherent to the human being, but it is far from being exclusive to it. On the contrary, from a much broader biological perspective, the microbiota is present in diverse locations of a wide range of species of the animal and vegetable kingdom. These would range from microscopic organisms to higher animals [2, 4].

*Address correspondence to this author at the Departamento de Bioquimica y Biologia Molecular, Facultad de Medicina y Enfermeria, Universidad de Cordoba, Avda. Menendez Pidal s/n, CP: 14004, Spain;
Tel: +34 957218268; Fax: +34957218229; E-mail: fm2tufi@uco.es

Microorganisms and substances derived from their metabolic activities are of great relevance to the development and functions of other phylogenetically superior living beings. This would be the case of *Caernorhaditis elegans*, which uses AWB chemoreceptors to drive away *Serratia marcescens*, which could destroy the eggs of this worm by digestion. Another case is that of the fly *Drosophila melanogaster,* which is repelled by geosmin (substance produced by the fungus *Penicillium* and by the bacterium *Streptomyces*), because if the fly were to ingest fruit infected by geosmin, it would die. Another example in insects is *Schistocerca gregraria* (lobster of the desert) that, in herding instinct situations, undergoes changes in behavior, as well as hormonal and genetic modifications, to enable it to develop communities. Such changes are produced by a response to guaiacol, which is synthesized by different bacteria: *Pantoea agglomerans, Klebsiella pneuominiae* and *Enterobacter cloacae* [5, 6].

In other higher beings, such as mammalians, similar situations can be verified. Herpestes auropunctatus, a mongoose of Indian origin, contains in its olfactory glands bacteria capable of producing short-chain fatty acids (SCFA), which serve as a communication tool between individuals of the same species. Another example in mammals could be the house mouse (Mus musculus), whose urinary tract contains bacteria with metabolic products that enable them to communicate with their congeners and with competing animals [7].

It could be said that the microorganisms that make up the microbiota have evolved towards being able to live in the host, having achieved a bilateral tolerance and even beyond that, both parts having been interweaved to develop functions in a coordinated and sometimes collaborative way [8, 9]. Such coexistence could bear some analogy with the theory that mitochondria were bacteria that evolved in conjunction with primitive cells. This hypothesis was proposed by Guerrero and Margulis, who claimed that the co-evolution of the original cell and the mitochondria phylogenetically ended up originating a single "symbiotic entity", which would be the cell ancestor of the cytological lineages of higher animals. Although both original elements (primitive cell and mitochondria) had different genomes, they came to live in a stable and balanced way, and can even function synchronously and harmonically [10].

In humans, the microbiota can be located in numerous areas and anatomic compartments, and can go from the skin cover (or an equivalent surface) to all the space that is in some way in contact with the outside environment. Therefore, at the tissue level, it usually presents lining epithelia: kerato-conjunctival surface, auditory ducts, respiratory mucosa (from oral cavity and nostrils, to tracheobronchial tree), urinary tract and vaginal cavity. Special mention should be made of areas with abundant capillary presence (scalp, armpits, genitals), as well as folds and rough or irregular areas, such as nail bed and groin [11, 12]. But, undoubtedly, the microbiotic location of the greatest relevance, both in quantity and in diversity, is the digestive tract, in which 90% of the known bacteria in the human body can be found [13].

The intestinal microbiota consists essentially of two bacterial families with a majority presence: *Firmicutes* and *Bac-* *teroides.* In the first family we could single out the genera *Clostridium, Lactobacillus* and *Ruminococcus*; the genera *Eubacterium, Faecalibacterium* and *Roseburia* could also be distinguished. In the second family, the genera *Prevotella* and *Xylanibacteria* are prominent [14]. There is a relatively constant proportion between both families, which when altered gives rise to situations called dysbiosis (also known as dysbacteriosis) [15].

There are two other major families of relevant bacteria, although they are less present: *Actinobacteria* (the major exponent of which is *Bifidobacterium*) and *Proteobacteria* (among which we should highlight *Escherichia* and *Desulfovibrio*). In addition to the above-mentioned bacterial families, the gut microbiota is also composed of viruses, protozoa, archaea and fungi [15, 16].

It can be observed how the composition of the microbiota presents variations in the different locations of the same organism. Thus, the oral cavity, the skin and the intestines of the same higher animal can present a completely different microbiota profile. Similarly, it can also be seen that, within the same tract (as in the digestive system), both the composition and the proportion of various microorganisms are changeable throughout it [1, 17]. That finding, as will be described later, is not a casual fact but, precisely because of it, it is possible for certain processes that are habitual in the normofunctioning organism to be carried out [17-19].

Although classic microbiologists had already advocated that certain germs normally inhabited various parts of the body, among the earliest scientific evidence Breznak's work, which described the existence of gut microbiota in termites, is noteworthy [2]. As early as the 20th century, in the 1960s and 1970s, Gibbons's research demonstrated a continuous change in oral microbiota throughout human life [20]. They had to wait two decades until Manning *et al.*, thanks to their studies in the human intestine, managed to contribute the subsequent salutary lesson on microbial research, pointing out the impact of microbiota on physiologic and pathophysiologic processes [21, 22].

Focusing on Gibbons's research, the changing nature of microbiota has been addressed. As previously mentioned, this property could be observed in the same individual throughout his/her life, but, beyond that, different microbiomes of the same person (oral, intestinal, cutaneous, *etc.*) may experience variations following a basal pattern, which will be influenced later by the different needs of that person at certain moments of his/her life [23, 24]. Such would be the case between what happens between birth and two months of age, a period in which the enterobacteria *Escherichia-Shigella-Klebsiella* predominate in the intestine. These produce metabolites, capable of creating a suitable habitat for subsequent intestinal colonization by other types of facultative aerobic bacteria. That is to say, in the first months of life the microbiota shows a qualitative change and the chronological order of appearance reveals that the first types of bacteria condition the habitat for the later ones. During these qualitative changes, both types of bacteria establish relations with the host, adapting themselves to his/her needs [25, 26].

There would also be external factors capable of modifying this microbiota, such as dietary habits in conjunction with the individual's energy requirements (in different health and disease states), and therefore with caloric expenditure. It is obvious to assume that diet, and everything that surrounds the nutritional side, has a determinant effect on the intestinal microbiota profile [17, 27, 28].

It has been demonstrated that there is an adaptation of microbiota to nutritional states, in combination with the metabolic needs of the subject. As we will explain in more detail later on, bacteria play a fundamental role in processes such as carbohydrate decarboxylation or protein deamination, as well as in the synthesis of vitamin K, like in the re-circulation of bile salts and various gastric and pancreatic juices. Among other agents capable of promoting intra-individual changes in microbiota, we should especially emphasize the use of antibiotics [27-29]. These stand out paradigmatically, so that the use of antibiotic therapy in certain moments of the life of an individual, especially at birth and in childhood, can have a determining influence on the later composition of the adult microbiota and, in relation to this, antibiotic treatment could interfere with the normal development and maintenance of structures and systems to which the microbiota is related [25, 26, 28].

Similar to the intra-individual changes in the above-mentioned microbiota, the existence of inter-individual variations is well known. Consequently, the quantitative and qualitative differences in microbiota composition are evident if we consider individuals in relation to their race and geographical setting and, more specifically, their lifestyles and socioeconomic and cultural levels [26-28]. An example of this can be observed in how neonates from Eastern countries show a higher proportion of *Proteobacterium,* while those from Western countries possess a higher proportion of *Actinobacterium* [30].

Recent studies carried out in healthy humans indicate that microbiota is usually influenced in a relevant way by factors such as the manner of birth and the maternal microbiota (both genito-urinary and recto-intestinal), with a close relationship between the birth canal and the newborn's gut microbiota [31-33].

Even more novel are studies that reveal the existence of various forms of microbiota in amniotic fluid, which have been found following several investigations aimed at identifying etiopathogenic mechanisms of chorioamniotis [25, 34]. Thereafter, these amniotic germs have been linked to the fetal microbiome and (later) to the neonatal microbiome [6]. Such a relationship would find a robust biological plausibility, given that the fetus swallows and excretes amniotic fluid during intrauterine life.

As has been suggested above, diet is another of the most influential factors in the development of microbiota. Its effect is felt from the first moments of life and it seems to be strongly influenced by the manner of feeding (breast milk or formula milk) [28]. A recent study relates the microbiota present in the colostrum of two populations of mothers fed with totally different diets and the development of different gut microbiota in their infants; one group corresponded to Italian women with a diet rich in animal proteins, sugar and fatty acids, while the other group was of women from Bu-

rundi with a diet based on legumes and cereals, with abundant fiber and few animal proteins [35].

The decisive imprint of the diet can also be noticed in later stages of the pediatric age, so that diets rich in simple sugars and low in carbohydrates of reduced use for the bacteria, result in changes in the microbiota that are able to be maintained permanently. Those changes are: i) a decrease in bacterial biodiversity; and ii) the possible extinction of some microbial families [27-29].

On some occasions, the words microbiota and microbioma are used interchangeably. This is incorrect, since the number and diversity of microbial strains is what we call microbiota, whereas the complexity and uniqueness of all the genetic material of the latter is what would be called microbiome [22]. It should be added that this genetic material is of the utmost importance, not only from a structural point of view, but also from a functional angle. Its study from this perspective is becoming increasingly accessible thanks to the progressive development of laboratory techniques, especially biotechnology ones, having reached the well-known era of "omics" (genomics, proteomics, transcriptomics, metabolomics, *etc.*) These techniques, in turn, are accompanied by scientific advances at other levels, such as information and communication technologies (ICTs) and computer sciences in general, both hardware and software. Based on these sciences there is bioinformatics, which enables a better management and interpretation of the information obtained by the above biotechnological techniques [36, 37].

By means of new molecular analysis techniques, it has been discovered that the bacterial genetic material that inhabits the human organism is 10 times greater than that of its body cells. That is, at a molecular level /we are more microorganism than human. Some authors consider the human microbiome to be our second genome [1, 36, 37]. This original perspective has led to new international projects. Thus, similar to one of the great challenges of the 20th century, the Human Genome Project, that of the 21st century is possibly the Human Microbiome Project (HMP) Consortium, started in 2008 under the auspices of the National Institute of Health (NIH) and several US universities [38]. The same year saw the start of its European equivalent, the MetaHIT (Metagenomics of the Human Intestinal Tract) project with the participation of 13 countries and supported by the Seventh Framework Program [39].

Knowledge of human microbiota has also benefited from large-scale studies promoted by other consortia, such as research into inflammatory bowel disease. An example of this is a recent study carried out within the GEM Project Research (Crohn's Disease Collaborative Network), which showed the change in microbiota throughout the world and how migratory processes had left a genetic trail in it. It also described its influence on the development of certain types of diseases, as well as ethnic and transcultural differences in dietary habits and lifestyles, to which microbiota has been evolutionarily adapting [40].

Over the last decade, scientific production focused on microbiota has grown exponentially, and this has generated most of the knowledge currently available on this subject. However, it has been estimated that only one third of the microorganisms that inhabit the human body are known. Nevertheless, those studied amount to double the total genome of the cells of the human body. Recently, the bacterial cell biomass of the intestine has been calculated and estimated to be around 1.5-2 kg. That is, taking into account the average body weight of an adult, the microbiota would represent a mass similar to that of the brain [7, 13].

The study of human microbiota is continuously providing new information. As a consequence, scientific literature offers new contributions on a permanent basis, such as the identification of new microorganisms in coexistence with those already known. Such is the case of the discovery of *Lagierella massiliensis* in human feces last year [41].

In the light of successive advances in the knowledge of the gut microbiota, it has been proposed that it could be categorized into two different perspectives: i) According to its taxonomic order, which in turn considers its kingdom and family, resulting in 3 different enterotypes: *Bacteroides* (type 1 enterotype), *Prevotella* (type 2 enterotype) and *Ruminococcus* (type 3 enterotype); ii) According to their function or activities developed within the host, that in turn considers their potential influence on nutrient metabolism, drug processing and the uptake of xenobiotics, as well as their local and systemic antimicrobial actions; the latter, therefore, participates in immunomodulatory processes, in the gastrointestinal barrier homeostasis and in the development and maintenance of the neuroendocrine axis [1, 15, 18, 27].

However, the microbiota does not always make beneficial contributions in the host or have a saprophyte role. In situations where the delicate balance between microbiota and the body's immune system is not well regulated, these microorganisms can become pathogens [5, 42].

2. MICROBIOTA IN HUMAN HEALTH AND DISEASE

Successive studies on the microbiota have shown that this is not an entity which is independent of the human body, but that it coexists with the latter in a constant state of communication and interrelation, based on substances and metabolites produced on both sides. As previously mentioned, the microbiota is found in practically all body compartments, in which each of them can perform one or more useful functions in physiologic states. In these cases, the microbiota inhabits a symbiotic state [4-6, 42].

However, the microbiota-host relationship is not always so harmonious, but, rather, under many circumstances, their symbiosis can be altered and lost. This may be due to the fact that microorganisms represent a pathological condition per se, or that the human body recognizes them as intruders with a hostile presence. Under such circumstances of imbalance, we are faced with the aforementioned dysbiosis or dysbacteriosis, which may lead to states of illness or situations of an uncertain significance as no harm or benefit can be identified for either side [5, 42].

We can observe numerous examples of microbiota in a state of balance or desbalance with the host, both locally and systemically. i) At the local level the absorption of many nutrients and the synthesis of vitamins (K_2, B_1, B_2 and B_8)

takes place thanks to bowel microorganisms; experiments in germ-free mice showed that in these animals a larger supply of these vitamins in the diet is necessary due to the lack of bacteria, whose enzymatic actions participate in the absorption of these nutrients. However, microbiota may also be an adverse entity and cause diseases such as enterocolitis. ii) At the systemic level, beneficial elements such as the relationship between certain intestinal bacteria and a decrease in total cholesterol or an increase in HDL-cholesterol; or harmful events such as bacteremia that can evolve into sepsis and even into the death of the host may be found [11, 14].

Among the roles attributed to microbiota, the following have been described: maintaining intestinal epithelial integrity, acting as a barrier against pathogens, intervening in the stimulation and development of the immune response, serving as an energy source, contributing to maturation and development of the central nervous system (CNS), as well as engaging in metabolic activities [17, 43-46]. These activities may include the aforementioned vitamin synthesis, bile salt transformation, xenobiotic metabolism and the production of short chain fatty acids (SCFA). They result from the fermentation of the microbiota and include propionate, butyrate and acetate, which interact directly and indirectly with the G protein coupled receptors. They are related to energy balance and metabolism of adipose, muscle-skeletal, and hepatic tissues [11, 14].

All of the above seems to indicate that the microbiota could be considered as one more organ of the economy. It may not be a solid one and may not match the already recognized definition of blood as a liquid organ, but it could represent another system that relates to the organism and whose variations can involve changes, both loco-regional and global ones [47].

This close relationship between microbiota and host as well as the different genomic composition of both, is what characterizes humans as holobiont organisms. The term holobiont is defined as being the set formed by a complex multicellular entity (animal or plant) and all its associated microorganisms [4, 6, 9].

In any case, it should be noted that the relationship between microbiota and host is bilateral, with a permanent feedback between them. This relationship would be contingent upon a determining element, which would be the immune system of the host. On these bases, the human species has evolved from a continuous balance between microbiota and body cells, even exchanging DNA with each other (and mRNA, as has been seen recently) [47-49]. The role of miRNAs in microbiota host interactions is beginning to be investigated. It is suspected there are many ways to interact between miRNA and gut microbiota, and their reciprocal role in influencing host immune system and related processes. For this proposal, two interesting approaches have emerged as interesting possibilities to study experimentally the interplays: i) use of engineered vectors; ii) by means of oral delivery of anti-miRNAs). It seems that the miRNA would be the main responsible for this bilateral relationship and that the host faecal miRNA even could regulate gut microbiota [47-49].

This would be placed in the context of the phylogenetic adaptation to its own needs and those of the environment In this conceptual framework the term 'phylosymbiosis' has been proposed, which alludes to the relations and functional effects of microbial communities throughout the evolutionary history of the host [4, 6, 9].

2.1. Impact on the Immune System

Peyer plaques are the biggest body defensive barrier against external agents. Structurally, they correspond to accumulations of lymphoid tissue and are located in the lamina propria of the small intestine, mainly in the ileum. They form a conglomeration of defensive cells that filter and modulate the interrelation with the commensal intestinal microbiota of the organism. In this way, a balanced response is established between the intestinal mucosa and the bacterial presence, which under normal conditions favors the correct maturation of the immune system. In fact, studies on germ-free mice show a decrease in the development of these defensive niches. The immune system, in turn, communicates with the nervous system through a bilateral relationship (feedback), as there is a close connection between the brain and the intestinal immune system, possibly through the enteric nervous system by means of signals that circulate through the bloodstream [4-6, 50].

This communication exists from the earliest stages of life, in which it has been observed that germ-free mice present a different development in the digestive tract (specifically of Peyer plaques), as well as a different functioning of innate and acquired immune responses. Exposure to certain antigens at crucial ages in life leads to the formation of regulatory T cells or T-regs cells (which modulate inflammation by IL-10) [12, 50, 51].

Regarding the above, it has been reported that the bacterial polysaccharide A is involved in the development of FoxP3+ and antigen-presenting cells (APCs), as well as maturation of Th-1-type helper (Th) cells, and Th-17. If these Th are present in a steady state after being exposed to a proinflammatory environment (in the presence of IL-12, IL-23, IL-1β or TGF-β3), they become involved in the immune response and produce IFN-γ (Fig. **1**). Analogously, Th-2 cells are encouraged to stimulate B-cells and Toll-like receptors (TLRs) and NOD-like receptors (NLRs) [51, 52].

Similarly, what could also occur (in parallel) is that, in the presence of certain types of bacteria, the processes of communication between generalized immunity and the CNS through immunochemical processes will be evident, resulting in the synthesis of certain types of proinflammatory cytokines, such as IL-6 and IL-1B. All these phenomena have been related to the development of neurodegenerative diseases [5, 51, 52].

Furthermore, the short chain fatty acids produced by the commensal microbiota of the digestive tract, exert anti-inflammatory actions on the immune system, favoring an increase in the production of IL-4 and IL-10 and thus reducing the leukocyte adhesion mediated by VCAM-1 molecules. They also modulate the function of regulatory T lymphocytes (T-regs), inhibiting the production of IFN-γ [51, 52].

Regarding the humoral immune response, the function that IgA carries out in the intestinal epithelium is worth mentioning. IgA is the predominant immunoglobulin in intestinal secretions (as in saliva), this being in the form of secretory IgA with most of it coming from a local synthesis and not from the circulatory torrent. The usual presence of microbiota in the intestine justifies the existence of permanent levels of IgA at this level. Among its functions are the inhibition of bacteria adhesion and the neutralization of enzymes, viruses and toxins. It can bind specifically to molecules present on the bacterial surface, mediating its binding to the intestinal epithelium, causing that binding to increase the affinity (of this complex) to mucin; this, in turn, facilitates the immobilization of the microorganism in the mucosal layer, thus facilitating its elimination. When IgA binds to a viral particle, it prevents the binding of the latter to the host cell by blocking specific receptors, and this binding can even occur within the epithelial cell at the time of transport of that IgA. Neutralization of enzymes and toxins can occur by blocking the binding site of the toxin with a receptor, or by conformational modification of this site. Germ-free mice have been reported to show a decrease in IgA synthesis, as did IgG [42, 51, 52].

The overall result of the actions of all these cytokines with anti and proinflammatory effects is usually beneficial to infections. But, as hinted earlier, an imbalance between the two effects may lead to pathological situations. Thus, it has been reported that lesions in the blood-brain barrier and in the choroid plexuses increase the barrier's permeability, allowing the passage of antigenic substances through it. Depending on the nature of the lesion, an immune stimulus is triggered (primarily at the expense of proinflammatory cytokines) that is capable of travelling through the vagus nerve and reaching distant anatomic regions [42, 43, 50-54].

Situations characterized by a proinflammatory environment have been related to the development of multiple conditions, such as inflammatory bowel disease, which, in turn, may be closely related to neurodegenerative disorders, such as multiple sclerosis (MS) [22, 31, 53, 54].

2.2. Inflammation, Oxidative Stress, Neuromodulation and Neurodegeneration

From an early age, our microbiota and the development of the nervous system are directed and coordinated, acting on angiogenesis, axonal growth, dendritic progression and synaptogenesis. It is in these stages in which these processes occur most and, therefore, there is an increase in neuroplasticity. This dynamic process is marked by the microbiota acquired from birth. But these interactions are not always so successful, which is why some neuropsychiatric disorders are established from very early ages [53, 54].

Throughout the different stages of life, neuronal plasticity is constantly changing. This also alters the microbiota of our body and allows for brain maturation, behavior improvement and cognitive enhancement processes [30, 31, 33].

The adult stage is related to a greater degree of diversity of microbiota, but with aging it loses that diversity, which coincides with the potential development of diseases of a neurodegenerative character typically related to senescence, such as Alzheimer's or Parkinson's disease [53-55].

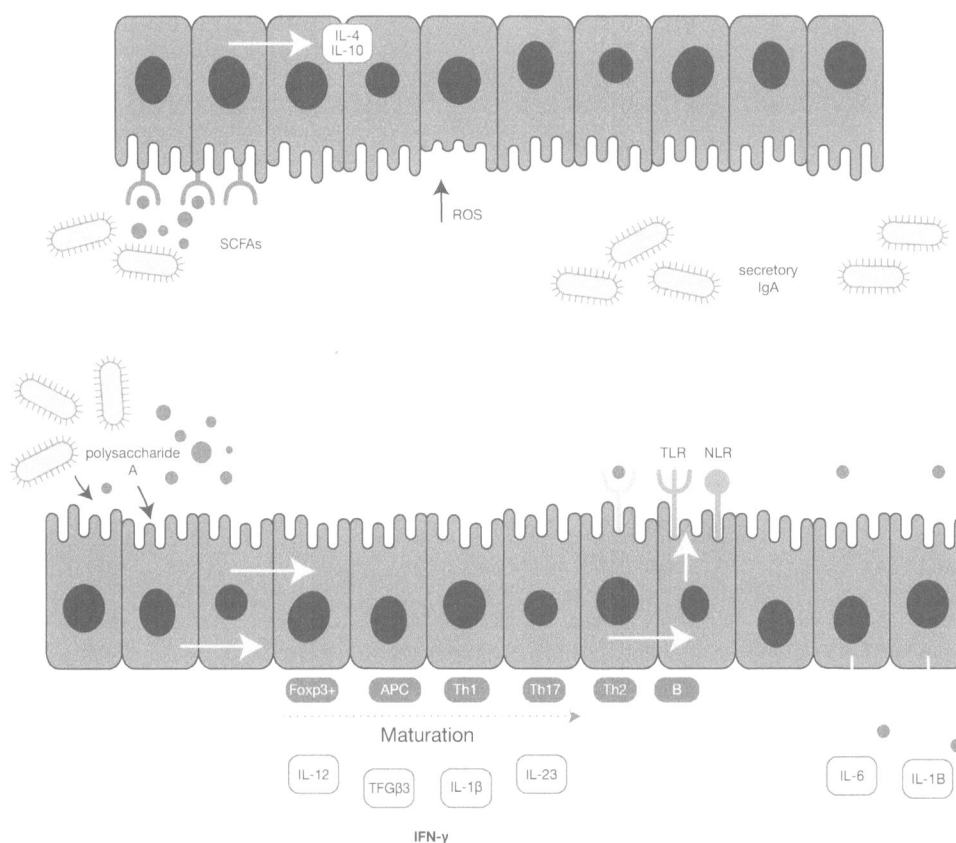

Fig. (1). Molecular and cellular pathways that happen on the host bowel-surface faced with microbiota.

The proinflammatory and anti-inflammatory processes resulting from the interactions between microbiota and the immune system, as mentioned, have been established in a delicate balance. Normally, the microbiota-epithelium interaction generates reactive oxygen species (as happens in the immunity-pathogen interaction when a cell disruption occurs), as well as nitrogen and sulfur, but all of them are counteracted by our own antioxidant system and immune response. Occasionally, our oxidative balance is negative and damage occurs in some of our tissues, with the development of known oxidative stress [22, 31, 56, 57]. This state can alter the epithelial barrier by modifying proteins, which can lead to a pathological situation in which intestinal microbiota (saprophyte or pathogen per se), can directly develop an infective state or, indirectly, initiate an autoimmune disease producing an excitation of the immune system that later results in an attack on anatomy structures. The latter has been related to the onset of neurodegenerative diseases, when the aforementioned structures attacked belong to the nervous system which, as has been previously hinted at, is intimately related to gut microbiota [54-57].

The presence of certain molecules in the immunochemical profile of the human being is essential in the nervous system for it to be able to respond to lesions of a diverse nature. Among these molecules, IL-4 and IL-10 can be highlighted as being essential anti-inflammatory cytokines for damage repair, as well as for the maintenance of some structures and recovery of homeostasis. These cytokines facilitate

communication between the intestine and the immune system, resulting in the recognition of the antigens inherent and non-inherent in the blood-brain barrier (composed of endothelial cells and astrocytes). These molecular interactions may or may not be facilitated, depending on whether the local homeostasis is intact or altered. Under normal conditions occurs a coordinated response of physiological systems occurs, which may include interactions with neuropeptides, neurotransmitters, hormones and immunomodulatory elements [51-54].

In neurodegenerative diseases, the migration of immune cells, cytokines, chemokines, neuroendocrine molecules and microbial products through this membrane that constitutes the blood-brain barrier has been demonstrated [42, 43, 51, 52].

2.3. Microbiota and CNS. Implications of the Microbiota on the Basis of the General Etiopathogenesis of Neuropathological Processes

In recent years, the relationship between the microbiota, and the nervous and endocrine systems has been grouped into what is called the brain-gut axis and the hypothalamic-pituitary-adrenal axis (HPA). These structures constitute the establishment of complex communication networks that play a crucial role in maintaining homeostasis. Regarding the nervous system, both the sympathetic and parasympathetic nervous systems are involved, both at the central (cerebrospinal) and peripheral (neuro-enteric) levels. These, in turn, are related to the immune and endocrine systems [31, 58].

The cerebellum and hippocampus (a key area in social behavior) are two of the regions that are most sensitive to changes in microbiota, showing variations in gene expression in experiments performed on germ-free mice [59].

One of the most important forms of communication between the brain and intestinal microbiota is the vagus nerve pathway, as previously mentioned. This nerve collects the afferent information from the viscera of our body; it is the one that is capable of activating intestinal microbiota itself through signals directed to the enteric nervous system. In turn, the brain responds by neuromodulating various parameters such as adiposity, immunity or energy balance. It also responds with electrical brain signals that directly affect the bowel muscles. Pathological states of anxiety or stress produce an ostensible activation of these processes, since the vagus nerve plays a fundamental role in them. Experiments performed on germ-free mice subjected to a vagotomy show a blockage of the ansyogenic mechanisms, thus demonstrating the importance of the contribution of the vagus nerve in the behavior of the subject [55, 60].

The microbiota plays a fundamental role in the metabolism of certain neurotransmitters. For example, serotonin (5-HT) and quinurenine are the product of tryptophan metabolism, in which some elements of microbiota (*Candida, Streptococcus, Escherichia* and *Enterococcus*) play an essential role (Fig. 2). Serotonin acts in the CNS and bowels, promoting gastrointestinal motility or pain perception. That is, changes in the microbiota, together with an insufficient intake of tryptophan, may lead to a decrease in cerebral serotonin and, as has already been described, could be related to depressive states, which, in the future, could make microbiota become a possible therapeutic target in depression [60, 61].

Another of the neurotransmitters related to microbiota is GABA, which is influenced by the presence of lactic acid producer bacteria. *Lactobacillus rhamnosus* and *Bifidobacterium* are some of the most important ones; their presence has demonstrated higher levels of GABA, as well as its carrier protein in the blood-brain barrier. This neurotransmitter acts on the vagus nerve, *i.e.*, it can modulate states of anxiety or depression through that pathway. Another example of a neurotransmitter related to the microbiota is acetylcholine, in the synthesis of which bacteria of the genus *Lactobacillus* are also involved [55, 60, 61].

Catecholamines adrenaline, noradrenaline and dopamine are also influenced by intestinal microbiota. Thus, the synthesis of dopamine has been related to the *Bacillus* family. Studies in germ-free mice showed a decrease in noradrenaline and dopamine levels in the intestinal lumen. Conversely, low tyrosine levels in these mice give an increase in brain catecholamines. These phenomena are reversible since it has been observed that, when performing an intestinal repopulation in this murine model, the situation normalizes [55, 58, 61].

The brain-derived neurotrophic factor (BDNF) plays a key role in memory and learning processes, and its synthesis has also been seen to be influenced by the intestinal microbi-

ota. Studies in mice treated with antibiotics demonstrate a reduction of this factor in the hippocampus. As it is known, its decrease alters the morphology and growth of neurons. As with catecholamines, the intestinal recolonization of these treated mice reverses the situation (though not completely), causing an increase of *BDNF* gene expression in that brain region [55, 58, 60].

The regulation of microglia (defensive cells of the nervous system) is also conditioned by microbiota, with a bilateral relationship between the two parts. The presence of peptides (synthesized by intestinal microorganisms or their constituents) can produce inflammatory processes in the nervous tissue, as well as a stimulus for the proliferation of microglia; which induce injuries in the CNS, which can originate neuropsychiatric disorders or neurodegenerative diseases [55, 58, 62].

From a neuroendocrine perspective, the bowel also relates to the nervous system through hormonal signals. The synthesis of certain proteins such as leptin, ghrelin, orexins or galanin, is of great relevance. They act directly on the CNS by modulating eating behaviors, energy balance, memory and anxiety states (In addition to the aforementioned role of the vagus nerve), as well as light-dark cycles and reproductive behaviors. Furthermore, the neuropeptide Y (NPY) is involved in the interrelations of the brain with the microbiota. NPY is one of the most potent orexigenic peptides found in the brain, with four functional types identified in humans. The Y1 and Y5 subtypes contribute to appetite stimulation, whereas Y2 and Y4 appear to act by inhibiting the feeling of hunger, which is an indirect way of producing satiety (they are therefore anorexigenic). Other neuronal systems of the brain (brain stem, nucleus accumbens and corticolimbic system) expressing NPY also intervene in food intake, through the regulation of appetite [24, 27, 59, 60].

3. SPECIFIC ROLE OF THE MICROBIOTA IN MENTAL AND NEUROLOGIC DISORDERS

3.1. Neuropsychiatric Disorders

In recent decades, the processes of dysbiosis between gut microbiota and the host have been linked to numerous diseases of high prevalence, such as inflammatory bowel disease, diabetes, cancer and cardiovascular diseases. In this context, this microbiota has been linked to neurologic pathologies and neuropsychiatric disorders [12, 22, 55, 58].

According to studies based on fecal analysis, associations have been found between the development of certain intestinal microbiota profiles and autistic spectrum disorders. Although the existence of a genetic component associated with the development of autism is known, this genotype could be predisposed to a dysfunction in the intestinal wall and in proteins of the blood-brain barrier from a very early age. This would interfere with the formation of the neuro-axonal network in certain behavioral areas of the brain and thus alter the normal neurodevelopment of the child [31, 55].

Intestinal-brain connections and interrelations are classically known. In routine clinical care, for example, in people with an irritable bowel syndrome among their usual symptoms (in addition to the typical digestive ones), it is observed

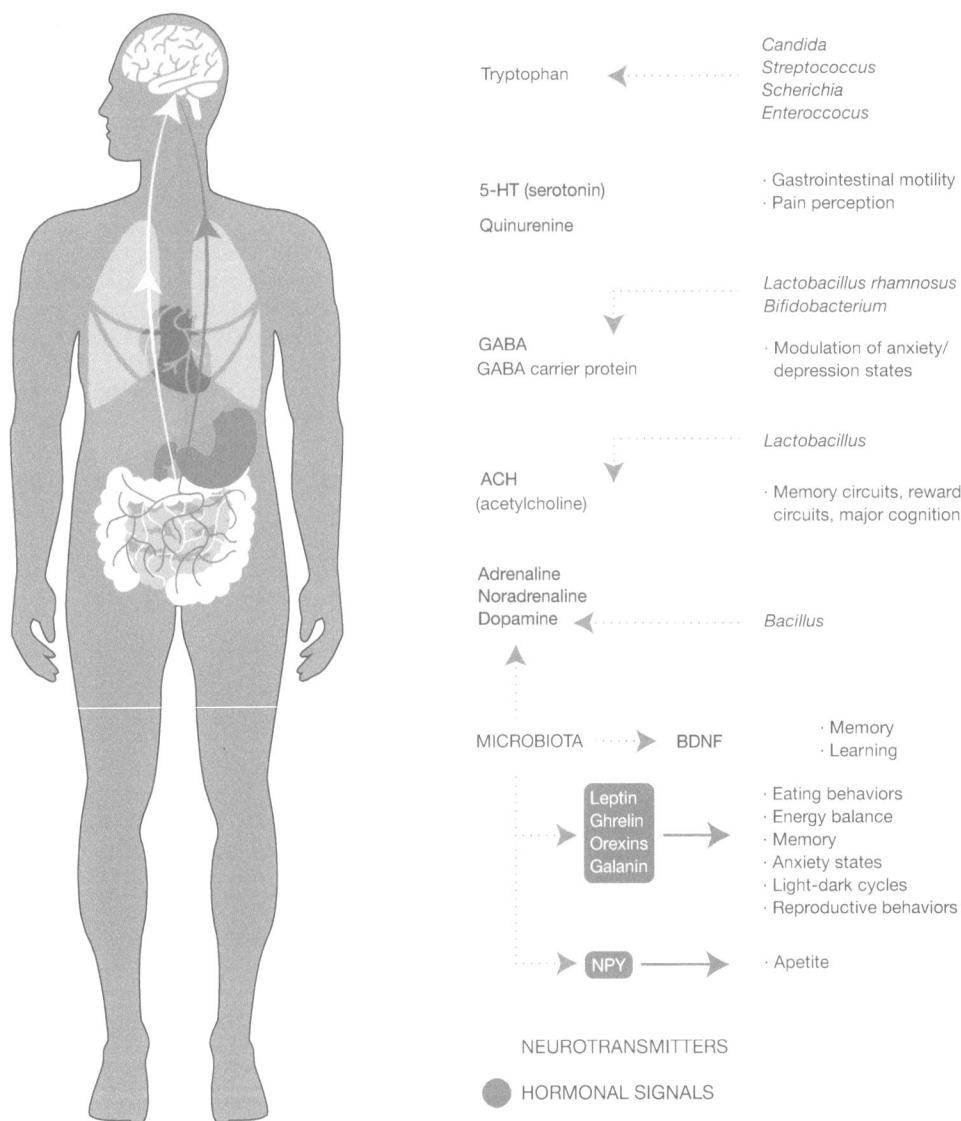

Fig. (2). Brain-gut-microbiota axis. Neurotransmitters and hormonal signals stimulated by the microbiota and triggered actions.

that they suffer from depression and anxiety. As a result of these and subsequent observations, the enteric nervous system has been defined as being a "second brain" because of its ability to function autonomously and communicate with the CNS, both through the parasympathetic nervous system (*via* the vagus nerve) and the sympathetic one. This intestine-brain axis, therefore, consists of a two-way communication between the CNS and the enteric nervous system, linking the emotional and cognitive centers of the brain with peripheral (digestive and immune) intestinal functions [63, 64].

The implications of these phenomena not only produce neuropsychic or intellectual consequences in the early stages of life. For example, in observational clinical studies in elderly subjects, it has been shown that latent toxoplasmosis may induce deficiencies in learning and cause alterations in central dopaminergic transmission [65].

From an epidemiologic perspective, an increase in the frequency of microbial-host dysbiosis has been observed in recent years. This fact may be partly related to the indiscriminate use of antibiotics and to the current hectic pace in developed societies, in which the consumption of precooked and fast food has increased, reducing the consumption of healthier diets and of a proven anti-inflammatory effect, as is the Mediterranean diet. These facts, in relation to the aforementioned implications between gut microbiota and the vagus nerve (conditioned in turn by states of anxiety and stress), have led to a higher incidence of pathologies related to deregulation of the intestine-brain axis. Consequently, the frequency of CNS diseases, such as cognitive disturbances and other pathologies such as nerve depression, has increased [65-68].

Depression is considered to be a disease in itself, with its own entity, although in many cases it is an epiphenomenon linked to an enormous amount of pathologies of a diverse nature. We can observe how in inflammatory bowel disease there is a relevant presence of depressive symptoms. Such symptoms are also related to other diseases such as multiple sclerosis, where depression is one of its characteristic features. The use of probiotics, particularly *Bifidobacterium infantis,* has exerted a protective effect against the damage of some mechanisms of response to psychic stress, such as reactive depression [61, 65].

Experimental models have confirmed the bilateral relationship between gut microbiota, and anxiety and depression. In one study, mice (with equal intestinal microbiota) were subjected to a process of maternal separation to cause them early stress. It was observed that mice that had been separated from their mother developed anxiety and depression with increased levels of corticosterone (stress hormone), just as they demonstrated intestinal dysfunction as a result of the release of acetylcholine. The experiment was repeated in germ-free mice and it was found that in the absence of intestinal bacteria, mice that were separated from their mother maintained altered levels of corticosterone and intestinal dysfunction, but showed no signs of anxiety or depression. After these results, it was discovered that when intestinal bacteria were transferred to the germ-free mice, after several weeks their metabolic activity changed, in addition to which the mice began to show anxiety and depression [69].

Clinical observations have also linked intestinal microbiota to other psychiatric entities, such as schizophrenia. As is already known, prematurity is a risk factor for the development of this disease; biological plausibility has been sought to verify this by means of the chronobiology of the intestinal microbiota in the neonate. In preterm infants the qualitative, quantitative and functional profile of this microbiota has been studied, as well as its stability, in situations of precocious microbial intestinal colonization. In general terms, preterm infants have low microbial intraindividual and high interindividual diversity. This difference is more marked if one considers the manner of birth. Thus, when comparing babies born vaginally with preterm infants to cesarean section, the latter present a smaller bacterial population of *Bifidobacterium* and *Bacteroides* and a larger one of *Clostridium difficile*. It is known that *Bifidobacterium* has positive effects on the developing brain, while the presence of the genus *Clostridium* is pathological. Some cases (both in schizophrenia and autism) have been associated with infections from *Clostridium difficile* and in which the latter's pathogenic effect is considered to be due to the production of a derivative of phenylalanine by this bacterium [70, 71].

The involvement of microbiota in the development of schizophrenic behavior has also been addressed by several experimental studies. Among these, one of the most important has been the model of maternal immune activation in the mouse. One such investigation showed that this activation generates an altered metabolic profile in the serum of the offspring of these mice. On administering an oral treatment with the human bacterium *Bacteroides fragilis,* the intestinal permeability and microbial composition became normalized, while reducing anxious type manifestations in the offspring. It has been found that germ-free mice present a similar behavior pattern to that of the schizoid human being and that

this pattern can be reversed if the intestine of these mice is repopulated in early stages of life. Interestingly, these behavioral alterations were more pronounced in males than in females, which is consistent with epidemiological data on schizophrenia [60, 61, 64].

Moreover, there is also evidence that the development of cognitive abilities happens in parallel with the postnatal microbial colonization of the intestine and the subsequent production of metabolites. Several studies have demonstrated that germ-free mice, compared to mice raised under natural conditions, present deficits in spatial memory and mechanical fitness, in addition to having lower levels of BDNF in the hippocampus [56-58]. This has been interpreted as being cognitive deficits. *Toxoplasma gondii* has also been implicated as an etiological factor of schizophrenia, its ability to decompensate gut microbiota already being known. Epidemiologically, this parasite has been postulated as an environmental risk factor for the development of schizophrenia. Its experimental inoculation in rodents causes behavioral alterations and promotes anxiety states [55, 58, 61, 64].

All these studies are prompting conceptual changes in the bases of behavioral genetics, so the question arises as to whether the genes of the microbiota should be paid more attention to (for their relevance and protagonism in the etiology of schizophrenia), than the schizophrenic patient's own genotype [72].

3.2. Prion Diseases

As the name implies, these diseases have their origin in prions. These are the causative agents of transmissible spongiform encephalopathies (TSEs), which need the participation of the pathogenic cellular prion protein (PrPsc), which, in turn, requires the presence of the physiological protein (PrPc) to propagate and replicate. Indeed, it has been shown that knock-out mice for PrPc do not develop disease if they are inoculated only with PrPsc [73].

The cellular prion protein (PrPc) is a membrane glycoprotein that is constitutively found in different organs of most of the animal species studied. It is especially abundant in the CNS. The scrapie prion protein (PrPsc or prion, which is a term derived from the acronym *PROteinaceous INfectious particle*) may be a different isoform and its presence is pathological. Both PrP isoforms are encoded by the same gene and have the same amino acid sequence, albeit with differences in their secondary structure. PrPc can be digested by proteinase K, whereas PrPsc may be only partially digestible [73, 74].

PrPsc therefore only appears in prion diseases and in the brain it reaches a concentration of between 10 and 20 times higher than PrPc. Sometimes, PrPsc accumulations appear in the form of plaques. Detection of the pathogenic isoform (PrPsc) is the 'gold standard' for the diagnosis of the disease [73-75].

Abrasion of the tongue has been shown to be a factor favoring the onset of these diseases. These can be suffered by both people and animals, and their prognosis is fateful, leading to the death of the subject [73-75].

In humans, prion diseases include: Creutfeldt-Jakob disease (CJD), fatal familial insomnia, Gerstmann-Sträussler-Scheinker disease, Kuru and familial spongiform encephalopathy associated with the PrP gene mutation [73].

Several studies suggest that these diseases are usually initiated by ingesting some food infected by prions, resulting in the subsequent invasion of the host through the digestive tract. Stool analyses of infected animals confirm the resistance of prions to the chemical changes inherent to digestion, as their protein structure remains intact in these feces. It appears that the β-pleated sheet structure of PrPsc is responsible for this protein being resistant to the action of gastric juices and other secretions of the digestive tract. Some papers suggest that in certain diseases such as Kuru, there could be an alternative route of invasion, such as infection of the oral cavity and, from there, it may spread through the cranial nerves [75, 76].

Prion infection affects the transduction of signals and, thereby, the maintenance of the myelin is also affected. Decreased serum concentrations of IL-4, IL-10 and IL-13 have been observed in infected subjects. An activation of the microglia and the astrocytes takes place in these subjects, affecting the circadian rhythms, all of which favor the neurodegenerative mechanisms [75, 77].

It is likely that, after its arrival in the digestive tract, possible alterations in the intestinal membrane would be the gateway of these prion proteins to the nervous system. After traversing the intestine, they may reach the enteric nervous system and travel through the vagus nerve until arriving at the CNS. A decrease in the protease activity of *Streptomyces, Bacillus* and other thermophilic anaerobic microorganisms (*Thermococcus, Thermosipho, Thermoanaerobacter*) has been reported in the colon of mice and hamsters infected with the proteic isoform PrPSc. In these, the aforementioned astrocytes and microglia cells activation has also been observed, increasing the expression of anti-inflammatory cytokines TGF-β, and PGE2 (prostaglandin E2) [75-77].

Most experimental studies on these diseases have been carried out on sheep, cows or hamsters, although they can also be found in *in vitro* models. In these, a relevant presence of prions was observed in Peyer plaques, which corroborates the key role that the microbiota plays in the activation of these defensive structures [75, 76].

Furthermore, the use of antibiotic therapy in the hamster has demonstrated a slower progression of the disease, increasing survival. This fact would also support the role of the microbiota in the development of these diseases [77].

3.3. Mitochondrial Diseases

Mitochondria is an essential organelle in the eukaryotic cell and, therefore, in the organism of all higher animals. Thanks to the mitochondrial respiratory chain, the energy supply necessary for metabolic processes can be made available. In humans, those known as mitochondrial diseases can be especially crippling (and even lethal) for the patients who suffer from them, as they compromise the obtaining of energy by the neuronal mitochondria, which also show a higher level of oxidative stress. This results in a molecular injury which encourages the death of neurons and can therefore

lead to the loss of motor and/or cognitive functions, more or less accentuated according to their localizations and the extension of CNS that becomes affected [78].

The human species is a holobiont, as stated above, whose constant relationship with microbiota is of paramount importance, assuming a bilateral impact in various areas of the anatomy and at multiple levels within its locations. Such is the case of the mitochondrial genome, which could reflect this impact both at the level of the enterocytes and of the bacteria that make up the intestinal microbiota. Alterations in microbiota-host relationships could lead to an imbalance between the mitochondrial and nuclear genomes leading to the development of diseases [79-81].

In this regard, the hypothetical origin of mitochondria has been pointed out, and they are assumed to come from an ancestry of bacterial lineage that coexists in symbiosis with cells of higher organisms. Based on this hypothesis, the aging of the subject or the etiopathogenesis of some pathologies have been related to alterations in mitochondrial biology [82, 83]. These alterations would be equivalent to the loss of the aforementioned symbiotic coexistence, thus becoming pathological for the host. Such pathologies would include entities as diverse as cancer or mitochondrial diseases themselves [83, 85]. The bases of all these disorders would be due to the existence of different mitochondrial phenotypes on the part of the hosts, which are able to interact in different ways with the microbiota, also subject to their different profiles. Therefore, diseases arising from these different interactions become dysfunctional and, as a result, the necessary microbiota-host equilibrium is broken [82-84].

3.4. Huntington's Disease

Huntington's disease is linked to a defect in chromosome 4, which causes an excessive repetition of the genetic sequence CAG (cytosine-adenine-guanine). It is a defect that increases in affected families as successive generations inherit it. Changes in personality and language, disorientation and loss of memory (even leading to dementia) are frequent among the symptoms presented [85, 86].

Certainly the most typical feature is the exaggerated movement of the limbs (choreic movements) and the appearance of sudden grimaces. On the other hand, patients with Huntington's disease present anxiety, stress and muscle spasticity with loss of reflexes [85, 86].

Dementia symptoms, as well as those related to emotional aspects (anxiety, for example) may be related to the composition and functionality of the microbiota. Although the specific literature on the microbiota in this entity is scant, it is possible that new knowledge on the functions of the brain-intestine-microbiota axis may also lead to new responses in Huntington's disease. As in other pathologies of this nature, although those responses fail to find the key to the cure of the disease, they may contribute to the improvement of their symptoms and signs, or slow down their progression [87].

3.5. Parkinson's Disease

Parkinson's disease (PD) is another type of movement disorder. It is due to an insufficient ability of the substantia nigra neurons to synthesize dopamine. Some cases are of genetic origin but most are sporadic. It would seem that the genetic basis actually confers a susceptibility to the disease, but it would require the presence of environmental factors to develop it. It is more common in men and usually begins at around 60 years of age, although there is an early form that manifests before the age of 40 [88].

Symptomatology usually begins insidiously in a hemibody. Subsequently, it extends to the contralateral hemibody. The most characteristic symptom of these patients is the tremor, which usually affects the hands and then the arms, legs, jaw and face. These patients also denote stiffness in the arms, legs and trunk, as well as bradykinesia and problems in balance and motor coordination. They may suffer non-motor effects, such as sleep disturbances and psychiatric disorders [88].

At the cellular level there is a deregulation of the glia. At the molecular level, biochemical interactions occur involving neurotoxins, neurotrophic factors and neurotransmitters [89].

In PD a protein of special importance appears: α-synuclein. This is a nuclear and synaptic protein, which is the main component of Lewy bodies in both sporadic and hereditary forms of PD (as well as Lewy body dementia). *In vitro* studies show that α-synuclein may exhibit distinct behaviors, such as different aggregation properties and toxic capacity, depending on the environment. In proinflammatory situations, the activation of the kappa-β factor increases its toxicity by altering its structural conformation (by changing its folding). Increased expression of the α-synuclein gene in the colon of patients with PD has been detected. The presence of phosphorylated α-synuclein has also been observed in colon biopsies of these patients (at the submucosal level), although not in healthy subjects. Possibly, α-synuclein aggregates, such as prions, are propagated to the CNS. Patients with a more variegated PD have higher levels of α-synuclein in the choroid plexus than in cases of PD of a mild or moderate intensity [88, 89].

Initially, α-synuclein aggregates appear in the vagus nerve and in the dorsal motor nuclei of the glossopharyngeal nerve. Subsequently, this protein migrates until, in advanced stages of the disease, it can be found in the pars compacta of the substantia nigra. In this area, a decrease in dopaminergic neurons is observed [88, 89].

Furthermore, structures of the olfactory bulb, the brainstem, and the autonomic nervous system can also be affected, as well as noting a decrease in cells in the cerebral cortex. Analogously, a dysfunction of the autonomic nervous system and of the enteric nervous system ensues. Braak's hypothesis, currently accepted, holds that PD begins in the enteric nervous system [90].

According to this hypothesis, the vagus nerve plays a fundamental role in the development of PD, allowing the expansion of Lewy bodies from the enteric nervous system to the CNS [88]. The process begins with an increase in the permeability of the intestinal mucosa and the subsequent accumulation (with cranio-caudal distribution) of these bodies in the submucosa and the myenteric plexus of the enteric nervous system. After this, the presence of Lewy bodies in the dorsal motor nuclei of the vagus nerve, which is charac-

teristic of the early stages of the disease, are already observed [90, 91].

The aforementioned increase in the permeability of the intestinal mucosa may also contribute to the abnormal diffusion of bacterial products. For this and other reasons that we will see below, similar to other neurodegenerative diseases, the gut microbiota shows an ostensible relation with PD [91-93]. In this disease, we should especially bear in mind that its specific medication may influence intestinal bacteria; thus, Levodopa is absorbed through the intestine and could alter the gut microbiota [94].

The study of microbiota in feces of PD patients reveals a different pattern than that of healthy people, in terms of diversity and microbial concentrations. Subjects affected by PD show a reduction of 77.6% of *Prevotellaceae* compared to non-affected individuals. The decrease in *Prevotellaceae* along with the increase in *Lactobacillus* has been associated with a decrease in ghrelin levels. This hormone regulates the nigroestrial dopaminergic function [91, 92].

The aforementioned decrease in *Prevotellaceae* may be related to a lower synthesis of SCFA such as propionate or butyrate, related to the activation and regulation of antimicrobial peptide (AMP) expression, which contributes to the stability of the intestinal mucosa membrane. The decrease in *Prevotellaceae* is also associated with lower mucus production, also inducing a greater permeability of the intestinal mucosa [91, 92].

Variants can also be found in the microbiota profile in relation to different PD phenotypes. In patients with postural instability and difficulty in ambulation, a decrease in concentrations of *Prevotellaceae* is observed along with an increase in *Enterobacteriae*, compared to patients with tremor. There is also a positive correlation between *Enterobacteriae* concentration and severity of motor impairment [93].

Constipation is one of the most prominent symptoms in PD. It is a risk factor possibly secondary to a slowed intestinal transit, which is observed along with the other manifestations typical of the degeneration of the enteric nervous system from early stages of the disease [88, 91-93].

3.6. Alzheimer's Disease

Alzheimer's disease (AD) is the dementia most known, and it produces degenerative CNS involvement. Although there is also an early (much less frequent) form that can set in after the age of 40, it usually appears after 65 years of age. Consequently, its incidence is increasing in developed countries in relation to increasing longevity. It affects the quality of life of the patients psychologically and even physically, at first the intellectual and cognitive functions begin to deteriorate, in advanced stages there is also a regression at the psychomotor level. Its evolution, therefore, is of a progressive character [95].

These clinical manifestations are related to the loss of cholinergic functions in hippocampal neurons. Histologically, AD is characterized by the presence of the protein deposits in the hippocampus and in the parietotemporal areas of the cerebral cortex. These lesions consist of neuritic plaques composed of extracellular deposits of β-amyloid protein (the so-called senile plaques, corresponding to laminae of this protein) and of interneuronal pellets formed by neurofibrils consisting of coiled filaments of the cytoskeletal tau protein. Hyperphosphorylation of this tau protein can also be observed [95, 96].

Its etiology is unknown, although the latest research seems to indicate that prionic-type processes are involved [92]. There are some genomic regions related to AD that participate in the immune response, inflammation, cell migration and lipid transport pathways. It has been observed how apolipoprotein E (APOE) modulates the lipid metabolism and aggregation of the β-amyloid protein. This is especially relevant at the cerebral level, since synaptic function is mediated by the receptors of this APOE. The gene encoding this apolipoprotein E has 3 alleles related to the possible risk of developing AD: ε-4 (high-risk), ε-3 (neutral) and ε-2 (protective) [96, 97].

AD has also been linked to non-genetic factors. These include the microbiota, which is able to regulate cognitive and behavioral functions through the known microbiota-gut-brain axis [96, 97].

It has been proven that the composition of the microbiota is stabilized in adulthood until it reaches a point of inflection in which the onset of inflammatory processes begins on the intestinal surface, losing that subtle balance between the host and the microbiota. Thus, in the event of a hypothetical disruption of the intestinal barrier, an increase in the inflammatory status would be caused, thereby altering the composition of the microbiota, both quantitatively and qualitatively. Among other consequences, a certain loss of gastrointestinal motility, nutrient absorption and local defensive capacity would begin, while increasing oxidative stress. This in turn involves of amyloid plaques formation processes [96-98].

Polyunsaturated fatty acids (PUFAs), such as Omega-3, are closely related to brain functions and neuronal physiology per se. A relevant intake of those fatty acids decreases the risk of developing AD and other neurodegenerative processes. PUFAs directly affect both the nerve tissue itself, and indirectly, favor changes in the composition of the microbiota [97, 98].

It has also been observed that coffee may exert a protective effect on the brain due to its abundance in polyphenols, which antagonize oxidative stress. Coffee consumption may also reduce the *Firmicutes/Bacteroides* ratio, which is related to an attenuation of the inflammatory status [97, 98].

A high intake of fats and refined sugars carries a greater risk of involvement of memory-associated brain areas (such as the hippocampus), thereby increasing the likelihood of developing dementias. It has been suggested that some diets especially rich in saturated fats could induce the accumulation of β-amyloid in the CNS and thus contribute to the development of AD. On the contrary, the Mediterranean diet is considered to be protective of this disease, due to its lipid-lowering and antioxidant effects [96-98].

Elevated levels of lipopolysaccharide (LPS) produce a proinflammatory situation and an increase in the β-amyloid protein in the hippocampus, as well as the appearance of cognitive deficits. An increase in BMAA (beta-methylamino-L-alanine, a neurotoxin that augments in states of anxiety or stress and or malnutrition, and in inflammatory bowel disease) may also be related to an increased risk of AD. Conversely, vitamin B_{12} is associated with an increased risk of developing dementia when its plasma levels are lowered [95, 97-100].

The neurotransmitter GABA, as discussed above, is related to the composition and activity of the microbiota. The involvement of the intestinal barrier, as well as an alteration in the quantity or quality of this microbiota, can reduce the levels of the neurotransmitter. Scant levels of GABA have been observed in the motor, frontal and temporal cortex of patients with AD [98-100].

It has been investigated the possible role of the gut microbiota in AD pathogenesis by studying the association of brain amyloid plaques with this microbiota taxa with pro- and anti-inflammatory activity. It turns out an increase in the quantity of *Escherichia/Shigella* (pro-inflammatory taxon) and a decrease in the presence of *Eubacterium rectale* (anti-inflammatory taxon), are possibly associated with a peripheral inflammatory state in patients with cognitive impairment and brain amyloidosis [101].

Moreover, NMDA receptors (N-methyl-D-aspartate, another neurotransmitter), are molecule protagonists in neuronal plasticity, learning and memory; the increase in these molecules provides greater neuroprotection. The use of antibiotics decreases the levels of these receptors in the hippocampus [98-100].

NMDAs are also lower in germ-free mice. These animals also show a decrease in the expression of the BDNF promoter gene, which also has neuroprotective effects, as already commented. The re-population of intestinal microbiota in these mice decreases the permeability of the blood-brain barrier and favors the up-regulation of the gene expression of 'tight junction proteins' (occlusive junctions or *zonula occludens*, constituted by a framework of proteins which approach the lipidic membranes of adjacent cells); those proteins confer impermeability to the epithelium, preventing the free flow of substances between cells [99, 100].

3.7. Amyotrophic Lateral Sclerosis (ALS)

Amyotrophic lateral sclerosis (ALS) is a neuromuscular disease that presents a selective degeneration of motor neurons, responsible for innervating the muscles involved in voluntary movement. As its name suggests, there is a sclerosis at the expense of an astrocytic proliferation (or gliosis) that affects the nerve fibers of the lateral part of the spinal cord, which causes muscle atrophy (or amyotrophy) as a result of the muscles ceasing to receive nerve stimuli. The consequence is a progressive muscle weakness that advances toward the patient's total paralysis, also affecting the ability to speak, chew, swallow and breathe. On the other hand, functions such as sensitivity and intelligence are not affected; nor are ocular movements, because they have higher resistance neurons [102].

ALS requires a fundamentally clinical diagnosis. At the tissue level, a hyperphosphorylated, ubiquitinated and cleaved form of TDP-43 may be found in motor neurons; this being the most important protein related to this disease. Only 20% of patients have a known hereditary component

So that most cases are due to environmental causes. Of these, it has been suggested that infectious etiology is most likely to be the cause of this condition [102-104].

An elevation of serum IL-17 has been found in patients with this disease. This interleukin increases in infections caused by bacteria and fungi. In ALS models produced in transgenic mice, IL-17 has been shown to be related to the activation of astrocytes and microglia [103, 104].

Recent studies in murine models of ALS reveal that there is an increase in intestinal permeability, as well as a lower presence of *Escherichia coli* and *Butyrivibrio fibrisolvens* in stool samples. It has been hypothesized that this increase in intestinal permeability could allow the passage of toxins that would reach the bloodstream, which would agree with the well-known role of LPS or endotoxins in the pathogenesis of this disease. Reduced levels of tight junction proteins have also been found in the tissues of the lumbar spinal cord as well as of the blood-brain barrier [105, 106].

3.8. Multiple Sclerosis (MS)

Multiple Sclerosis (MS) is characterized by the progressive demyelination of CNS axons and neuronal degeneration. Its etiology is unknown and probably multifactorial, with non-hereditary and hereditary causes, such as a genetic predisposition related to 2 HLA alleles DRB1* 1501 and DQ6 [107, 108].

Its clinical manifestations are characterized by recurrent episodes of neurological dysfunctions such as fatigue, numbness, loss of coordination, loss of vision, bladder and sphincter dysfunction, pain and nerve depression [107].

Its incidence has increased progressively in recent years, the man to woman ratio being 1:3. This last fact suggests that its genesis could be influenced by hormonal factors. Among other etiological elements, MS has been associated with Epstein Barr virus (EBV), alcohol, smoking, latitude, vitamin D (with its important immunomodulatory effect of T-regs lymphocytes), vitamin A, leptin, sodium intake, high body mass index in adolescence, and infection by helminths and by *Helicobacter pylori* [107, 109]. In recent years, the "hygiene hypothesis" in the origin of this and other neurodegenerative diseases [107, 110, 111] has also become particularly relevant.

This hypothesis was proposed in 1989 by David Strachan and, in short, it advocates the pertinence of human exposure to allergens and infectious agents from early life, in order to achieve adequate maturation of their immune system during growth. Proceeding the opposite way would give rise to typical conditions in developed societies, such as allergic or autoimmune nature diseases. Therefore, the increased frequency of these processes may be due to socio-cultural hygienic habits that drastically reduce the exposure of children to allergens and germs [111].

It is known that MS carries objectivable alterations at the cellular and humoral level. Histologically, glial scars, demyelination, loss of oligodendrocytes and axonal damage can be observed. It is known that there is a large autoimmune component, with a relevant implication of CD8+ and CD161+ T-proinflammatory cells, as well as an increase in T-helper and IL-17 [112, 113].

Inflammation of the CNS could produce a stimulus in the Peyer plaques, and, as a result, this would increase the permeability of the intestinal wall, thus altering its structure. This increased penetrability would facilitate the passage of macromolecules, toxins and bacteria. Patients with MS have an altered intestinal permeability, as well as a deficit in the activation mechanisms of absorption in the lumen of the intestine [112, 113].

Recent studies have shown that patients with MS show differences in the diversity and proportion of the microbiota compared to healthy individuals. The genera *Faecalibacterium, Prevotella* and *Anaerostipes* are diminished in MS. All these butyrate-producing microorganisms act protectively in inflammatory environments, so that their reduction leads to pathologies. Such is the example of *Faecalibacterium prausnitzii,* which shows scarce levels in inflammatory bowel disease [109, 110, 114].

Patients affected by MS have a significant increase in bacteria of the phylum *Euryarchaeota* (of the genus *Methanobrevibacter,* related to inflammatory processes) due to their capacity to recruit inflammatory cells and activate dendritic cells), and phylum *Verrucomicrobia* (of the genus *Akkermansia,* with anti-inflammatory properties and immunomodulatory agents by producing increased expression of genes from antigen-presenting cells to B cells, in addition to triggering complement activation). On the other hand, *Collinsella* and *Slackia* (Actinobacterias) and *Prevotella* (Bacteroides) are diminished in these patients. Similarly, they have a lower proportion of *Clostridium perfringens* type A than healthy people [109, 114, 115].

Variations in intestinal microbiota may also arise as a function of the therapy to which MS patients are subjected. Bacteria of the genus *Sarcina* are decreased in the treated patients compared to the untreated ones. If they are treated with immunomodulators, the microbiota alterations typical of MS are normalized. In contrast, patients treated with interferons do not show any significant changes in their microbiota [114-116].

One of the signs that frequently appears in MS is optic neuritis. This is due to an autoimmune phenomenon directed against the aquaporin-4 protein (AQP4) and mediated by Th-17 cells. In addition to the appearance of optic neuritis, an increase in gastrointestinal antibodies has been detected, specifically against a protein similar to that produced by *Clostridium perfringens* [107, 117].

Experimental autoimmune encephalomyelitis (EAE) represents the animal model most commonly used in the study of MS. It can be said that EAE is the murine equivalent of MS in the human species. In EAE models it has been observed how some segmented filamentous bacteria promote the expansion of Th-17 lymphocytes and the production of IL-17 in the intestine and of Th-17 in the spinal cord. Oral administration of *Bacteroides fragilis* causes a spread of CD4 T-regs of the FoxP3+ type, which inhibit the development of autoimmune processes against CNS structures [112, 113].

In phagocytes of primates affected by demyelinating lesions, peptidoglycan from the wall of bacterial cells has been detected. It appears to be related to inflammatory processes and interacts with the protein kinase 2 receptor. In turn, the muramyl dipeptide (which is a component of this peptidoglycan) produces an activation of NOD2 and NLRP3 in the microglia. The presence of RNA and bacterial DNA in the human brain, particularly from proteobacteria, suggests that along with the inflammatory mechanisms there is a morphological disruption that leads to demyelination [113, 116].

A clear association has also been found between the presence of bacterial material and the immune response mediated by NF-kB (nuclear factor, enhancer of kappa light-chains from activated B cells), which is related to synaptic plasticity and memory processes, as well as neuroinflammatory and degenerative phenomena [112].

Furthermore, the EAE models have shown that vaccination with the antigenic factor of the colonization (CFA/I) of *Escherichia coli* by means of oral immunization with *Salmonella typhimurium* strains, has made the disease less severe and it shows a more benign evolution. After this vaccination, a smaller number of foci with inflammatory infiltrate appear in a gray and white substance of the spinal cord, with decreased expression of IFN-γ secreting T cells and increased secretion of IL-4, IL-10, IL-13 and TGF-β. These anti-inflammatory actions associated with the vaccine may be achieved through the involvement of lymphocytes T-regs-FoxP3+ [112, 113].

The use of broad-spectrum oral antibiotics prior to the induction of EAE improves its clinical course, while the serum levels of IL-6, IL-17, IFN-γ, TNF-α and the Th-17 cell count decrease. It is also observed that the antibiotic prophylaxis prior to EAE, implies that the mice modify the expression of B cells inducing the B CD5+ subpopulation [112, 116].

In research in which *Bacteroides fragilis* polysaccharide A (PSA) was administered, this lipopolysaccharide was also found to be a factor antagonizing the severity of EAE. In the presence of PSA, Toll-like receptor 2 (TLR2) induces the dissemination of CD4+ and CD39+ T lymphocytes, which can result in an immunomodulation of T lymphocytes in general and T-regs-FoxP3+ in particular [112, 113, 116].

Germ-free mice have a form of attenuated disease with lower levels of IFN-γ and IL-17 in the gut and marrow. This form is characterized by having an immune response with increased T-regs-FoxP3+ and a reduced Th-1/Th-17 ratio at the CNS level. These microbiota-free mice also show lower levels of antibodies against the myelin oligodendrocytic glycoprotein (MOG), which can increase after intestinal recolonization. The presence of MOG provides an antigenic stimulus known as the etiological factor of MS; in fact, the induction of EAE can be achieved by inoculation of MOG [116, 117, 119].

The use of probiotics (specifically *Bifidobacterium animalis*) in lactating mice prior to the MOG inoculum has also been linked to a decrease in the severity and duration of clinical signs of EAE, although this has only been observed in male mice [120].

4. MICROBIOTA THERAPEUTIC PROJECTION AND PROSPECTS

The microbiota could be manipulated or handled in order to modify it, knowing full well that it is closely related to the neurological entities addressed above. If we therefore consider the microbiota as a therapeutic target, its management would be one more resource to approaching this type of disease. The first course of action on the intestinal microbiota would be nutritional or dietary strategies.

4.1. Nutritional Strategies

As mentioned earlier, it is known that food and lifestyles are closely related to caloric expenditure and all of this influences the subject's microbiota. It is also known that diets high in fiber are recommended for maintaining good health. The individuals that follow these diets show in their microbiota a greater presence of certain bacterial genera, such as *Bacteroides* (*Prevotella* and *Xylanibacter*), and a smaller proportion of other genera, such as *Firmicutes* and *Enterobacterias*. This would increase the *Bacteroides*/*Firmicutes* ratio, which is related to lower dysbiotic activity [121].

In contrast, some current diets (common in Western countries) have high amounts of saturated fats, animal proteins and refined sugars, as well as low proportions of cereals and fiber. All this provokes an increase in situations of intestinal dysbiosis and pathologies of an inflammatory character. Such a situation can have a generalized effect, leading to chronic diseases of very diverse natures, such as diabetes, metabolic syndrome or rheumatoid arthritis [122, 123].

These diets, in addition to their qualitative aspects, carry a quantitative problem such as their implicit high caloric content, which is also not recommended for the health of the nervous system. It has been observed how the antimicrobial peptide REG3G- gamma expression is decreased in high calory diets [122, 123].

This is where the Mediterranean diet is particularly relevant. It has metabolic benefits (such as its lipid-lowering effect, lowering LDL-cholesterol), antioxidant nature, and also anti-inflammatory properties, which are apparently due to its ability to inhibit proinflammatory ILs and TNF-α. Perhaps its most remarkable consequence at the brain level is the decrease in lipoperoxides and oxidative stress in general, thus protecting against these neurodegenerative agents [124].

This diet is characterized by the constant presence of fruit, vegetables, olive oil, cereals and nuts. Thus, a considerable source of vitamins, antioxidants, mono and polyunsaturated fatty acids and, of course, fiber is available. These components would contribute to a greater proportion of the microbiota strains that promote anti-inflammatory activity [28, 124].

To all this we should add the synergies of vitamin D, which, among its multiple pleiotropic actions, has a recognized anti-inflammatory and immunomodulatory activity Deficient states or problems in vitamin D metabolism, have been specifically related to some of these diseases, such as MS, ALS, Huntington's disease and various mental illnesses [125]. This vitamin contributes decisively to the absorption of calcium at the intestinal level. At this same level, vitamin

D itself would also be absorbed (although only a small proportion of this molecule would enter the body with the intake, since the majority would come from cutaneous synthesis after stimulation by solar ultraviolet radiation). It should be noted that the above-mentioned digestive absorption of calcium and vitamin D would be conditioned, in turn, by the presence of intestinal microbiota. For this, and for many other reasons, it is advisable to maintain an adequate status of this vitamin [125-127].

Other strategies of the nutritional scope, are the incorporation into the diet of several products: i) probiotics; ii) prebiotics; iii) symbiotic; and iv) postbiotics.

i) Probiotics are, according to the World Organization of Gastroenterology, living microorganisms. They are bacteria or yeasts that are present in certain foods (especially dairy), medications, or dietary supplements. Their intake in a sufficient amount is capable of producing health benefits. Those most commonly used belong to the species *Lactobacillus* and *Bifidobacterium.*

Foods that typically contain probiotics are yoghurts, ice cream, black sugar-free chocolate, fermented cabbage (sauerkraut), pickled gherkins, yeasts such as kefir, and commercial fermented milks using the above-mentioned *Bifidobacterium, Lactobacillus* or combinations of other probiotics.

These substances are able to modulate the gastrointestinal barrier by increasing the production of mucin. Among their positive effects, we can find: maintenance of the intestinal barrier, production of SCFA and stimulation of intestinal gluconeogenesis [128].

They also intervene in the immune response, activating T-regs lymphocytes and inhibiting dendritic cells. As a consequence, the production of IL-12, TNF-α (of a proinflammatory nature) is decreased and the synthesis of IL-10 and β-TFGF (of anti-inflammatory actions) is increased.

Probiotics also have beneficial effects at other levels, such as in the synthesis and absorption of vitamins, antioxidants and defensins. They have also acted protectively against hypercholesterolemia [128, 129].

In addition to these effects at the molecular level, the use of probiotics also leads to clinical manifestations. Thus, treatment with *Lactobacillus rhamnosus* has demonstrated its ability to attenuate anxiety and depression. *Lactobacillus helveticus* also reduces anxious states and mitigates memory deficits. Treatment with *Mycobacterium vaccae* also decreases anxiety and activates cognitive functions. Other research shows that the intake of milk enriched in probiotics also causes an improvement in cognition and mood in healthy people. In a pilot study, a reduction in their level of anxiety was noted in patients with chronic fatigue syndrome treated with *Lactobacillus casei. Bacteroides fragilis* has been tested in an analogous way in autistic patients, producing a symptomatic improvement [130].

ii) Prebiotics are nondigestible substances that favor the selective growth of beneficial gut bacteria. They correspond to carbohydrates found in the composition of various vegetables and fruit. They are used by probiotics as a food substrate. In this way, they favor the growth of *Bifidobacterium* and *Lactobacillus,* in addition to enhancing bacterial prote-

olytic activity. The largest sources of prebiotics can be found in: garlic, onions, artichokes, escarole and leeks.

The two prebiotics most studied are: inulin and fructooligosaccharides (FOS). Both can appear naturally in some foods or be added during their manufacturing process. FOS has shown positive effects on the intestinal barrier [128, 129].

It has been reported that the consumption of the prebiotic substances galactol or galactooligosaccharides (GOS), increases the production of IL-10 anti-inflammatory cytokines, reducing the production of proinflammatory toxins such as IL-1, IL-6 and TNF-α. Similarly, patients taking xylooligosaccharides (XOS), showed a diminution in the synthesis of IL-1β, IL-8, IL-12 and TNF-α. *In vitro* studies demonstrate how the use of prebiotics produces effects on the synthesis of cytokines and on the immune system in general. The combination of several prebiotics and probiotics has also demonstrated their ability to modify the microbiota, which, in turn, corresponds to the observation of changes at the neurochemical level, with different repercussions at the clinical level [130].

iii) Symbiotics are products that have been enriched with both probiotics and prebiotics, while providing both components. Their goal is that when they reach the intestine, probiotics do so accompanied by those substances (prebiotics) that help their growth and colonization. The natural symbiotic food model is breast milk, since it contains both lactic bacteria (*Lactobacillus* and *Bifidobacterium*) and fructooligosaccharides and nucleotides that also favor the development of *Bifidobacterium.* For this reason, infant milks have been incorporating symbiotics into their formulations to resemble breast milk. In addition, as with prebiotics and probiotics, some symbiotic food supplements are presented in capsules or powder [129, 131].

iv) Postbiotics are substances produced by probiotics, exerting metabolic and immunomodulatory effects on the host. They are soluble factors generated by the metabolism of probiotics and released into the extracellular medium. They correspond to new compounds containing metabolites or purified bacterial components. They also provide positive health effects, with the advantage that they are designed and elaborated to perform specific functions.

Some authors have proposed a new group of functional foods: *paraprobiotics.* These are characterized by the use of non-viable elements of a microbial origin (inactivated microorganisms or cell fractions), which have demonstrated potential benefits for human or animal health and, theoretically, have the advantage of being safer and more stable products [129].

4.2. Stool Transplantation

Stool transplantation (FMT, Fecal Microbiota Transplantation) was started in China in the fourth century by Ge Hong. He used what he called "yellow soup" in patients with diarrhea. In the 16th century an oral solution was also used to treat diarrhea, fever, pain, constipation and vomiting [132, 133].

Already in contemporary times, FMT use was tested during World War II in soldiers who had dysentery. But it was not until 1958 that patients with pseudomembranous colitis due to *Micrococcus pyogenes* began to be treated with FMT; in this case it was done with enemas. Years later (specifically in 1989), it was used in *Clostridium difficile* infections *via* different methods of administration [132, 133].

Some studies in experimental models suggest that FMT may be useful as a treatment for inflammatory bowel disease or irritable bowel syndrome. It has also been observed that intestinal repopulation of germ-free mice leads to an increase in IL-10 levels [133].

Today, FMT is in the developmental phase. Different forms of application are being optimized and numerous clinical trials targeting various diseases are being carried out. The common goal is to restore the normality of microbiota to reverse certain pathophysiologic processes and, thus, to facilitate are return to health. Solutions of feces conveyed in saline solution, water or milk, have been tested. The administration of heterologous feces by enemas has been shown to be more effective than recolonization by gastroscopy, nasogastric tube, or oral capsules. Frozen stool specimens are commonly used for all these forms [133, 134].

In clinical research, gastrointestinal diseases represent the area where the potentialities of stool transplantation have been verified most. The most widespread use, currently, is the treatment of recurrent infection by *Clostridium difficile*. Promising results have been achieved, reaching a cure rate of more than 90% in some studies [134, 135].

It has been postulated that the FMT therapeutic action mechanism in patients infected by *Clostridium difficile* could be based on different actions of the transplanted microbiota: i) competing for nutrients; ii) inhibiting the toxigenic activity of this bacterium; iii) modulating metabolites and transforming bile acids; and iv) interacting with the immune system, regulating it and thus preventing *Clostridium difficile* invasion [135, 136].

Stool transplantation has also been tried in other digestive diseases. In patients with ulcerative colitis, some studies show symptomatic remission rates of around 63%. Furthermore, it has been shown that FMT combined with fiber intake is an effective option as a therapy for constipation [134].

Fecal transplants have also been performed as part of the therapeutic approach to some metabolic diseases. A group of pathologies on which a significant number of studies have been performed is related to diabetes, metabolic syndrome and obesity. In some patients, FMT treatment has shown up to a 75% decrease in peripheral insulin resistance. Stool transplantation has also been tested in autoimmune diseases, such as Hashimoto's thyroiditis or idiopathic thrombocytopenic purpura [134].

FMT has also been tested in pathologies such as multiple sclerosis, Parkinson's disease, myoclonic dystonia and neuropsychiatric disorders such as autism, being fully aware of the transcendence of the microbiota-bowel-brain axis in the origin, development and maintenance of numerous neurological entities such as autism [134, 137]. In this latter disease, stool transplantation leads to symptomatic improvement, both in murine models and in clinical trials with children [138].

4.3. Prospects

Identifying the role of the microbiota in the etiology and pathogenesis of numerous diseases (digestive and non-digestive) can make this a relevant element for a better knowledge and approach to these diseases. This fact could lead to the design and implementation of new strategies in which some elements of the microbiota can participate in the diagnosis or treatment of pathologies of a diverse nature.

It is logical to think that they will be able to increase the potentials of the use of the microbiota (as a diagnosis tool or therapeutic resource) and that it will be possible to perfect the currently known utilities. This will be in terms of the advances in the knowledge of microbiota itself, which will depend, in turn, on the development of all the scientific areas in some way related to it (fundamentally those concerning biotechnology, such as bioinformatics, genomics, proteomics and nanomedicine) [36, 37, 139].

As can be seen, at the present moment, there are many potentialities in the use of the microbiota as a therapeutic target, most of them probably being based on dietary or nutritional approaches, which have already been discussed. In fact, these approximations are those most studied because they are the most physiologic and easy to apply. In the context of nutrigenetics and nutrigenomics, we are inclined to think that the manipulation of the microbiota could be oriented towards preventing, palliating, or even reversing certain pathologies. The manufacture of new, genetically modified foods would also move in this direction. Thus, some of the multiple consequences of the gene-diet interactions could be directed towards tackling certain diseases. They would be indirect actions, mainly because they would be mediated by the impact of diet on the immune system and/or on the microbiota itself. For this reason, devising personalized diets as an additional resource in some neurodegenerative diseases could have a future usefulness, especially when the genetic component or susceptibility of each of these diseases is better known [140, 141].

Analogously to the handling of elements outside the human organism, such as food, we might think of direct manipulations on the microbiota itself. More selectively than current stool transplantation, strategies for the implantation or potentiation of beneficial microorganisms could be designed, as well as the exclusive destruction of harmful microorganisms. To the extent that genetic engineering increases its potential, bacteria are capable of antagonizing or destroying other undesirable microorganisms by direct action (increasing the synthesis of their endotoxins) or indirectly (by modifying their antigenicity and thus interfering with the immune response). The differential labeling of certain microorganisms of the microbiota by means of nanoparticles would allow them to act on them, restrictively [139, 142]. Recent studies show that bacteria react against nanoparticles, which can be included in the diet. Zhano *et al.* have shown a reaction to tiny particles of titanium dioxide, zinc oxide and cerium dioxide, which produce changes in the synthesis of SCFA, thus inhibiting inflammatory mechanisms [143].

Microbiota and its derivate products in the human organism could also be manipulated. These would include the previously suggested immune system procedures that could be focused on both local and systemic immunity. From this perspective, manoeuvers could be devised on Peyer plates or on circulating lymphocytes [144, 145]. Specific strategies could also be designed for the intestinal mucosa or the enteric nervous system. All of these manipulations would be closely related to the biotechnological advances previously described.

CONCLUSION

This makes us think that the development of various forms of cell therapy, gene therapy and new nanomaterial could be used in actions directed towards: the microbiota, the interactions of the microbiota with the host, and, more specifically, interventions on the brain-gut-microbiota axis [146].

LIST OF ABBREVIATIONS

AD	=	Alzheimer's Disease
ALS	=	Amyotrophic Lateral Sclerosis
BDNF	=	Brain-Derived Neurotrophic Factor
CNS	=	Central Nervous System
EAE	=	Experimental Autoimmune Encephalomyelitis
FMT	=	Fecal Microbiota Transplantation
GABA	=	Gamma-Aminobutyric Acid
IFN	=	Interferon
IL	=	Interleukin
MOG	=	Myelin Oligodendrocytic Glycoprotein
MS	=	Multiple Sclerosis
NPY	=	Neuropeptide Y
PD	=	Parkinson's Disease
PrPc	=	Cellular Prion Protein
PrPsc	=	Pathogenic Cellular Prion Protein
SCFA	=	Short-Chain Fatty Acids
TGF-β	=	Transforming Growth Factor Beta

CONSENT FOR PUBLICATION

Not applicable.

CONFLICT OF INTEREST

The authors declare no conflict of interest, financial or otherwise.

ACKNOWLEDGEMENTS

Authors thank Ms. Heather Thoelecke for helping us with editing.

REFERENCES

[1] Jandhyala SM, Talukdar R, Subramanyam C, Vuyyuru H, Sasikala M, Reddy DN. Role of the normal gut microbiota. World J Gastroenterol 2015; 21(29): 8787-803.

[2] Gibbons RJ, Socransky SS, Sawyer S, Kapsimalis B, Macdonald JB. The microbiota of the gingival crevice are of man. II. The predominant cultivable organisms. Arch Oral Biol 1963; 8: 281-9.

[3] Rosengaus RB, Zecher CN, Schultheis KF, Brucker RM, Bordenstein SR. Disruption of the termite gutmicrobiota and its prolonged consequences for fitness. Appl Environ Microbiol 2011; 77(13): 4303-12.

[4] Shapira M. Gut Microbiotas and host evolution: scaling up symbiosis. Trends Ecol Evol 2016; 31(7): 539-49.

[5] Rolhion N, Chassaing B. When pathogenic bacteria meet the intestinal microbiota. Philos Trans R Soc Lond B Biol Sci 2016; 371: 1707.

[6] Gilbert SF, Bosch TC, Ledón-Rettig C. Eco-Evo-Devo: developmental simbiosis and developmental plasticity as evolutionary agents. Nat Rev Genet 2015; 16(10): 611-22.

[7] Eisthen HL, Theis KR. Animal-microbe interactions and the evolution of nervous systems. Philos Trans R Soc Lond B Biol Sci 2016; 371(1685): 20150052.

[8] Ley RE, Lozupone CA, Hamady M, Knight R, Gordon JI. Worlds within worlds: evolution of the vertebrade gut microbiota. Nat Rev Microbiol 2008; 6(10): 776-88.

[9] Kisseleva EP. Innate immunity underlies symbiotic relationships. Biochemistry (Mosc) 2014; 79(12): 1273-85.

[10] Guerrero R, Margulis L, Berlanga M. Symbiogenesis: the holobiont as a unit of evolution. Int Microbiol 2013; 16: 133-43.

[11] Shafquat A, Joice R, Simmons S, Huttenhower C. Functional and phylogenetic assembly of microbial communities in the human microbiome. Trends Microbiol 2014; 22(5): 261-6.

[12] Muszer M, Noszczynska M, Kasperkiewicz K, Skurnik M. Human microbiome: when a friend becomes an enemy. Arch Immunol Ther Exp (Warsz) 2015; 63(4): 287-98.

[13] Rajilic-Stojanovic M. Function of the microbiota. Best Pract Res Clin Gastroenterol 2013; 27(1): 5-16.

[14] Schroeder B, Bäckhed F. Signals from the gut microbiota to distant organs in physiology and disease. Nat Med 2016; 22(10): 1079-89.

[15] Althani AA, Marei HE, Hamdi WS, et al. Human microbiome and its association with health and diseases. J Cell Physiol 2016; 231(8): 1688-94.

[16] Ly M, Jones MB, Abeles SR, et al. Transmission of viruses via our microbiomes. Microbiome 2016; 4(1): 64.

[17] Staley C, Weingarden AR, Khoruts A, Sadowsky MJ. Interaction of gut microbiota with bile acid metabolism and its influence on disease states. Appl Microbiol Biotechnol 2017; 101(1): 47-64.

[18] Dave M, Higgins P, Middha S, Rioux KP. The human gut microbiome: current knowledge, challenges, and future. Asian Pac J Allergy Immunol 2016; 34(4): 249-64.

[19] Breznak JA. Symbiotic relationships between termite and their intestinal microbiota. Symp Soc Exp Biol 1975; 29: 559-80.

[20] Manning BW, Cerniglia CE, Federle TW. Metabolism of the benzidine-based azo dye Direct Black 38 by human intestinal microbiota. Appl Environ Microbiol 1985; 50(1): 10-5.

[21] Lynch SV, Pedersen O. The human intestinal microbiome in health and disease. N Engl J Med 2016; 375(24): 2369-79.

[22] Greenhalgh K, Meyer KM, Aagaard KM, Wilmes P. The human gut microbiome in health: establishment and resilience of microbiota over a lifetime. Environ Microbiol 2016; 18(7): 2103-16.

[23] Thaiss CA, Levy M, Korem T, et al. Microbiota diurnal rhythmicity programs host transcriptome oscillations. Cell 2016; 167(6): 1495-510.

[24] Blaser MJ, Dominguez-Bello MG. The human microbiome before birth. Cell Host Microbe 2016; 20(5): 558-60.

[25] Cong X, HendersonWA, Graf J, McGrath JM. Early life experience and gut microbiome. Adv Neonatal Care 2015; 15(5): 314-23.

[26] Proctor C, Thiennimitr P, Chattipakorn N, Chattipakorn SC. Diet, gutmicrobiota and cognition. Metab Brain Dis 2017; 32(1): 1-17.

[27] Mischke M, Plösch T. More than just a gut instinct-the potential interplay between a baby's nutrition, its gut microbiome, and the epigenome. Am J Physiol Regul Integr Comp Physiol 2013; 304(12): R1065-9.

[28] Maukonen J, Saarela M. Human gut microbiota: does diet matter? Proc Nutr Soc 2015; 74(1): 23-36.

[29] Kuang YS, Li SH, Guo Y, et al. Composition of gut microbiota in infants in China and global comparison. Sci Rep 2016; 6: 36666.

[30] O'Mahony SM, Stilling RM, Dinan TG, Cryan JF. The microbiome and childhood diseases: focus on brain-gut axis. Birth Defects Res C Embryo Today 2015; 105(4): 296-313.

[31] Prince AL, Chu DM, Seferovic Antony KM, Ma J, Aagaard KM. The perinatal microbiome and pregnancy: moving beyond the

vaginal microbiome. Cold Spring Harb Perspect Med 2015; 5(6): 178.

[32]   Chu DM, Ma J, Prince AL, Antony KM, Seferovic MD, Aagaard KM. Maturation of the infant microbiome community structure and function across multiple body sites and in relation to mode of delivery. Nat Med 2017; *(in press).*

[33]   Kacerovsky M, Vrbacky F, Kutova R, *et al.* Cervical microbiota in women with preterm prelabor rupture of membranes. PLoS One 2015; 10(5): e0126884.

[34]   Drago L, Toscano M, De Grandi R, Grossi E, Padovani EM, Peroni DG. Microbiota network and mathematic microbe mutualism in colostrum and mature milk collected in two different geographic areas: Italy versus Burundi. ISME J 2016; *(in press).*

[35]   Xiong W, Abraham P, Li Z, Pan Ch, Hettich RL. Microbial metaproteomics for characterizing the range of metabolic functions and activities of human gut microbiota. Proteomics 2015; 15(20): 3424-8.

[36]   Lagier JC, Khelaifia S, Alou MT, *et al.* Culture of previously uncultured members of the human gut microbiota by culturomics. Nat Microbiol 2016; 1: 16203.

[37]   Human Microbiome Project Consortium. A framework for human microbiome research. Nature 2012; 486(7402): 215-21.

[38]   Li J, Jia H, Cai X, *et al.* An integrated catalog of reference genes in the human gut microbiome. Nat Biotechnol 2014; 32(8): 834-41.

[39]   Turpin W, Espin-Garcia O, Xu W, *et al.* Association of host genome with intestinal microbial composition in a large healthy cohort. Nat Genet 2016; 48(11): 1413-7.

[40]   Traore SI, Khelaifia S, Dubourg G, Sokhna C, Raoult D, Fournier PE. "Lagierella Massiliensis", a new bacterium detected in human feces. New Microbes New Infect 2016; 14: 53-5.

[41]   Honda K, Littman DR. The microbiota in adaptive immune homeostasis and disease. Nature 2016; 535(7610): 75-84.

[42]   Cholewa-Waclaw J, Bird A, von Schimmelmann M, *et al.* The role of epigenetic mechanisms in the regulation of gene expression in the nervous system. J Neurosci 2016; 36(45): 11427-34.

[43]   Min YW, Rhee PL. The role of microbiota on the gut immunology. Clin Ther 2015; 37(5): 968-75.

[44]   Yan J, Herzog JW, Tsang K, *et al.* Gut microbiota induce IGF-1 and promote bone formation and growth. Proc Natl Acad Sci USA 2016; 113(47): 7554-63.

[45]   Ridler C. Bone: gut microbiota promote bone growth *via* IGF1. Nat Rev Endocrinol 2017; 13(1): 5.

[46]   Guinane CM, Cotter PD. Role of the gut microbiota in health and chronic gastrointestinal disease: understanding a hidden metabolic organ. Therap Adv Gastroenterol 2013; 6(4): 295-308.

[47]   Masotti A. Interplays between gut microbiota and gene expression regulation by miRNAs. Front Cell Infect Microbiol 2012; 2(2): 137.

[48]   Liu S, da Cunha AP, Rezende RM, *et al.* The host shapes the gut microbiota *via* fecal microRNA. Cell Host Microbe 2016; 19(1): 32-43.

[49]   Thomas H. Gut microbiota: host faecal miRNA regulates gut microbiota. Nat Rev Gastroenterol Hepatol 2016; 13(3): 122-3.

[50]   Kubinak JL, Round JL. Do antibodies select a healthy microbiota? Nat Rev Immunol 2016; 16(12): 767-74.

[51]   Kim D, Yoo S-A, Kim W-U. Gut microbiota in autoimmunity: potential for clinical applications. Arch Pharm Res 2016; 39 (11): 1565-76.

[52]   Rosser EC, Mauri C. A clinical update in the significance of the gut microbiota in systemic autoimmunity. J Autoimmun 2016; 74: 85-93.

[53]   Bienenstock J, Kunze W, Forsythe P. Microbiota and the gut-brain axis. Nutr Rev 2015; 73 Suppl 1: 28-31.

[54]   Dinan TG, Cryan JF. Gut instincts: microbiota as a key regulator of brain development, ageing and neurodegeneration. J Physiol 2017; 595(2): 489-503.

[55]   Sampsons TR, Mazmanian SK. Control of brain development, function, and behaviour by the microbiome. Cell Host Microbe 2013; 17(5): 565-76.

[56]   Sánchez-López F, Tasset I, Agüera E, *et al.* Oxidative stress and inflammation biomarkers in the blood of patients with Huntington's disease. Neurol Res 2012; 34(7): 721-4.

[57]   Túnez I, Sánchez-López F, Agüera E, Fernández-Bolaños R, Sánchez FM, Tasset-Cuevas I. Important role of oxidative stress biomarkers in Huntington's disease. J Med Chem 2011; 54(15): 5602-6.

[58]   Maqsood R, Stone TW. The gut-brain axis, BDNF, NMDA and CNS disorders. Neurochem Res 2016; 41(11): 2819-35.

[59]   Luczynski P, Whelan SO, O'Sullivan C, *et al.* Adult microbiota-deficient mice have distinct dendritic morphological changes: differential effects in the amigdala and hippocampus. Eur J Neurosci 2016; 44(9): 2654-66.

[60]   Borre YE, Moloney RD, Clarke G, Dinan TG, Cryan JF. The impact of microbiota on brain and behaviour: mechanisms & therapeutic potential. Adv Exp Med Biol 2014; 817: 373-403.

[61]   Sherwin E, Sandhu KV, Dinan TG, Cryan JF. May the force be with you: the light and dark sides of the microbiota-gut-brain axis in neuropsychiatry. CNS Drugs 2016; 30(11): 1019-41.

[62]   Rea K, Dinan TG, Cryan JF. The Microbiome: a key regulator of stress and neuroinflammation. Neurobiol Stress 2016; 4: 23-33.

[63]   Ridaura V, Belkaid Y. Gut microbiota: the link to your second brain. Cell 2015; 161(2): 193-4.

[64]   Ochoa-Repáraz J, Kasper LH. The second brain: is the gut microbiota a link between obesity and central nervous system disorders? Curr Obes Rep 2016; 5(1): 51-64.

[65]   Dinan TG, Cryan JF. Gut-brain axis in 2016: brain-gut-microbiota axis - mood, metabolism and behaviour. Nat Rev Gastroenterol Hepatol 2017; 14(2): 69-70.

[66]   Neufeld KA, Kang N, Bienenstock J, Foster JA. Effects of intestinal microbiota on anxiety-like behavior. Commun Integr Biol 2011; 4(4): 492-4.

[67]   Kelly JR, Kennedy PJ, Cryan JF, Dinan TG, Clarke G, Hyland NP. Breaking down the barriers: the gut microbiome, intestinal permeability and stress-related psychiatric disorders. Front Cell Neurosci 2015; 9: 392.

[68]   Mangiola F, Ianiro G, Franceschi F, Fagiuoli S, Gasbarrini G, Gasbarrini A. Gut microbiota in autism and mood disorders. World J Gastroneterol 2016; 22(1): 361-8.

[69]   De Palma G, Blennerhassett P, Lu J, *et al.* Microbiota and host determinants of behavioural phenotype in maternally separated mice. Nat Commun 2015; 6: 7735.

[70]   Pyndt JB, Krych L, Pedersen TB, *et al.* Investigating the long-term effect of subchronic phencyclidine-treatment on novel object recognition and the association between the gut microbiota and behavior in the animal model of schizophrenia. Physiol Behav 2015; 141: 32-9.

[71]   Caso JR, Balanzá-Martínez V, Palomo T, García-Bueno B. The microbiota and gut-brain axis: contributions to the immunopathogenesis of schizophrenia. Curr Pharm Des 2016; 22: 6122-33.

[72]   Dinan TG, Borre YE, Cryan JF. Genomics of schizophrenia: time to consider the gut microbiome? Mol Psychiatr 2014; 19: 1252-7.

[73]   Will RG, Ironside JW. Sporadic and infectious human prion diseases. Cold Spring Harb Perspect Med 2017; *(in press).*

[74]   Scherbel C, Pichner R, Groschup MH, *et al.* Degradation of scrapie associated prion protein (PrPSc) by the gastrointestinal microbiota of cattle. Vet Res 2006; 37(5): 695-703.

[75]   Scherbel C, Pichner R, Groschup MH, *et al.* Infectivity of scrapie prion protein (PrPSc) following *in vitro* digestion with bovine gastrointestinal microbiota. Zoonoses Public Health 2007; 54(5): 185-90.

[76]   Böhnlein C, Groschup MH, Maertlbauer E, Pichner R, Gareis M. Stability of bovine spongiform encephalopathy prions: absence of prion protein degradation by bovine gut microbiota. Zoonoses Public Health 2012; 59(4): 251-5.

[77]   Donaldson DS, Mabbott NA. The influence of the commensal and pathogenic gut microbiota on prion disease pathogenesis. J Gen Virol 2016; 97(8): 1725-38.

[78]   Alston CL, Rocha MC, Lax NZ, Turnbull DM, Taylor RW. The genetics and pathology of mitochondrial disease. J Pathol 2017; 241(2): 236-50.

[79]   Trinchese G, Cavaliere G, Canani RB, *et al.* Human, donkey and cow milk differently affects energy efficiency and inflammatory state by modulating mitochondrial function and gut microbiota. J Nutr Biochem 2015; 26(11): 1136-46.

[80]   Mottawea W, Chiang CK, Mühlbauer M, *et al.* Altered intestinal microbiota-host mitochondria crosstalk in new onset Crohn's disease. Nat Commun 2016; 7: 13419.

[81]   Garagnani P, Pirazzini C, Giuliani C, *et al.* The three genetics (nuclear DNA, mitochondrial DNA, and gut microbiome) of longevity in humans considered as metaorganisms. Biomed Res Int 2014; 2014: 560340.

[82] Zorov DB, Plotnikov EY, Silachev DN, *et al.* Microbiota and mitobiota. Putting an equal sign between mitochondria and bacteria. Biochemistry (Mosc) 2014; 79(10): 1017-31.

[83] Saint-Georges-Chaumet Y, Edeas M. Microbiota-mitochondria inter-talk: consequence for microbiota-host interaction. Pathog Dis 2016; 74(1): 096.

[84] Novak EA, Mollen KP. Mitochondrial dysfunction in inflammatory bowel disease. Front Cell Dev Biol 2015; 3: 62.

[85] Baksi S, Bagh S, Sarkar S, Mukhopadhyay D. Systemic study of a natural feedback loop in Huntington's disease at the onset of neurodegeneration. Biosystems 2016; 150: 46-51.

[86] Nopoulos PC. Huntington disease: a singles-gene degenerative disorder of the striatum. Dialogues Clin Neurosci 2016; 18(1): 91-8.

[87] Degroote S, Hunting DJ, Baccarelli AA, Takser L. Maternal gut and fetal brain connection: increased anxiety and reduced social interactions in Wistar rat offspring following peri-conceptional antibiotic exposure. Prog Neuropsychopharmacol Biol Psychiatry 2016; 71: 76-82.

[88] Yang Y, Tang BS, Guo JF. Parkinson's disease and cognitive impairment. Parkinsons Dis 2016; 2016: 6734678.

[89] Menges S, Minakaki G, Schaefer PM, *et al.* Alpha-synuclein prevents the formation of spherical mitochondria and apoptosis under oxidative stress. Sci Rep 2017; 7: 42942.

[90] Nandipati S, Litvan I. Environmental exposures and Parkinson's disease. Int J Environ Res Public Health 2016; 13(9): 51-62.

[91] Vizcarra JA, Wilson-Perez HE, Espay AJ. The power in numbers: gut microbiota in Parkinson's disease. Mov Disord 2015; 30(3): 296-8.

[92] Scheperjans F. Can microbiota research change our understanding of neurodegenerative diseases? Neurodegener Dis Manag 2016; 6(2): 81-5.

[93] Felice VD, Quigley EM, Sullivan AM, O'Keeffe GW, O'Mahony SM. Microbiota-gut-brain signalling in Parkinson's disease: implications for non-motor symptoms. Parkinsonism Relat Disord 2016; 27: 1-8.

[94] Tateno F, Sakakibara R, Yokoi Y, *et al.* Levodopa ameliorated anorectal constipation in de novo Parkinso"s disease: the QL-GAT study. Parkinsonism Relat Disord 2011; 17(9): 662-6.

[95] Naj AC, Schellenberg GD. Alzheimer's Disease Genetics Consortium (ADGC). Genomic variants, genes, and pathways of Alzheimer's disease: an overview. Am J Med Genet B Neuropsychiatr Genet 2017; 174(1): 5-26.

[96] Wang D, Ho L, Faith J, *et al.* Role of intestinal microbiota in the generation of polyphenol derived phenolic acid mediated attenuation of Alzheimer's disease β-amyloid oligomerization. Mol Nutr Food Res 2015; 59(6): 1025-40.

[97] Pistollato F, Sumalla Cano S, Elio I, *et al.* Role of gut microbiota and nutrients in amyloid formation and pathogenesis of Alzheimer disease. Nutr Rev 2016; 74(10): 624-34.

[98] Hu X, Wang T, Jin F. Alzheimer's disease and gut microbiota. Sci China Life Sci 2016; 59(10): 1006-23.

[99] Alkasir R, Li J, Li X, Jin M, Zhu B. Human gut microbiota: the links with dementia development. Protein Cell 2017; 8(2): 90-102.

[100] Chakraborty A, de Wit NM, van der Flier WM, de Vries HE. The blood brain barrier in Alzheimer's disease. Vascul Pharmacol 2017; 89: 12-8.

[101] Cattaneo A, Cattane N, Galluzzi S, *et al.* INDIA-FBP Group. Association of brain amyloidosis with pro-inflammatory gut bacterial taxa and peripheral inflammation markers in cognitively impaired elderly. Neurobiol Aging 2017; 49: 60-8.

[102] Tefera TW, Borges K. Metabolic dysfunctions in amyotrophic lateral sclerosis pathogenesis and potential metabolic treatments. Front Neurosci 2017; 10: 611.

[103] Scheperjans F. Can microbiota research change our undestanding of neurodegenerative diseases? Neurodegener Dis Manag 2016; 6(2): 81-5.

[104] Fang X. Potential role of gut microbiota and tissue barriers in Parkinson's disease and amyotrophi lateral sclerosis. Int J Neurosci 2016; 126(9): 771-6.

[105] Moling O. Increased IL-17, a pathogenic link between hepatosplenic schistosomiasis and amyotrophic lateral sclerosis: a hypothesis. Case Reports Immunol 2014; 2014: 804761.

[106] Zhang YG, Wu S, Yi J, *et al.* Target intestinal microbiota to alleviate disease progression in amyotrophic lateral sclerosis. Clin Ther 2017; 39(2): 322-36.

[107] Olsson T, Barcellos LF, Alfredsson L. Interactions between genetic, lifestyle and environmental risk factors for multiple sclerosis. Nat Rev Neurol 2017; 13(1): 25-36.

[108] Escribano B, Tunez I. Gut microbiota and central nervous system condemned to understand each other: their role in multiple sclerosis. MOJ Cell Sci Report 2014; 1(2): 00005.

[109] Mielcarz DW, Kasper LH. The gut microbiome in multiple sclerosis. Curr Treat Options Neurol 2015; 17(4): 344.

[110] Jangi S, Gandhi R, Cox LM, *et al.* Alterations of the human gut microbiome in multiple sclerosis. Nat Commun 2016; 7: 12015.

[111] Strachan DP. Family size, infection and atopy: the first decade of the "hygiene hypothesis". Thorax 2000; 55 Suppl 1: S2-10.

[112] Colpitts SL, Kasper LH. Influence of the gut microbiome on autoimmunity in the central nervous system. J Immunol 2017; 198(2): 596-604.

[113] Branton WG, Lu JQ, Surette MG, *et al.* Brain microbiota disruption within inflammatory demyelinating lesions in multiple sclerosis. Sci Rep 2016; 6: 37344.

[114] Buscarinu MC, Cerasoli B, Annibali V, *et al.* Altered intestinal permeability in patients with relapsing-remitting multiple sclerosis: A pilot study. Mult Scler 2016; *(in press)*.

[115] Chen J, Chia N, Kalari KR, *et al.* Multiple sclerosis patients have a distinct gutmicrobiota compared to healthy controls. Sci Rep 2016; 6: 28484.

[116] Forbes JD, Van Domselaar G, Bernstein CN. The gut microbiota in immune-mediated inflammatory diseases. Front Microbiol 2016; 7: 1081.

[117] Miyake S, Kim S, Suda W, *et al.* Dysbiosis in the gut microbiota of patients with multiple sclerosis, with a striking depletion of species belonging to Clostridia XIVa and IV Clusters. PLoS One 2015; 10(9): e0137429.

[118] Wang Y, Kasper LH. The role of microbiome in central nervous system disorders. Brain Behav Immun 2014; 38: 1-12.

[119] Arndt A, Hoffacker P, Zellmer K, Goecer O, Recks MS, Kuerten S. Conventional housing conditions attenuate the development of experimental autoimmune encephalomyelitis. PLoS One 2014; 9(6): e99794.

[120] Kobayashi T, Kato I, Nanno M, *et al.* Oral administration of probiotic bacteria, Lactobacillus casei and Bifidobacterium breve, does not exacerbate neurological symptoms in experimental autoimmune encephalomyelitis. Immunopharmacol Immunotoxicol 2010; 32(1): 116-24.

[121] Mayorga RL, González VR, Cruz Arroyo SM, *et al.* Correlation between diet and gut bacteria in a population of young adults. Int J Food Sci Nutr 2016; 67(4): 470-8.

[122] Natividad JM, Hayes CL, Motta JP, *et al.* Differential induction of antimicrobial REGIII by the intestinal microbiota and Bifidobacterium breve NCC2950. Appl Environ Microbiol 2013; 79(24): 7745-54.

[123] Everard A, Lazarevic V, Gaïa N, *et al.* Microbiome of prebiotic-treated mice reveals novel targets involved in host response during obesity. ISME J 2014; 8(10): 2116-30.

[124] Del Chierico F, Vernocchi P, Dallapiccola B, Putignani L. Mediterranean diet and health: food effects on gut microbiota and disease control. Int J Mol Sci 2014; 15(7): 11678-99.

[125] Fernandes de Abreu DA, Eyles D, Féron F. Vitamin D, a neuroimmunomodulator: implications for neurodegenerative and autoimmune diseases. Psychoneuroendocrinology 2009; 34 Suppl 1: S265-77.

[126] Barbáchano A, Fernández-Barral A, Ferrer-Mayorga G, *et al.* The endocrine vitamin D system in the gut. Mol Cell Endocrinol 2016; *(in press)*.

[127] Clark A, Mach N. Role of vitamin D in the hygiene hypothesis: the interplay between vitamin D, vitamin D receptors, gut microbiota, and immune response. Front Immunol 2016; 7: 627.

[128] Pandey KR, Naik SR, Vakil BV. Probiotics, prebiotics and synbiotics- a review. J Food Sci Technol 2015; 52(12): 7577-87.

[129] Shokryazdan P, Jahromi MF, Navidshad B, Liang JB. Effects of prebiotics on immune system and cytokine expression. Med Microbiol Immunol 2017; 206(1): 1-9.

[130] Liu X, Cao S, Zhang X. Modulation of gut microbiota-brain axis by probiotics, prebiotics, and diet. J Agric Food Chem 2015; 63(36): 7885-95.

[131] Sandhu K, Sherwin E, Schellekens H, Stanton C, Dinan TG. Feeding the microbiota-gut-brain axis: diet, microbiome, and neuropsychiatry. Transl Resp 2016; 179: 223-44.

[132]   Baron TH, Kozarek RA. Fecal microbiota transplant: we know its history, but can we predict its future? Mayo Clin Proc 2013; 88(8): 782-5.

[133]   Vindigni SM, Surawicz CM. Fecal Microbiota Transplantation. Gastroenterol Clin North Am 2017; 46(1): 171-85.

[134]   Choi HH, Cho YS. Fecal Microbiota Transplantation: current applications, effectiveness, and future perspectives. Clin Endosc 2016; 49: 257-65.

[135]   Konturek PC, Koziel J, Dieterich W, *et al.* Successful therapy of Clostridium difficile infection with fecal microbiota transplantation. J Physiol Pharmacol 2016; 67(6): 859-66.

[136]   Staley C, Hamilton MJ, Vaughn BP, *et al.* Successful resolution of recurrent clostridium difficile infection using freeze-dried, encapsulated fecal microbiota; pragmatic cohort study. Am J Gastroenterol 2017; *(in press).*

[137]   Evrensel A, Ceylan ME. Fecal microbiota transplantation and its usage in neuropsychiatric disorders. Clin Psychopharmacol Neurosci 2016; 14(3): 231-7.

[138]   Frye RE, Slattery J, MacFabe DF, *et al.* Approaches to studying and manipulating the enteric microbiome to improve autism symptoms. Microb Ecol Health Dis 2015; 26: 26878.

[139]   Aljuffali IA, Huang CH, Fang JY. Nanomedical strategies for targeting skin microbiomes. Curr Drug Metab 2015; 16(4): 255-71.

[140]   Goni L, Cuervo M, Milagro FI, Martínez JA. Future perspectives of personalized weight loss interventions based on nutrigenetic, epigenetic, and metagenomic data. J Nutr 2016; *(in press).*

[141]   Ferguson JF, Allayee H, Gerszten RE, *et al.* American heart association council on functional genomics and translational biology, council on epidemiology and prevention, and stroke council. Nutrigenomics, the microbiome, and gene-environment interactions: new directions in cardiovascular disease research, prevention, and treatment: a scientific statement from the American Heart Association. Circ Cardiovasc Genet 2016; 9(3): 291-313.

[142]   Mercier-Bonin M, Despax B, Raynaud P, Houdeau E, Thomas M. Mucus and microbiota as emerging players in gut nanotoxicology: the example of dietary silver and titanium dioxide nanoparticles. Crit Rev Food Sci Nutr 2016; *(in press).*

[143]   Zhao Y, Li L, Zhang PF, *et al.* Regulation of egg quality and lipids metabolism by Zinc Oxide Nanoparticles. Poult Sci 2016; 95(4): 920-33.

[144]   Chen Y, Song K, Eck SL. An intra-Peyer's patch gene transfer model for studying mucosal tolerance: distinct roles of B7 and IL-12 in mucosal T cell tolerance. J Immunol 2000; 165(6): 3145-53.

[145]   Bonaccorsi I, Buda C, Campana S, *et al.* Th17 skewing in the GALT of a Crohn disease patient upon Lactobacillus rhamnosus GG consumption. Immunol Lett 2016; 170: 95-7.

[146]   Sun J, Chang EB. Exploring gut microbes in human health and disease: pushing the envelope. Genes Dis 2014; 1(2): 132-9.

CONFERENCE REPORT

183rd American Association for the Advancement of Science Annual Meeting, Boston MA, USA Feb 16-20, 2017

"Serving Society through Science Policy"

Hari S. Sharma[1,*], Stephen D. Skaper[2], and Aruna Sharma[1]

[1]*International Experimental CNS Injury & Repair (IECNSIR), Department of Surgical Sciences, Anesthesiology & Intensive Care Medicine, University Hospital, Uppsala University, SE-75185 Uppsala, Sweden;* [2]*Department of Pharmaceutical and Pharmacological Sciences, University of Padua, Largo "E. Meneghetti" 2, 35131 Padua, Italy*

The 183rd annual meeting of the American Association for the Advancement of Science (AAAS) was held in the Hynes Convention Center, Boston, MA, USA from Feb 16 to 20, 2017. This year's theme was "*Serving Society through Science Policy*", and attracted more than 20,000 participants from around the world including students, basic and industrial researchers, policy makers, healthcare specialists, environmentalists, engineers, space scientists, lawmakers and government officials from both the USA and abroad. Family science activities to promote a greater awareness of science for school children - as well as the general public - was once again a key event. More than 1000 families participated in this open science fair. The key developments in science with regard to medicine and health perspectives, policy decision, neuroscience research and related disciplines are summarized below.

Thursday, February 16

The 1st day started with a special session organized by WesleyNexux Inc. (Bethesda, MD) on the "Wicked Problem" of climate change: what is it doing to US and us? This was followed by a seminar on scientist motivation, support and challenges for public engagement organized by Jessica Sickler (Pittsburgh, PA) comprising 3 speakers. Tracey Hollaway (Madison, Wisconsin) talked on connecting NASA data with user needs as a case study in public engagement.

Promoting meaningful public engagement: how and why to get scientists involved was discussed by Ezra Markowitz (Amherst, MA). Sriram Sunderarajan (Ames, Iowa) presented instilling a "Broader Impact" identity at Iowa State University. The other notable special session was the Bioscience Entrepreneurship organized by the AAAS. An afternoon key seminar was held on 'The online scientist: Social media and public engagement', organized by Erika Shugart (Bethesda, MD) in which 3 speakers presented their views. Raychelle Burks (Austin, TX) discussed 'Scientist online: Visibility, vagaries and victories'. 'Communicating science online: Scientist-media interactions' was the topic of Sara Yeo (Salt Lake City, Utah). Nsikan Akpan (Arlington, VA) spoke on 'Please watch: Navigating the social video snake pit'. The day closed with the AAAS President's Address by Barbara Schaal (St. Louis, MO), followed by a lavish presidential reception for all delegates at the Hynes Convention Center.

Friday, February 17

On 2nd day of the congress 4 special sessions and 2 seminars were held. The section "**Biology & Neuroscience**" comprised of 5 symposia, 3 of which were held on the 17th and 2 the next day. On 17th February Jane Roskmas (Vancouver, BC, Canada) and Terrence Sejnowski (La Jolla, CA) organized a symposium entitled 'Innovative neurotechnologies and strategies from BRAIN initiatives', with 3 speakers. Novel approaches to high-speed imaging of neural activity in the behaving brain were discussed by Elizabeth Hillman (Vancouver, BC, Canada). Sarah Stanley (New York, NY) presented on 'Remote regulation of neural activity. Imaging

*Address correspondence to this author at the International Experimental CNS Injury & Repair (IECNSIR), Department of Surgical Sciences, Anesthesiology & Intensive Care Medicine, University Hospital, Uppsala University, SE-75185 Uppsala, Sweden; Tel/Fax: +46 18 24 38 99; Cell: +46 70 2011801; E-mail: Sharma@surgsci.uu.se

1871-5273/17 $58.00+.00

a human in motion'. The ambulatory microdose positron emission tomograph scanner was discussed by Julie Berfczynski-Lewis (Morgantown, VA). 'Optical nanoscale imaging: Unraveling the chromatin structure-activity relationship' was the theme of the 2nd Symposium organized by Vadim Backman (Evanston, IL). Xiaowei Zhuang (Cambridge, MA) demonstrated super resolution imaging of chromatin organization in individual chromosomes. Leonard Mirny (Cambridge, MA) elaborated on physical models of chromosomal domains, while Hao Zhang (Evanston, IL) presented on label-free super resolution imaging of chromatin structure and dynamics. The 3rd and final symposium focused on 'Science, ethics and engagement of the governance of gene drives: It takes a village', and was organized by Keegan Sawyer and Andrey Thevenon (Washington DC). Speakers included James P. Collins (Tempe, AR) discussing 'What are gene drives? How do they work? Why are they important?' Elizabeth Heitman (Nashville, TN) talked about informing the development of responsible governance with responsible science. Lastly, Jason Delborne (Raleigh, NC) discussed 'Incorporating public engagement in research and governance'.

In relation to AAAS and public policy another important scientific session was organized by Aidan Gilligan (Brussels, Belgium) and Peter Gluckman (Auckland, New Zealand), on 'A new blueprint for the ethics and principles of science policymaking'. Four speakers presented on a range of viewpoints. Julian Kinderlerer (Cape Town, South Africa) discussed 'Why science into policy has never been about "Truth" only: Our initiative's story', followed by Wilson Compton (Bethesda, MD) on 'What should we expect from the scientific community?' Michael Kazatchkine (Geneva, Switzerland) next discussed 'What we expect from the policymaking community?', with the session closing on Kathrin O' Hara's (Ottawa, Canada) talk on 'What we expect from the public, industry, media and interest group community?'

Shifting perspectives on dementia, science and health policy was the subject of a session under Medical Science and Public health program, organized by Ann Lam (Washington DC) and built around 3 talks. Rhoda Au (Boston, MA) presented 'Roads to dementia prevention: leveraging the past and enabling the future', followed by Jessica Langbaum (Phoenix, AZ) talking on 'The need for national engagement in Alzheimer's disease prevention strategies'. The final presentation, 'Alzheimer's disease: Prevention through dietary interventions' was discussed by Neal D. Barnard (Washington DC). Microbes and Humans: Effects on Health, Disease and Society was another session put together by Janet Rossant (Toronto ON, Canada), with talks by B. Brett Finlay (Vancouver BC, Canada) on the role of microbes in early childhood, followed by 'Deciphering the diet-microbiome-metabolism axis (Eran Elinav, Rehovot, Israel), and Hendrik Poiner (Hamilton, Canada) covering 'The benefits of time travel: Reconstructing ancient genomes and microbiomes'.

The highlights of the day include 3 topical lectures, and 1 plenary lecture. Alta Charo (Madison, WI) delivered 1st topical lecture on Human Gene Editing: Recommendations from US National Academics. Daniel Nocera (Boston, MA) delivered his talk on Global Energy Challenge. Solutions from Science to technology transition. John P. McGovern Award Lecture in the behavioral Sciences was given by Henry L. Roediger III (St. Louis, MO) entitled Making it Stick: The Science of Successful Learning.

The day's scientific sessions concluded with a plenary lecture by Naomi Orskes (Boston, MA) on 'The Scientist as Sentinel'.

AAAS Awards and Prizes 2017. Special Events

The evening of the 17th was dedicated to the awarding of AAAS annual prizes on various categories. The AAAS Phillip Haugue Abelson Prize went to Ioannis Miaoulis, Museum of Science (Boston, MA). The Science Diplomacy Award was presented to Grace Naledi Mandisa Pandor from the Ministry of Science and Technology, South Africa. The Award for Scientific Freedom and Responsibility was bestowed on Kurt Gottfried of Cornell University (Ithaca, NY). Suzanne Gage (Liverpool, UK) received the AAAS Early Career Award for public engagement with science. Richard Tapia (Rice University, Huston, TX) received the Public Engagement with Science Award. The AAAS Mentor Award went to Ami Radunskaya of Pomona College (Claremont, CA) and the AAAS Mentor Award for Lifetime Achievement was given to Margret Werner-Washburne, University of New Mexico (Albuquerque, NM).

Saturday, February 18

The 3rd day of the meeting continued the session "**Biology & Neuroscience**" organized around two additional symposia. 'RNA splicing at 40: Reflecting on scientific progress, policy and social justice' was the topic of the 4th Symposium organized by Pinna G. Abir-Am (New Haven, CT), with talks by Pinna G. Abri-Am on 'Historical perspectives on scientific anniversaries: Science policy to social justice', Louise Chow (Birmingham, AL) on 'Discontinuation of genes and regulation of high eukaryotic gene expression', and Ruth Sperling (Jerusalem, Israel) on 'From virus structure to spliceosome function via RNA splicing'. The 5th symposium, on 'The neuroscience of time and memory, was organized by Sheena Josselyn (Toronto, ON, Canada), with presentations by Howard Eichenbaum (Boston, MA) on 'Time, cells and memory', Alcino Silva (Los Angeles, CA) on 'Hippocampal engrams and time', and Sheena Josselyn (Toronto, Canada) on 'Temporal context and emotional memory'.

Other key highlights of this day were topical lectures delivered by Venki Ramkrishnana, 2009 Nobel Laureate in Chemistry (London, UK) speaking on 'Potential and risks of recent developments in Biotechnology'. Leila Takayama

(Santa-Cruz, CA) next discussed 'Robotics: Towards a more human-centered future', followed by Susan Lindee (Philadelphia, PA) on 'The rise of the genome: Genetics after the bomb'.

The day ended with lavish international reception at the Presidential Tower of the Skywalk Observatory, presented by the UK Research Council.

Sunday, 19 February

The 4th day of the meeting started with a session on 'Assessing the impact of medical marijuana: The grass could be greener' organized by Staci Gruber (Baltimore, MD). 'Cannabis pharmacovigilance: Lessons from a living laboratory' was presented by Mark Ware (Montreal, Canada), followed by Ryan Vandrey (Baltimore, MD) talking on 'Cannabis research and policy: Lessons from the lab and field'. Staci Gruber (Belmont, MA) then discussed 'Marijuana on the mind: Assessing the impact of medical marijuana'. The topical subject of 'Serving aging societies globally through science, technology and innovation policy' was organized by Naoki Saito and Kuniko Urashima (Tokyo, Japan), with participation by Luke Georghiou (Manchester, UK) discussing 'Integrating health and social care to cope with an aging population: Innovation challenges', followed by 'Immigration, medical research and robots: US science and technology policy for an aging society' given by David Hart (Arlington, VA), and then Nares Damrongchai (Bangkok, Thailand) discussing 'Internationalization of aging in Thailand and the importance of biomedical innovation'.

Erin Faulconer (Seattle, WA) organized a symposium on 'Big data synthesis in health policy' with talks by Abraham Flaxman (Seattle, WA) on 'Global burden of disease: Determining priorities on a global scale', followed by Scott Dowell (Seattle, WA) who discussed 'Big data needs for informing childhood investment policies'. Finally, Geospatial analysis: Distributing resources and interventions at a subnational level was presented by Peter Gething (Oxford, UK).

The day ended with a plenary lecture by S. James Gates Jr. (Baltimore, MD) on 'Who talked about science and evidence-based policymaking'. This was followed by the Bill and Melinda Gates Foundation: Open Access to Scientific Research Reception for all delegates with the message of free and immediate access to research findings for the future of scientific innovation.

Monday, 20 February

A highlight of the day was a Meeting with Science Editors special event where Jeremy M. Berg, Editor-in-chief of Science hosted a reception for all delegates with coffee and light refreshment. In this reception the Science family of journals was discussed with ethics of scientific publication at the final concluding session of the meeting.

Poster Sessions

One important facet of the annual AAAS meeting are the poster sessions, which are divided into Student and General Poster sessions on several themes in the categories of Animal Science, Cellular Science, Environmental Science, Medicine, Brain and Behavior, Cellular and Molecular Biology, Medicine and Public Health, along with the physical, chemical, ecology, plant and computer sciences.

Selected key poster presentations in the neurosciences are summarized below.

February 17

Friday's poster session was devoted to the American Junior Academy of Science (AJAS) with 11 posters in Animal Science, 12 in Cellular Sciences, and 16 from the medicine section (apart from chemistry, earth science, engineering and other branches of science). Among the more interesting neuroscience-related posters were those: describing the effect of gabapentin on Dugesia Tigrina's nervous system (Allison Kohl, Nebraska Academy of Science, Lincoln); using caffeine and taurine to improve memory retention in Dugesia Dorotcephala (Alex Jayyosi, Massachusetts Academy of Science, Worcester); studying the effects of toluene on memory retention in Planaria (Tal Usvyatsky, New Jersey Academy of Science, Piscataway); window to the brain using retinal biomarkers to diagnose Alzheimer disease (Archana Murali, Minnesota Academy of Science, St Paul); the effects of polyphenols in spices on the aggregation of amyloid beta peptide 1-40 (Swathi Srinivasan, Ohio Academy of Science); combinatorial effects of bitter melon and temozolomide on glioma cells (Farheen Zaman, Virginia Academy of sciences, Fredericksburg).

February 18

This day's poster session comprised of general session (8), Brain and Behavior (17), and Medicine and Public heath (46). The student poster session dominated the day. Among the general posters some notable results related to neuroscience include: deconstructing depression (Per Svensson, Solna, Sweden); nanodelivery of drugs for neuroprotection in sleep deprivation-induced brain pathology (Aruna Sharma, Uppsala University, Sweden); a preliminary study showing that alcohol and carbon nanoparticles exacerbate nicotine neurotoxicity (Suraj Sharma, Uppsala University); neuroprotection in Alzheimer disease by nanodelivery of neprilysin with cerebrolysin (Hari Sharma, Uppsala University); evidence showing cerebrolysin reduces neuron-specific UCHL1 and brain pathology in Alzheimer disease (Dafin Muresanu, Cluj-Napoca, Romania); effects of waterpipe water on reward, antinociceptive and locomotor activity in rats (Ahmad Altarif, Irbid, Jordan).

Some key developments relating to Brain and Behavior posters included: Sox17 transgenic mice revealed functional suppression of beta-catenin in neuroprotection (Kimberly

Cruz, Washington, DC); a tool for diagnostic and staging synucleinopathies (Claire Erikson, Columbus, OH); neuro-protective efficacy of P7C3 compounds in models of Huntington disease (Lance Heady, Iowa City, IA); the role of dopamine D2 receptors in modulating alcohol-related behaviors (Vanessa Kob, Kingston, RI); evidence for peripheral actions of calcitonin gene-related peptide in migraine-like behavior (Anne Ojo, Twickenham, UK); exploring Drosophila HIFA regulation in neuronal cell mitochondrial retro-grade signaling (Amara Thind, Irvine, CA); neuronal cell activity patterns predict cortical viability in a rodent model of ischemic stroke (Ellen Wan, Irvine, CA).

Overall the 183rd AAAS meeting was a highly highly successful even in which more than 20,000 delegates participated. The 184th AAAS annual meeting is scheduled for Austin, TX from February 15-19, 2018. All interested are welcome!

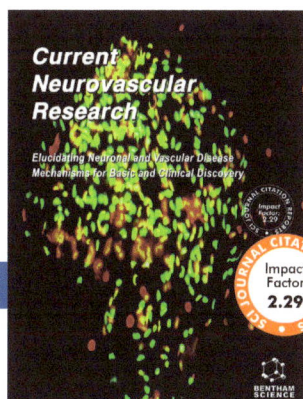

Current Neurovascular Research

Editor-in-Chief:
Kenneth Maiese
USA

Impact Factor 2.29

About the Journal

Volume 14, 4 Issues, 2017

The journal serves as an international forum publishing novel and original work as well as timely neuroscience research reviews in the disciplines of cell developmental disorders, plasticity, and degeneration that bridges the gap between basic science research and clinical discovery. Current Neurovascular Research emphasizes the elucidation of disease mechanisms, both cellular and molecular.

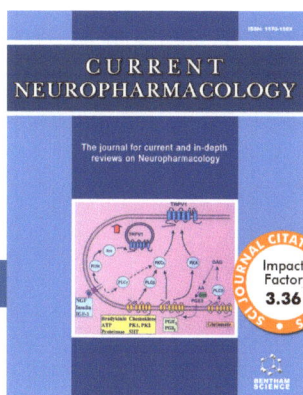

Current Neuropharmacology

Editor-in-Chief:
T.E. Salt
UK

Impact Factor 3.36

About the Journal

Volume 15, 8 Issues, 2017

Current Neuropharmacology aims to provide current, timely and comprehensive reviews and guest edited issues of all areas of neuropharmacology and related matters of neuroscience. The reviews cover the fields of molecular, cellular, and systems/behavioural aspects of neuropharmacology and neuroscience.

BENTHAM SCIENCE *Publishers of Quality Research*

www.benthamscience.com

For Subscriptions
Contact: subscriptions@benthamscience.org

For Advertising & Free Online Trials
Contact: marketing@benthamscience.org

Abstracted/Indexed in: Science Citation Index Expanded, Journal Citation Reports/Science Edition, Current Contents®-Clinical Medicine, Neuroscience Citation Index®, BIOSIS, BIOSIS Previews, BIOSIS Reviews Reports and Meetings, MEDLINE/PubMed, Scopus, EMBASE/Excerpta Medica, Chemical Abstracts Service/SciFinder, PsycINFO, ProQuest, ChemWeb, Google Scholar, MediaFinder®-Standard Periodical Directory, Cabell's Directory, Genamics JournalSeek, PubsHub, J-Gate, CNKI Scholar, Suweco CZ, TOC Premier, EBSCO, British Library and Ulrich's Periodicals Directory

Impact Factor: 2.506 (2016 SCI Journal Citation Reports)